Handbook of
Unusual and Unorthodox
Healing Methods

J. V. Cerney, A.B., D.M., D.P.M.

Parker Publishing Company, Inc.

West Nyack, New York

Library of Congress Cataloging in Publication Data

Cerney, J. V.
   Handbook of unusual and unorthodox healing methods.

   Includes index.
   1. Physical therapy. 2. Massage. 3. Hydrotherapy.
4. Fasting. I. Title. [DNLM: 1. Therapeutic Cults--
Popular works. WB890 C415h]
RM701.C47   615'.8   75-23270
ISBN 0-13-382739-9.

Dedicated to my son Jim

What This Book Can Do for You

"I'd had all the modern care available," explained Jack D. "I'd made the expensive rounds of clinics, hospitals and eminent authorities but my aches and pains continued. I'd had surgery, literally tons of pills and potions and shots and I was dragging the bottom of the human race. Even my personality did a nosedive. Instead of getting better, I got worse. Instead of getting a raise at the office, I got fired. My wife left me. The kids were farmed out to relatives. It seemed like the end of the world had come. Then I started taking treatments that some folks said were unorthodox and unusual. Today, after using them, I no longer look or feel like the wrath of God had been visited upon me. I'm back in the human race, back on the job, even my family's back and I feel great! Old-fashioned remedies created a whole new beginning for me!"

Are *you* looking for home remedies to restore health? Does it matter if these remedies, these methods and procedures are not new?

If you *are* looking for such remedies, this book is for you! The methods and procedures that follow in this text are not new. They have been called unusual and unorthodox. Some of them are thousands of years old. Some were considered "just passing fads" but the remarkable thing about all of them is that they have continued to persist down through time when many another so-called modern treatment has fallen by the medical wayside. So read carefully. Then re-read it and keep it handy as a desktop consultant.

It's All Briefed
for Easy Reading

This book is divided into sections. Each section is devoted to an area considered somewhat unorthodox in modern medicine today. The sections are as follows: *Section I* tells the story of those amazing "Z" zones that not only treat you, but can be used to diagnose your own problems. *Section II* is composed of healing agents called herbs, cell salts, raw juice and fasting. *Section III* has to do with physical therapy procedures you can use in your home, procedures such as *somatherapy*, the body cure, *spinal concussion, percussion, vibration* and *aquatonics*.

Each of these sections, if you read them carefully with an open mind—and without prejudice—can give you a whole new concept about human care during illness. Unorthodox as these procedures may be in the light of "modern medicine," they will intrigue as well as astound you in their effectiveness when properly used.

All I ask is that you don't expect overnight cures. Miracles never happen overnight although they do happen every day of your life. Where immediate results are not obtained, do not blame the book. You may have misread it or misdiagnosed your problem or misused the instructions given. In any case, read with care, because you are going to find that if just *one* procedure—of the many in this book—helps you back to health, this book will be the greatest investment you ever make.

J.V. Cerney, A.B., D.M., D.P.M.

Contents

What This Book Can Do for You   7

SECTION A

Chapter One   17

"Z" ZONE ALARM POINTS and the amazing health role they play. . . Five key tests that can change the course of your life . . . how to test yourself for illness. . . How to get rid of fatigue through Trigger Point therapy. . . How to generate energy with "Z" Zones at your very finger tips. . . The ice technique and how to use your "Z" Zones to restore health.

SECTION B

**NEW HEALTH THROUGH HERBS,
CELL SALTS, RAW JUICES
and FASTING**

C h a p t e r   T w o   **59**

NEW HEALTH THROUGH HERBS, or *Phytotherapy,* is within your command. . . How to save doctor bills and what to do. . . Best-by-Test herbal remedies you can use at home and exactly what to do: *ADRUE* for dyspepsia, *AGRIMONY to quell a child's cough, AMERICAN SENNA* for cathartic action, *ANGELICA* to relieve that nervous headache, *ASPEN* and a way to stop diarrhea, *BALSUM* of *PERU* for leg ulcers, *BLACKBERRY* as a cure for indigestion, *BLESSED THISTLE* as the remedy to induce vomiting, *BLACK COHOSH* the remedy for rheumatism, *BLUE COHOSH* for "female complaints," *BUCHU BERRIES* and how to get rid of urinary problems, *BUCKBEAN* as the treatment for "shingles," *BUSH HONEYSUCKLE* as the remedy for poison ivy, *CALIFORNIA LAUREL* to make muscle cramps disappear, *CAPSICUM* to clear up that alcoholic party, *DILL* for gas and dyspepsia, *ELDER* for bruises, pleurisy, gout, *EUCALYPTUS* for head colds and stomach ulcers, *FENNEL* for colic, *GENTIAN* as a cure for severe diarrhea, *GINGER* for toothache, headache, neuralgia, *JUNIPER* for dropsy and diseases of the skin, *LEEK* for burns,

C h a p t e r   T w o *(Continued)*

ulcers, insect bites, *MARSHMALLOW* as the treatment for swelling, itching and burns, *MUSTARD* to stop pain, *ONION* for colds and croup, *PEPPERMINT* and how to use it for "heartburn," nausea, vomiting and gas, *PLEURISY ROOT* for chest pain, acute rheumatism, and the teething baby, *PRINCE'S PINE* for sciatica, chronic rheumatism and gout, *PUMPKIN* for urinary problems, *RED CLOVER* to neutralize gastric acidity and purify the blood, *RED RASPBERRY* for cankers, proud flesh, sore mouth and burns, *SAGE* for quinsy and the felling of tiredness, colds and coughs, *SKUNK CABBAGE* for asthma and catarrh, *SLIPPERY ELM* the treatment for frostbite, wounds and burns, *SPEARMINT* for piles and stopping vomiting and nausea, *THYME* for headaches, *VIRGINIA SNAKE ROOT* for snake bite, fever and colds, *WILD CHERRY* for intermittent fever, diarrhea and dysentery, *WITCH HAZEL* for hemorrhoids, ulcers and external tumors, *ALLIGATOR PEAR* as your treatment for neuralgia.

C h a p t e r   T h r e e   **77**

MAGIC MINERALS CALLED "CELL SALTS" and an amazing route to health. . . Blood, your master conveyor belt to health. . . . The power of cell salts are in your own hands. . . Twelve amazing cell

C h a p t e r   T h r e e *(Continued)*

salts that make your life worth a
fortune . . . the treatment key and how you
can use it to restore health. . . How to
know when you should use *Potassium
chloride* . . . *Sodium chloride* imbalance
and what it does to you. . . *Calcium sulfate*
and how to treat kidney problems, neuralgia and "colds". . . *Sodium sulfate* and
how its absence brings on distinctive pains
and how to treat them. . . *Potassium sulfate* the magic mineral that conquers dizziness, headaches, toothaches and pain in the
extremities. . . *Calcium phosphate,* the
great tissue restorer and how it works in the
blood. . . *Iron phosphate* and what its absence does to the heart and circulation. . .
Potassium phosphate and the little miracles
it brings about. . . *Sodium phosphate* and
how to use it against gout, catarrh, dyspepsia and rheumatism. . . *Magnesium phosphate* and how its deficiency brings on
muscle cramps and other pain. . . *Calcium
fluoride* and its magnificent role in
health. . . *Silica* and how it assists bone
growth, controls infection and assists
healing. . . Foods to eat if these magic
minerals are not commercially available.

C h a p t e r   F o u r   **111**

RAW JUICES and CONCENTRATED
LIQUID HEALTH . . . How raw vegetables provide instant goodness. . . How to

C h a p t e r   F o u r   *(Continued)*

use raw juices to live longer and better. . .
The vegetable juices you can use to help
yourself back to health: *ALFALFA* juice
and the mystery of chlorophyl . . .
ASPARAGUS, the health-giving alkaloid
element. . . *BEET* juice, the great blood
builder. . . *CABBAGE* juice and how to use
it to reduce as well as cleanse your
body. . . *CARROT* juice the great
"cleanser," healing aid and resistance
builder. . . *CELERY* juice, the calcium-
rich route to body rehabilitation and
growth. . . *CUCUMBER* juice, the natural diuretic (kidney cleanser) . . .
DANDELION juice, the million-dollar
tonic. . . *ENDIVE* juice, the vitamin-rich
vegetable that fights eye problems and is
good for the heart. . . *LETTUCE* juice, the
secret to hair restoration and brain
vitality. . . *PARSLEY* juice, the kidney
cleanser . . . *GREEN PEPPER* juice to improve your nails and rid stomach gas. . .
POTATO juice, the skin blemish
remover. . . *SPINACH* juice and how it
cleans the intestinal tract. . . *TOMATO*
juice and the magic it works for kidney and
bladder problems. . . *TURNIP* juice, the
tooth hardener.

C h a p t e r   F i v e   **125**

FASTING, the miracle method to achieve a
longer and healthier life. . . How to use

Chapter Five *(Continued)*

fasting to cleanse the body . . . The answers to problems on fasting . . . What to
do, what to expect, how to go about it. It's
all here in this chapter!

SECTION C

**The Section that teaches you
how to treat pain through
Physical Therapy**

Chapter Six   **141**

SOMATHERAPY and the magic of soft-
tissue manipulation to relieve pain. . .
What it is, how it brings relief, key nerve
centers you use to restore health. . . Your
SPINAL COLUMN and how to relieve discomfort and pain and the procedures to
use. . . Your *NECK* and the circle and
stroke technique to achieve personal
relaxation. . . Your *SHOULDERS* and the
key trigger points to use. . . Your
ABDOMEN and what to do. . . Your
SKULL and the thumb pressure procedure. . . Your *FACE* and the trigger points
at your finger tips. . . Your *EYES* and how
to use cold applications after soft tissue
manipulation. . . How to use heat . . . Fifteen problems you can treat at home and
what to do (asthma, bed wetting, bronchitis, catarrh, "colds," constipation, ex-

C h a p t e r   S i x *(Continued)*

tremity cramps, diarrhea, earaches, gastritis, headache, hemorrhoids, insomnia, laryngitis, lumbago, sciatica, sprains and strains).

C h a p t e r   S e v e n   **173**

CUPPING and SKIN-ROLLING for pain relief. . . What it is and the equipment to use to get results. . .

C h a p t e r   E i g h t   **179**

CONCUSSION, PERCUSSION and VIBRATION, and how to use them effectively for health. . . *Concussion* and how it works, how it's applied and a special chart that tells you where. . . *Percussion,* the unorthodox way to health, and what to do. . . *Vibration* and how it's done, its purpose and what it can do just for you. . .

C h a p t e r   N i n e   **189**

HEALING   WITH   WHITE   CLAY PACKS. . . The mystery of mud and what it does. . . How to apply it, what happens

C h a p t e r   N i n e *(Continued)*

> to the skin, and its many uses. . . including
> how to use it to get rid of headaches.

C h a p t e r   T e n   **193**

_____

> *AQUATONICS* . . . the Water Way to
> Health. . . Nine magic accomplishments
> by using it and how a housewife used it
> successfully when all else failed. . . How it
> affects the spinal cord and nervous
> system. . . How to cure *depression*. . .
> How to alleviate "change of life". . .
> What to do about neuralgia, sciatica,
> neurasthenia and neuritis, whiplash injury
> and "colds." This amazing chapter and
> those that precede it are how-to-do-its in the
> quiet of your own home.

Index   **209**

_____

CHAPTER 1

"Z" Zone Alarm Points and the amazing health role they play in your life

Would you gamble thirty seconds of your life to be able to look forward to a future of health—thirty seconds to make some million-dollar tests that will astound you? Would you gamble a miracle-making-moment to guarantee that you will greet each day with a smile? Would you take another half minute to prove a point about the wonderfulness of "Z" zones and how they deal with one of the most magnificent human systems ever devised?

Good! Then this chapter and those that follow will teach you how to use your own body as a diagnostic aide. You won't need a college degree to open up a whole new world of self-understanding as well as self-help, and the following five key tests will not just astonish and fascinate you but help you with your current health problems as well.

"Z" ZONES . . . .
MILLION-DOLLAR KEYS
TO THE DOOR OF HEALTH

Revealed for the first time in these pages are some jealously guarded professional secrets. They are million-dollar keys to the door of health, methods to determine your state of well-being, how-to-do-its to help yourself feel that little bit better. Unusual? Unorthodox? Let's find out.

It's All There . .
At Your Finger Tips

Nature's own delicate mechanisms permit you to witness a natural phenomenon when they are set into action. Nature's own computer systems demonstrate vasomotor (blood vessel, skin and muscle) and autonomic nerve reactions. To demonstrate the how and why of these amazing methods, here are five self-tests that not only open the doorway to better understanding of yourself, but improve personal health as well.

FIVE KEY TESTS
That May Change the Course of Your Life

(1) *The Spinal Vasomotor Reaction Test*
    that reveals how you can gauge the state of your health.

(2) *The Abdominal Pulse Test*
    and how you can make pain disappear beneath your very finger tips.

(3) *The Chinese "Alarm Point" Test*
    and the unique system that points up your physical condition each day.

(4) *The Umbilicus Trigger-Point Test*
    and how you can use it efficiently each day.

(5) *Tension Test-Centers*
     and the role they play.

NOTE: All of these tests have to do with human "Z" zones, those unique spotlighted control areas that not only influence your health but can change your way of life as well . . . trigger points to help you stay younger, live longer and have what you want out of life as well.

SIGHT LINES
INTO THE STATE OF HUMAN HEALTH

Mrs. John K., a fine woman with a big family, tried to keep her children happy and healthy at all times. With this in mind she asked me one day, "Is there any way I can judge the condition of my children's health rather than wait until they get sick? Are there any tests I can make or do?" My answer to her was the following.

The Spinal Vasomotor Reaction Test

Instructions

With the subject stripped to the waist place your left and right index fingers just below the base of the skull. With firm pressure make a sweeping glide down the back on each side of the spinal processes. With both fingers parallel to each other make a firm excursion from the base of the skull all the way to the base of the spine (see Figure 1). Stand back! Watch! An amazing phenomenon takes place! Watch the skin react and see something you've never observed before!

**Before Your Eyes
. . a Phenomenon**

Tim R. sat in my office watching the examination of his wife with great interest. Marion R. was one of those sickly persons who goes

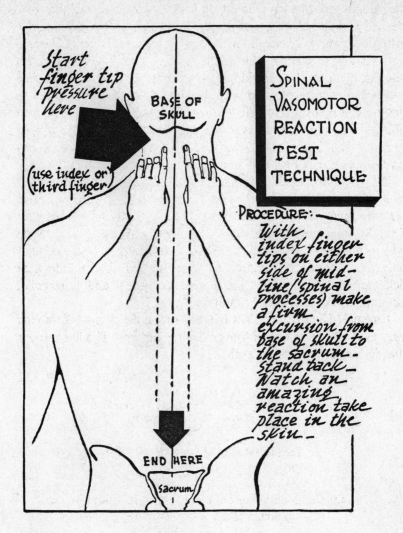

Start finger tip pressure here

(use index or third finger)

BASE OF SKULL

SPINAL VASOMOTOR REACTION TEST TECHNIQUE

PROCEDURE:

With index finger tips on either side of mid-line (spinal processes) make a firm excursion from base of skull to the sacrum. Stand back. Watch an amazing reaction take place in the skin.

END HERE

Sacrum

Figure 1

20

the rounds of doctors without end. She was underweight, flat-chested and flat-hipped, had no children, a sour disposition and a vitriolic tongue to blame the world for her physical misery. She was not just low in energy. Her estimate of doctors was low because none of them had helped rid her of her personal miseries. Her face and her eyes were clouded with disdain of the testing that was in progress. But not so Tim. He was watching avidly. His eyes popped open wider as the spinal vasomotor reaction took place. He wanted to know what in the world was happening when Marion's skin was reacting as it did. So I explained. Here's what I told him.

"If you have made a properly firm excursion down Marion's back, a change takes place beneath your finger tips. You use one of Nature's own diagnostic instruments and you can use it day after day. An intimately related action takes place between skin, blood vessels and nerve supply all the way down those two spinal lanes of pressure on the skin. It's a cunning mechanism. It's an extremely delicate mechanism called the *autonomic system* and as standard equipment it comes already built in."

Unusual? Unorthodox? Yes indeed, but on the skin—before your very eyes—appears one of four revealing patterns. The illustrations that follow demonstrate just this.

(1) Two parallel RED lines in the wake of your
finger tip pressure (Figure 2).

(2) Two parallel WHITE lines of pallor
(Figure 3), or it may be a . . .

(3) Combination of both red and white lines or
splotches (Figure 4) . . .or the

(4) Skin may remain unmarked (Figure 5).

How Your Vasomotor System
Tells an All-Revealing Story

In explaining the "Z" zones to Tim I said, "Three powerful factors are brought immediately to light. *First*, the skin reaction is an indicator of the general state of health.

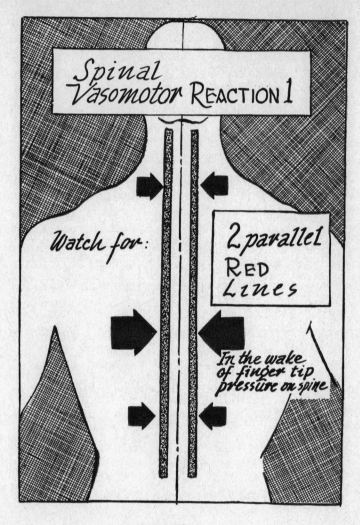

Figure 2

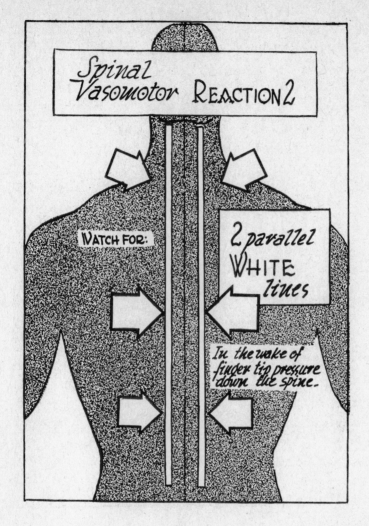

Figure 3

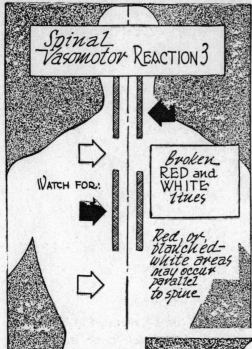

Figure 4

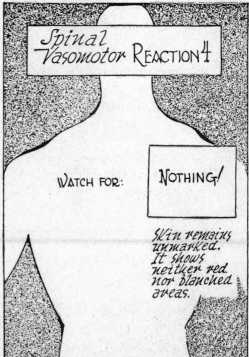

Figure 5

24

Second, it exemplifies the stability of the nervous system and how well the blood vessels just beneath the skin are capable of reacting to the finger tip pressure that has just passed over them. *Third,* it gives a clue as to the condition of intestinal organs as well as the spinal cord.''

Test One

The Spinal Vasomotor Test
How It Works . . . What It Tells You

This thirty-second test isn't just to see pink lines, white lines, or splotches on the skin. It's important because:

When:

(1) *those lines are red or pink* (on a Caucasian or Oriental skin) *it indicates the spinal cord underneath is anemic* and organs fed by these nerves are in similar condition.

When:

(2) *skin lines are blanched white* the spinal cord is congested or glutted with blood. The organs that these nerves feed, on the other hand, are anemic and sick.

When:

(3) *variegated lines appear* they are telling you that the nerve supply to the spinal cord, skin of the back and organs is very unstable.

When:

(4) *the skin goes unmarked* it tends to indicate that the individual's physiology and nerve supply are in relatively good condition.

These are positive and negative reactions on the skin and *you* have the capability to make the test and bring out the tattletale evidence that is a signpost to physical health! Mrs. John K. used this method on her big family and found it worked.

What These Million-Dollar
Vasomotor Reactions Mean to You

In the wake of finger tip pressure on each side of the spinal column, red lines appearing on the skin of the back indicate that there is congestion in the internal organs that these nerves feed. Get this matter exactly in mind because it's the whole physiological secret! I repeat, when doing this test on a friend or member of your family, if the lines on the skin are red or pink the internal organs interconnected by the same nervous system are not healthy. They are hyperemic or engorged with blood. This is your signal that organs are functioning improperly, inadequately, that they may be congested, that they are relaying a message to you and that's exactly what this test is all about. It's the *autonomic nerves* at work (see Figure 6).

According to Yoshio Nakatani, M.D., the brilliant Japanese advocate of the Ryodaraku acupuncture system, when any stimulation is applied to the human body or its surfaces a reaction occurs somewhere in the body. In other words, when stimulation is applied, this excitement passes along sensory nerves to the spinal column and finally the brain. The response to this signal goes back out and passes along the efferent nerves (motor, autonomic nerves via the sympathetic and parasympathetic nervous systems) and a reflex occurs in the outer skin. Sounds complicated, doesn't it? As complex as it sounds, it's simple to do. It's your "Z" zones at work, those very significant tattletale signposts that tell you about a person's state of health in a few seconds' time.

With This in Mind
Here's Why the "Z" Zones Work

As I explained all this to Tim and his wife I told them about how John R. complained of chest pain. His heart was sick. Coronary vessels feeding it were inefficient. Because his heart was not getting its normal blood supply, it became desperate and sent distress signals out over the nerve to the spinal cord. At the fourth thoracic vertebra where the nerve makes entrance to the cord was an area of pain. I call it an "ouch" or "hot" spot. In illness or nonhealth these ouch spots appear on your back as well. In John R.'s case additional pain shot into his left shoulder and down his arm. This is called a "reflex" pain and the cause of this pain is called "*angina pectoris.*"

If you still don't understand how this mechanism works, let's make another million-dollar test. Let's help you convince yourself about nervous system controls and how pressure points or another kind of "Z" zone can not only be diagnostic and help tell you what your problem is but can be used for treatments also.

$\boxed{\textbf{Test Two}}$

The Abdominal Pulse Test
and How to Make Belly Pain
Disappear Between Your Finger Tips

For the next remarkable test lay your hand on your own abdomen. Feel for pulsations. Feel your sides, up, down. Did you try the solar plexus area just beneath the tip of the breastbone?

If you have no pulsations anywhere in your abdomen that you can feel, then you are in fairly good shape. None of the bad physiological signposts are showing up. There are no local belly problems to set up a pounding pulse. Or, you may have a heavy fat pad through which you can't feel anything but more fat. So let's go deeper. Lie on your back. Relax your abdomen. Bury your finger tips deep in that belly fat. Can you feel pulsations? How about your umbilicus? How about the area to the left or right of your belly button?

Here's the Next Vital Step

If you *do* locate a pulsation, have a friend run his or her finger tips firmly down either side of your spinal column. Somewhere, from the shoulder blades down, he or she will find an area of pain or an "ouch" spot. You'll say, "Why does *that* hurt?" Note that the ouch spot is usually on the anatomical side of the belly pulsation.

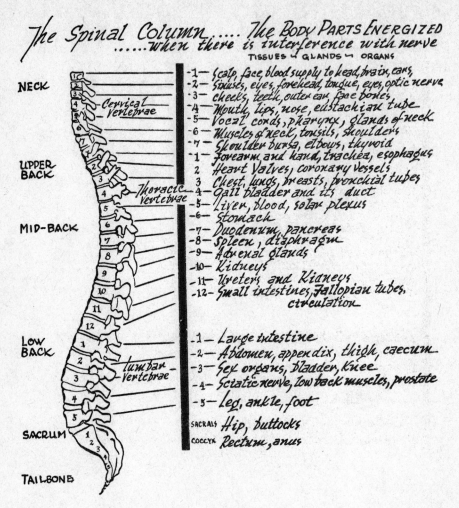

The Spinal Column..... The Body Parts Energized
...... when there is interference with nerve

TISSUES ~ GLANDS ~ ORGANS

NECK
Cervical Vertebrae

- 1 — Scalp, face, blood supply to head, brain, ears,
- 2 — Sinuses, eyes, forehead, tongue, eyes, optic nerve
- 3 — cheeks, teeth, outer ear, face bones
- 4 — Mouth, lips, nose, eustachian tube
- 5 — Vocal cords, pharynx, glands of neck
- 6 — Muscles of neck, tonsils, shoulders
- 7 — Shoulder bursa, elbows, thyroid

UPPER BACK
Thoracic Vertebrae

- 1 — Forearm and hand, trachea, esophagus
- 2 — Heart valves, coronary vessels
- 3 — Chest, lungs, breasts, bronchial tubes
- 4 — Gall bladder and its duct
- 5 — Liver, blood, solar plexus

MID-BACK

- 6 — Stomach
- 7 — Duodenum, pancreas
- 8 — Spleen, diaphragm
- 9 — Adrenal glands
- 10 — Kidneys
- 11 — Ureters and Kidneys
- 12 — Small intestines, fallopian tubes, circulation

LOW BACK
Lumbar Vertebrae

- 1 — Large intestine
- 2 — Abdomen, appendix, thigh, caecum
- 3 — Sex organs, bladder, knee
- 4 — Sciatic nerve, low back muscles, prostate
- 5 — Leg, ankle, foot

SACRUM
SACRALS — Hip, buttocks
COCCYX — Rectum, anus

TAILBONE

Figure 6

28

..... *AILMENTS THAT MAY OCCUR*
supply or *Meridians*

AILMENTS

Headaches, nervousness, insomnia, high B.P.
Deafness, earache, blindness, sinus trouble
Acne, eczema, neuralgia, neuritis
Allergies (hay fever), adenoids, catarrh
Laryngitis, hoarseness, "sore throat"
Tonsilitis, croup, stiff neck, pain in arms
Colds, goiter, bursitis
Asthma, cough, pain in forearm & hands
Heart problems, chest pain
Pleurisy, pneumonia, bronchitis, influenza
Gall bladder problems, shingles, jaundice
Liver problems, low B.P. anemia, arthritis
Stomach problems, indigestion, dyspepsia
Ulcers, diabetes, gastritis
Hiccough, stomach problems
Allergies, (hives etc)
Hardening of arteries, kidney trouble, tiredness
Acne, boils, eczema, autointoxication
Rheumatism, gas in bowel, sterility

Colitis, constipation, diarrhea, herniation
Cramps, acidosis, appendicitis, Varicose Veins
Bladder problems, knee pain
Lumbago, sciatica, pain on frequent urination
Swelling: legs, feet, poor circulation, coldness

Spinal curvature, sacroiliac problems
Hemorrhoids, itching, pain on sitting.

While your friend is pressing hard on the "button" or sore spot, keep your hand on the belly pulsation. Note the remarkable phenomenon that takes place. If your friend is pressing the right button, *the pulsation and discomfort around it will diminish and actually disappear beneath your finger tips* just as it has done for my office patients for thirty years.

In this test and treatment is another practical example of the "Z" zones at work. It's another example of how your very finger tips can make pain go away!

Two proof-positives are not enough? You're still not convinced? All right, then let's continue using your body as a diagnostic key. Let's check what the Chinese call *alarm points*.

Test Three

Alarm Points . . .
and How Traditional Chinese
Used Them to Gauge Conditions of Health

Study Figure 7. Note how nerve structures from the spinal cord are connected to internal organs and body parts as well as to the brain. This human electronic complex and its subelectrical systems feed all the body's component parts and is constantly on the alert. It's alert even while we sleep. As we learned earlier, when there is an ailment in the internal organs the message of nonhealth or sickness is relayed to that outer surface called the skin. These areas are tender to the touch. Orientals call these areas *acupuncture points*, and it is into these points that the Chinese doctor applies a needle and *you can apply your finger tip*. If anywhere along this network of nerves and blood vessels the circuit has been short circuited by disease, trauma (injury), infection or other causes, these "Z" zones hurt when pressed. What is amazing about these same areas of hurt is that they are also points to trigger a cure and pressure is all you need.

The V.M. Test and Alarm Points
Work for You with Lightning Speed

Keeping these physiological secrets in mind, let's make another excursion down your subject's back. Use your finger tips down the spine once more. Watch that amazing vasomotor reaction. It's almost instantaneous and that's just how fast that stimulus is traveling to all organs fed by the nerve supply. That's also how fast it works when you apply finger tip therapy to an alarm point. With just finger tip pressure you trigger a vasomotor reaction and become immediately aware of the condition of the organs connected with that nerve supply. Think about that phenomenon! At your very finger tips is the best computer system in the world and you can witness it at work every day of your life!

But How Can You Test Yourself?

You can't very readily run a test on your own back. So you go to more convenient areas such as the abdomen and chest. As with man-made computers, Nature builds into your body a warning signal or system. These diagnostic signposts are immediately at hand. The old Chinese masters thousands of years ago called these signposts "alarm points" and Nature put them conveniently within reach (see Figure 8).

Eleven Alarm Points Are on
Your Chest and Belly

Of the eleven alarm points on your chest and abdomen all are significant and purposeful. Each tells a story. Learn to understand the amazing story they have to tell.

What Are Alarm Points?

Alarm points are areas of sensitivity in and under the skin. In animals and man they are always in the same location. After studying these areas in Chinese medicine I began to realize, as will you, how these alarm points or "Z" zones can be used not just for diagnostic purposes but also for treatment (see Figure 8).

Tim watched the examination of his wife with avid interest. He studied the alarm point chart on the wall and then watched as I investigated these same points on his wife's chest. I told them both:

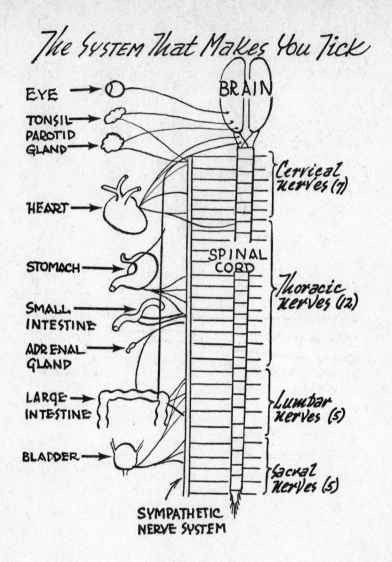

The System That Makes You Tick

EYE → ◯   BRAIN

TONSIL →

PAROTID
GLAND →

    } Cervical nerves (7)

HEART →

SPINAL
CORD

STOMACH →

    } Thoracic nerves (12)

SMALL
INTESTINE →

ADRENAL
GLAND →

LARGE
INTESTINE →

    } Lumbar nerves (5)

BLADDER →

    } Sacral nerves (5)

SYMPATHETIC
NERVE SYSTEM

Figure 7

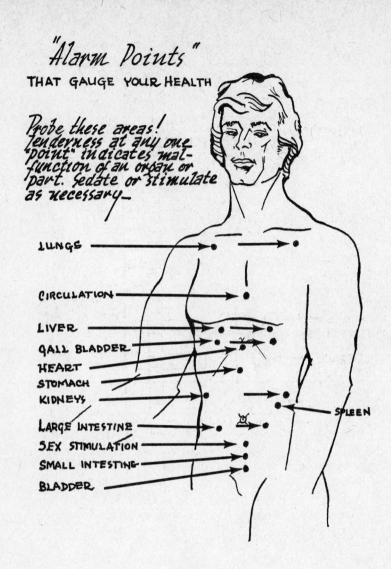

"Alarm Points"

THAT GAUGE YOUR HEALTH

*Probe these areas!
Tenderness at any one
"point" indicates mal-
function of an organ or
part. Sedate or stimulate
as necessary—*

LUNGS

CIRCULATION

LIVER

GALL BLADDER

HEART

STOMACH

KIDNEYS

SPLEEN

LARGE INTESTINE

SEX STIMULATION

SMALL INTESTINE

BLADDER

Figure 8

"Probe these points each morning. Get them definitely under your finger tips. Then ask yourself: (1) *Is this point painful on shallow pressure* or (2) *Is it painful on deep pressure?*" This makes a big difference, so be careful in your checkup. Stick to the following guidelines.

Guidelines for Testing
Your Alarm Points

To determine your state of health or someone else's health, each day test your alarm points. As you noted in Figure 8 they are conveniently within reach on the chest and abodmen. In making this test note the following important factors:

POINT 1:

> When your finger tip is placed lightly on the alarm point and it elicits pain, it means that the organ with which it intercommunicates (through the autonomic nervous system) is HYPOACTIVE (not working the way it should).

POINT 2:

> If no pain is elicited on light pressure, but deep-down pressure finds an area of hurt, it indicates the interconnecting organ is HYPERACTIVE (working too hard).
>
> **NOTE: The eminent British medical authority Felix Mann indicates that tenderness on deep pressure is indicative of acute disease.**

POINT 3:

> When no pain is experienced on either deep or superficial palpation (touch), that's the time to be happy. That's a red-letter day because all organs and parts are A-OK. They are operational without complication. That's the day you feel great, the day you play your best golf or bridge, sell your biggest insurance policy, perform your greatest role, and who could ask for anything more? Isn't that thirty-second test worth a million to you?

NOTE: As a guide use all alarm check points daily! After treating them, re-check them once more. When sensitivity is gone, Nature's own wonderful warning system tells you that healing or recovery has begun!

Three Important Factors to Remember About Alarm Points

Before letting you in on the next remarkable but unorthodox Oriental secret, there are three major points I want you to remember:

(1) *Your diagnostic alarm points are also used for treatment!* Remember that although the alarm button is expressing itself it does not always mean that a specific organ is at fault. For example, if the *liver* alarm point is tender to touch, don't arbitrarily blame the liver. Any tissue serviced by the nerve to the liver may be at fault and is expressing itself by way of a reflex pain. Anything that changes normal activity lights up the alarm signal.

(2) *The more chronic the ailment along the nerve involved, the more sensitive these alarm points are on deep pressure.*

(3) *These same alarm points may make themselves known by becoming red or warm to the touch!*

How an Alarm Point Points Up Problems of the Chest

The next time you have a cold check your alarm points. What is astounding about the chest alarm point is that *it tells you immediately that something, somewhere, in the respiratory system has gone wrong.* When a person with asthma, emphysema, tuberculosis or pneumonia are having, or about to have, their particular problem, these alarm points become immediately sensitive.

Check Your Alarm Points Each Morning!

Listen to the message your alarm points can give you each day. Use this unorthodox technique to predict your physical condition.

Apply pressure gently on each area, then heavily. Note the degree of pain, if any, elicited. As indicated earlier, the degree of pain on pressure is the tattletale sign of the condition of the organ or parts fed by that nerve. It also determines the degree and kind of pressure necessary for treating the problem.

The Two Key Rules
in "Z" Zone Treatment

Rule One: *Sedate* all points that show pain on *light* pressure.

Rule Two: *Stimulate*, or tonify (press hard), all points where there is pain on *heavy* pressure.

> **NOTE: (once more) A painful "alarm point" means a painful organ or part in the "Z" zone area being tested. WHEN PAIN SUBSIDES IN A SKIN TRIGGER POINT DURING TREATMENT, IT MEANS THAT THE PROBLEM IN THE CORRESPONDING ORGAN HAS BEGUN TO SUBSIDE! Nature once again has let you know, through the "Z" zones of the autonomic nervous system, your state of bodily health. By God's own processes you are not only warned but are given a way to treat your health problems as they arise!**

Is this all beginning to make sense now? Good! Let's get on with it! Let's talk about another type of "alarm point." These we'll call *trigger points* because they are recognized as such in Western medicine, and yet they continue to have unusual and unorthodox connotation. . . trigger points of treatment for self-application.

The Purpose of Treating
"Trigger Points," Otherwise
Known as "Z" Zones

In the treatment of *trigger points* with pressure (finger tip), the purpose is to *release local contraction of muscle, blood vessels, spasm or constriction of other soft tissues. It breaks a vicious cycle*

occurring in the local short-circuited nerve supply. Treatment im-
proves lymphatic drainage. It steps up blood supply, releases waste
products that have collected in local area in amounts sufficient to
cause discomfort and pain. It brings about that "Oh boy, I feel so
much better" feeling.

The magic of *trigger points* is that they release tension. When
triggers release, the pain stops. Pain coming from distant points
stops. Suddenly the feeling of tiredness and strain is gone. To
achieve this feeling of well-being, use your *trigger points* daily and
when properly applied you will be ready to get up and go almost on
command.

Where Are These Trigger Points Found?

All trigger points are located under the skin, in muscles, along the
nerve bodies, sometimes over closed venous valves. As triggers
they control the patterns of pain we experience from day to day. As
indicated earlier, these "Z" zones, or triggers, may be locally painful and yet be sponsored by something wrong elsewhere in the body.
This we remember is a "reflex pain."

To effectively control these patterns, the trigger has to be dis-
solved or resolved. The Chinese accomplish this by inserting a
needle or using a finger tip. You and I can use finger tip pressure to
break the physiological arc that closes the door to health and normal
function. Just press the button! Nature does the rest!

Each Trigger Has a Zone of Influence

Jake L. pitched slowball for his company softball team. As a
result he developed pain in his shoulder and upper right arm. It got
so bad he couldn't get his hand up to comb his hair or wash his face.
This otherwise healthy young man's pitching was done for the sea-
son. Or so it seemed until we started treating his "Z" zones.

One tender trigger point was found in front of his right shoulder.
This trigger point radiated a pattern of aggravation over the deltoid

shoulder muscle and the external surface of the upper arm. I used pressure on these "Z" zones and the aching shoulder muscles stopped hurting. Golfers, housewives, as well as baseball pitchers may all use this method Jake went back to his pitching once more.

Let's take another example: You will find an important trigger point at the angle of your thumb and index finger. This trigger not only controls the thumb. Thousands of years ago the Chinese found this point to be a key point for treating insomnia, headaches, eyestrain, head colds, toothaches, asthma, sinus problems and facial problems.

My wife had an abscessed tooth. The dentist was not available. Her pain was excruciating and aspirin didn't even touch the problem of pain. I put pressure on the hand trigger point and surprise lit my wife's face. "It's unbelievable!" she exclaimed. "The pain's going away!" The trigger point concerned may be seen in Figure 17. You can use the same simple process on yourself and you won't believe it until it happens to you.

Test Four

The Umbilicus . . . Testing
Center for Reflex Arcs

Let's make a fourth big test that provides another million-dollar key to the doorway of your health. For this purpose we can use the umbilicus as a valuable and easily accessible testing station. Stick the tip of your index finger into your belly button. Make a circling motion around its periphery. Note one or two areas of tenderness. Push deeper. Note where the pain radiates. This is significant. Why? The pain radiates to the organ or part that is sick and all you have to do to determine this is to press your umbilicus. Remember, the belly button is not just a testing center. It is a treatment point as well. It is a "Z" zone. Unusual? Unorthodox? Yes, but it works and I have proven it over and over again.

FATIGUE
and How to Get Rid of That Tired Feeling
by Using Your Trigger Points

Everyone today is in a state of unnatural tension. All tension is not bad. Some of it is even good. But when boredom enters the picture that's when tension leads to fatigue. It leads to exhaustion and disease. To help yourself to longer life free of these giant-killers, I advocate *trigger point* pressure with ice as a supplement. All you have to do is apply ice to the trigger points and I'm going to show you exactly where. This unusual method has been used for over 5,000 years. By using this particular version of the technique you rid yourself of fatigue. Hard work will no longer bother you because you will generate energy to cope with it. To awaken natural dynamos within yourself all you have to do is press these magic "buttons" with something as simple as a finger and a cube of ice. Remember, this fabulous treatment is at your very finger tips!

Trigger Point
Energy-Generating Technique
and How to Do It

Marion D. opened up a whole new way of life with just her finger tips and a cube of ice. Marion is a proud woman. She was married four times, and every one of her marriages ended in disaster and more children. Thin, tired, anemic, gaunt of face, feminine charms withered by her struggle, she held down two jobs and just barely managed to keep her family's head above financial waters. Fatigue? She was tension up to here!

Her four teenaged children were nothing but trouble. One of her unmarried daughters was pregnant. Another was a drug addict shooting heroin into her arm. Both boys had police records, and Marion, when she wasn't running to the police station and the juvenile authorities, was trying to keep her family together. The tension, the fatigue following in the wake of all this kept mounting until she was simply a bundle of nerves, a sack of hurt waiting to explode, and if it hadn't been for the *Trigger Point Energy-Generating Technique** she would never have made it. This treatment not only released her fatigue, but made her feel like a woman again. Her body began to fill out. Her appetite returned. Her tensions dissipated and she was capable of meeting emergencies once more.

In brief, I'm going to give you this fabulous technique to use on yourself. It is not a toy! It is not an untried newcomer. Failure in this technique occurs only due to its misuse. If you would release your tensions, if you would raise your energy level by stimulating the natural dynamos of your body, stick to the rules of the "Z" zones. Utilize your thumb and ice on these very important and unorthodox pressure points that have brought health to untold millions of Orientals over thousands of years.

How Ice-Supplemented Trigger-Point Energy-Generating Technique Works

Ice Therapy Procedure

Place a thumb on each trigger point designated in Figure 9. Make a rotary motion, with pressure, for fifteen seconds. Then apply the ice cube. Keep it moving in tiny circles. Simply press into the "point" for a half minute. Place the warmth of your palm temporarily on the cold spot. Then repeat the ice procedure once more.

Key Tension Release Points to Get Rid of Fatigue and Restore Health

The Feet

Trigger Point Position:

1. On the bottom of the foot behind the fourth metatarsal head (Figure 10).

---

*Also, see: Cerney J. V. *Acupuncture Without Needles*. (West Nyack, N.Y.: Parker Publishing Company, Inc., 1974).

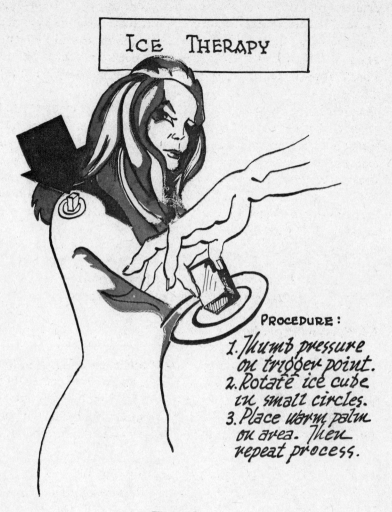

Figure 9

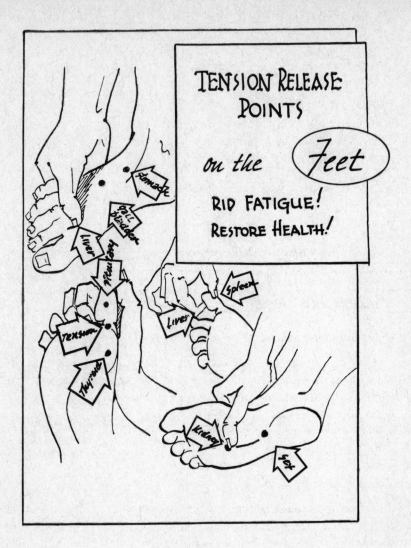

Figure 10

42

2. Grasp the big toe. Squeeze it. Search it for painful areas. Press until the hurt is gone.

The Ankle

Trigger Point Position:

Grasp the Achilles tendon between the thumb and index finger. Locate the exact sore point. Treat with pressure and ice cube as directed (Figure 11).

The Leg

Trigger Point Position:

Locate sore areas in the calf of your leg. Treat each painful area as indicated (Figure 12).

The Knee and Thigh

Trigger Point Position:

Find the sore areas as indicated on the chart (Figure 13). You will be amazed at the zones of hurt you didn't even know were there. You will be more amazed when the hurts disappear under treatment, your tension releases and your fatigue dissipates.

The Low Back

Trigger Point Position:

If you can't reach behind and feel your own back, have someone locate the release points for you. In the low back, on either side of the lumbar vertebrae, you will locate key points that relieve hip tension and sciatic distress (Figure 14). Treat with rotary pressure of your thumb tip or knuckle. Apply ice with the same rotary motion. Because of the heaviness of the muscles in this area, the pressure must be accentuated a bit. After treatment extend your legs. Stretch! Breathe deeply as you do this. Note the warmth flooding throughout your body. When this reaction occurs, fatigue areas in your body begin to relax. It's at this point that you get rid of the age-makers.

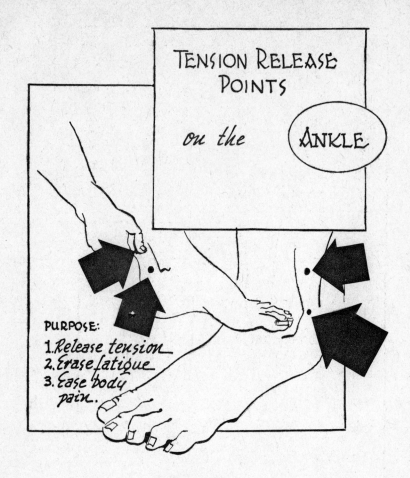

Figure 11

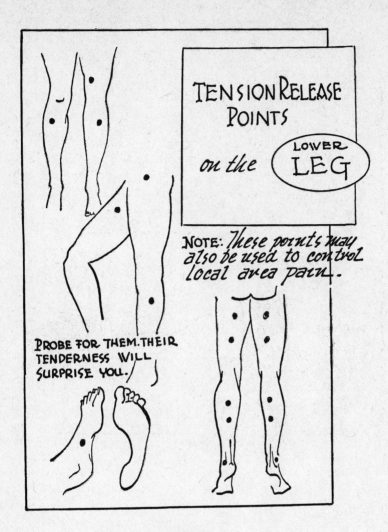

Figure 12

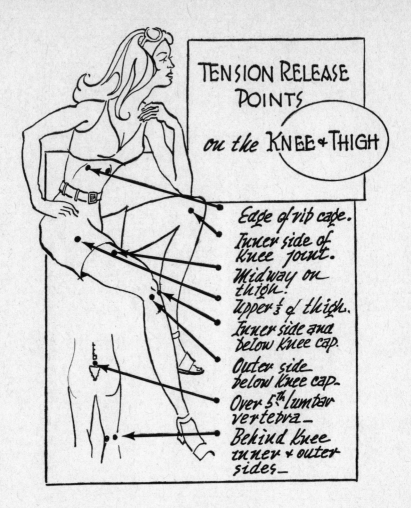

Figure 13

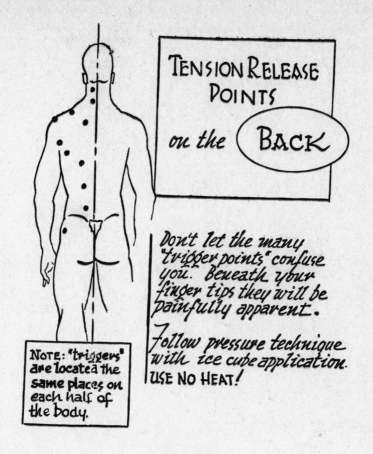

Figure 14

You will be dispelling toxic waste stored at all points of tension.

How can you do this at work or on a bus? Simply double your two fists, place them behind you into the key zones of hurt and lean back. If you are lying in bed this may be done with golf balls under the points of hurt. It's that simple.

The Neck

Trigger Point Position:

Check the areas at the base of your skull. Note that some of them are extremely tender on pressure. Sink your thumb into each of these "Z" zones (Figure 15). Follow the pressure technique by leaning back in an easy chair with an ice bag at the base of your skull or back of your neck. You will be pleased by the relief this brings.

The Shoulder

Trigger Point Position:

When shoulder stiffness or pain limits the function of your arm, you will find nodules of tension in your upper back just above the scapula. Locate and treat as prescribed (Figure 16).

The Arm and Hand

Trigger Point Position:

Test the area between the fingernail and the first joint (Figure 17). Probe. Is it tender? Test each finger in turn by grasping it between the index finger and thumb of the opposite hand. Twirl the finger around and around. Then check the *heart point*. This point is located on the heart line, palmside, just below the fourth and fifth interdigital web. This spot indicates tension in your heart, according to the Orientals, and twirling the third finger is beneficial to people with high blood pressure. Follow this procedure with dunking your finger tips in a glass of ice water. Follow this measure with checking for the trigger point between the index finger and thumb. Probe deeply.

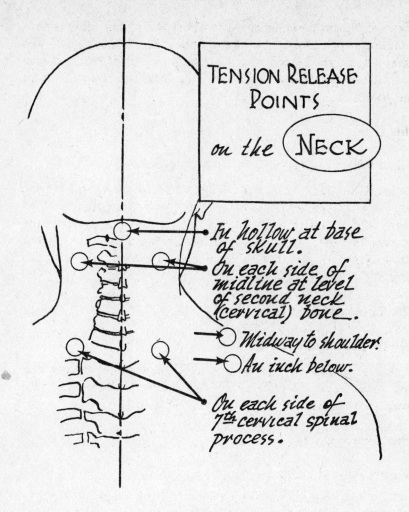

TENSION RELEASE
POINTS

on the (NECK)

In hollow at base
of skull.

On each side of
midline at level
of second neck
(cervical) bone.

Midway to shoulder.

An inch below.

On each side of
7th cervical spinal
process.

Figure 15

49

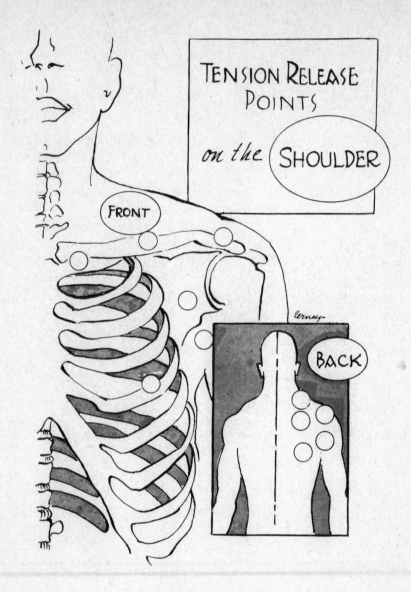

Figure 16

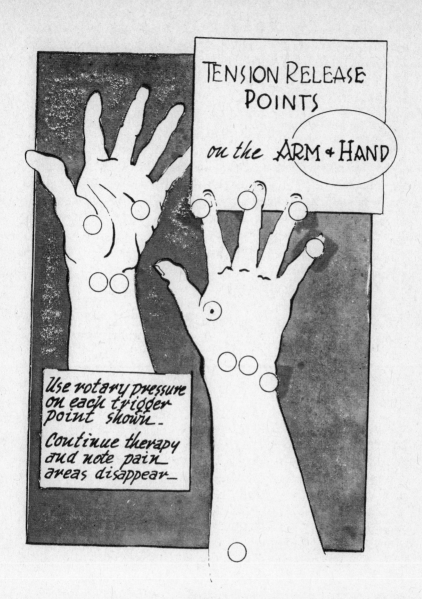

Figure 17

51

Sensitivity at this point indicates tension in your bowel. Even more than that, if you treat this area the loss of tension will result in added hours of comforting sleep.

The Abdomen

Trigger Point Position:

It has been said that "most human ailments begin in the gut," and when you are tense it is the abdomen that is first to be affected. To erase abdomen tension, put pressure on the painful area in your solar plexus as marked in Figure 18. This is a "Z" zone power switch. Respect it as such. Then move down a couple of inches on your abdomen toward the belly button. Press. Does this area hurt? Repeat the treatment. Apply ice. This may accentuate or reveal pain you didn't even know was there. Next descend to the navel. Repeat the procedure at one-inch intervals all the way down to the crotch. This treatment not only releases abdominal tension but stimulates the organs within. It's part of an overall basic health rejuvenation program.

The Chest

Trigger Point Position:

Run your finger tips across your chest in a seek-and-find mission. Locate each "ouch" spot. Verify its position in Figure 19. You may even locate some that are unique to you and not indicated in the illustration. Treat each trigger point with rotary pressure and an ice cube. Note how your chest begins to feel more at ease, how it's actually easier to breathe deeper. As indicated in the illustration, seek out each key "Z" zone and treat.

Facts to Note About Tension and How to Test for It

Mental and physical tension always leave their mark. For example, when the abdomen is affected by tension, it may manifest itself as *colitis* (inflamed and irritated intestine) with diarrhea followed alternately with constipation as well as other discomforts. Tension

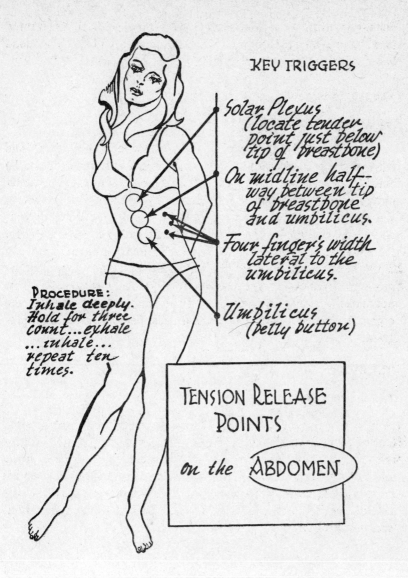

KEY TRIGGERS

Solar Plexus
(locate tender
point just below
tip of breastbone)

On midline half-
way between tip
of breastbone
and umbilicus.

Four finger's width
lateral to the
umbilicus.

Umbilicus
(belly button)

PROCEDURE:
Inhale deeply.
Hold for three
count...exhale
...inhale...
repeat ten
times.

TENSION RELEASE
POINTS

on the ABDOMEN

Figure 18

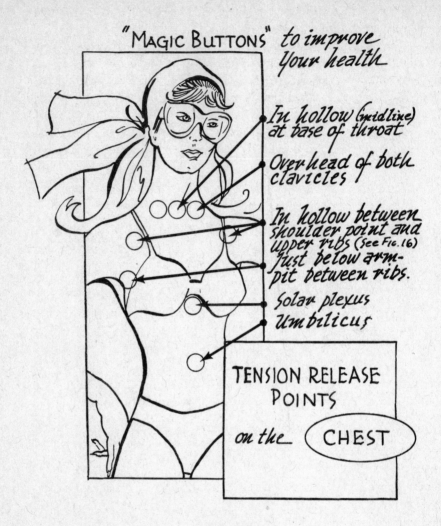

Figure 19

may reveal itself in the eyes or as a stomach ulcer. It may express itself as a pain in the neck or head.

To determine whether you have any of these tensions, just reach back to the hollow under each ear. This is just behind the angle of the jaw. Does it hurt? You bet it does! This is a signpost of tension. But it's something more. It's also a treatment trigger point for headaches and sinus problems. In other words, by treating these "Z" zones you can create little miracles of your own. Press these magic buttons. Do it daily! It may change the course of your life.

NEW HEALTH THROUGH HERBS, CELL SALTS, RAW JUICES and FASTING

Chapter 2:
  New Health Through Herbs (Phytotherapy)

Chapter 3:
  Magic Minerals Called "Cell Salts"

Chapter 4:
  *Raw Vegetable Juices . . . Concentrated
    Liquid Health*

Chapter 5:
  *Fasting . . . and How to Do It
    Without Hurt*

New Health Through Herbs (Phytotherapy)

How to Save Doctor Bills
and What to Do

It has been said often enough that, "If families would familiarize themselves with herbs, and their medicinal properties, as well as their uses, many doctor bills would be saved."

Herbs, no matter what fancy modern names are given them today and no matter how unorthodox they are said to be, continue to be the treatment of choice by those who know their value. Herbs *can* restore health. By knowing how to use herbs you may save yourself a lot of doctor bills along the way. By using herbs, you use Nature's way and there is no better way to go.

Herbs and Their Values
Have Often Been Discovered
by Accident

English medical men, hearing of the astonishing results with dropsy by a woman practitioner in Shropshire, England, investigated her cure. They found her using herbs. One of the herbs was *foxglove*, and out of her bag of healing herbs came the modern drug called *digitalis*, the drug destined to treat people efficaciously across the world. The herbal discoveries of the Orientals thousands of years ago, the discoveries of Paracelsus, Celsus and Hippocrates, often came about by accident. But in discussing herbs with you now there's nothing happenstance, nothing hit-and-miss. We're dealing strictly with known facts. We're dealing with herbs and their values that are available for use.

Most Herbs Are Available
at Health Food Stores

Most good and useful medications come from plant life. Today these herbs are available at health food stores and some drugstores. Some of these natural remedies can be purchased in dried form, extract, or other preparations. Many of them grow wild in rural areas, some in urban areas. For information on their growth, see your librarian. This text will not identify herbs by appearance or growing site. What I'm interested in is giving you a quick way to know what to do for yourself with herbs when you have a time of need. I won't use technical language, Latin terminology, or complicated applications. Just learn to use herbs. Learn how to use them and when. In this chapter I give you forty-one herbs you may use in self-application, herbs that have proven themselves through the centuries, herbs that may be an answer to common health problems when you need it most.

**Best-by-Test
HERBAL REMEDIES
You Can Use at Home**

ADRUE . . . Remedy
for Dyspepsia

Dyspepsia is an old-fashioned word and old-fashioned folks like myself continue to use it. *Dyspepsia* merely means faulty digestion. It's a symptom, not a disease. It has many causes. There may be excessive acid in the stomach. Dyspepsia may be brought on by too much alcoholic beverage. It may occur with heart disease, or result from failure of bile to enter the small intestine. It may even be brought on by hysteria.

With Geoffrey K. it was the pressure of his job that did it. For the most part he was a healthy young man, but every time he ate he was filled with gas and his abdominal pain became unbearable. He stopped eating to avoid pain. His weight dropped fantastically. One doctor suggested that Geoffrey had a malignancy. Another put him through extensive hospital tests and came up with nothing. I told Geoffrey about *adrue*. He used it. His stomachache disappeared. He obtained *adrue* at the health food store, made tea and boiled it down and then took twenty to thirty drops three times daily. He also obtained a new job. Between the *adrue* and the change of occupation his problem was solved. There has been no recurrence since.

AGRIMONY . . . and how
It Quelled a Child's Cough

Coughing is Nature's way of getting rid of waste matter in the respiratory system. Little Janie D. coughed and coughed and coughed until the whole family was upset. She kept them awake all night and worried them all day. Her face turned blue. The family physician tried everything in his bag of tricks and little Janie was taking all of these remedies when her mother called my office. An examination of the child revealed a cervical subluxation (a neck bone out of its normal position in the spinal column). An adjustment of that neck bone stopped the original conflict but didn't stop the chronic cough pattern. This was solved when Janie's mother made a decoction* from the root of the *agrimony* plant. She sweetened it with honey and gave Janie a cupful four times a day. In two days all vestiges of the cough were gone.

AMERICAN SENNA . . .
Nature's Best Remedy
for Cathartic Action

A cathartic is an active purgative. Movement of the bowel may or may not be accompanied by pain. Mrs. F.R. was constipated. She had been constipated for years until *American senna* was suggested to her as a remedy. To make her own fresh cathartic, Mrs. F.R. made a decoction of the leaves and pods of the *senna* plant. She placed one tablespoonful of this liquid in a half pint of hot water and drank it each morning. The cleansing was prompt and efficient.

ANGELICA . . . and How
It Relieves Nervous Headaches

Angelica is a gentle herb with an effective action. Not only good for nervous headaches, *angelica* is also good to get rid of flatulence (gas on the stomach), creates appetite and in general raises one's spirits. Road engineer John P. had lots of headaches on his job. When the pressure was on, on came the headache. John complained he was consuming "aspirin by the ton" and wanted something with fewer side effects. *Angelica* was recommended. He was instructed

---

*A *decoction* is a liquid preparation made by boiling an herb with water for a considerable time. Boiling or simmering the decoction over a long period of time may convert it into a thick syrup.

on how to make an infusion,* or tea, of the leaves and drink the
solution as needed. Where *angelica* powder was available he used a
half teaspoonful in a wineglass of hot water. He was cautioned to
never use the fresh roots of the angelica plant.

ASPEN . . . as a Way
to Stop Diarrhea

Diarrhea is Nature's way of expelling foreign or obnoxious material from the intestinal tract. The stool becomes fluid when peristalsis (wavelike movement of the bowel) is increased. Infections,
drugs, alcohol, food, change of water, or even milk may bring it on.
Mental stress may do it. Diet also plays a role.

Tim R. had diarrhea. He had it bad. According to Tim he spent
more time in the bathroom than out. I asked him if he'd ever seen an
aspen tree. "Sure," he said. "We have one in our backyard.
Why?"

With great doubt Tim went home and gathered bark from his
aspen tree. He made what is called a tincture* and placed ten drops
of it in sherry wine. His diarrhea stopped within hours. I put him on
a food-control program on which he ate only lean meat, white fish,
poultry, cooked apples, milk puddings with arrowroot, toast and
cereals. He was not permitted to have whole wheat, buttermilk,
whey, dry toast, tea, coffee, or cocoa. He was told to avoid oatmeal
and all fibrous foods that are hard to digest. If his diarrhea persisted
he was told to go on an all-protein diet and eat foods that had been
put through a sieve to make them simpler to digest. Because of
aspen and controlled diet Tim has not had a recurrence since.

The bark of the *aspen* tree may be made into powder form,
decoctions or tinctures. Start with a small amount. Determine the
exact quantity you need by adding to each dose. This way you get to
know what your own personal dosage may be.

Infusions are made by steeping herbs in hot water below the boiling point to get their active
ingredients. Tea is an example.

*A *tincture* is made from herbs that have been dried, chopped, and pounded into a pulp and
soaked. Two ounces of alcohol, plus two ounces of water, are added to each ounce of herb.
Let this stand for eight to fourteen days in a cool, dark place. Pour off the top liquid. A
teaspoonful of glycerin is added to each four ounces of this liquid to make an effective
tincture.

BALSAM of PERU . . .
and How It Cured an Elderly
Woman of Leg Ulcers

Maude J. was in her seventies. She had leg ulcers the like of which I hadn't seen for years. She had gone the route from famous clinic to clinic in distant large cities as well as to all the doctors in our town. She had deep, large varicose ulcers that were rank, dirty, full of pus and were currently in the ugly process of sloughing off a skin graft that had just been performed at the cost of $3,000. Maude was bitter about it all. She complained about her legs, but most of all she felt guilty about exhausting the family savings, her children's included. Everything was gone and she still had her problem. The ulcer caverns continued to yawn up from her ankles.

After using physical therapy and an Unna Boot on her legs, I told her about *balsam of Peru*. She obtained it and took ten to twenty drops internally every day and applied a fifty percent strength preparation of it to the ulcerous areas. With Nature's herbal remedies, the ulcer stopped smelling. Little islands of healing began to make their appearance. The infection disappeared. It was a "little miracle" according to Maude and it worked. Within months the wounds were healed. Today she has only scar tissue and happy words for *balsam of Peru*.

> **NOTE:** Balsam of Peru is also effective taken internally for chronic bronchitis, eczema, and dysentery.

BLACKBERRY . . .
as a Cure for Indigestion

In addition to making wine from the berries, *blackberry* plants provide other good things. One of them is the herbal quality that is good for treatment of the bowel and its complaints. In Peter R.'s case, he was told to grind dried blackberry roots into powder if his health food store didn't have powder, that he could also make a tea, or decoction, from the roots by crushing them and placing one ounce of this material in a pint of water. After soaking this for twelve hours, he was to take two tablespoonfuls of the fluid three times daily. Peter did as instructed. His bowel problem retreated.

His food started digesting. Side effects, such as headaches and sluggish feelings, disappeared almost immediately. It was hard to believe but it happened.

BLESSED THISTLE
. . . Remedy to Induce Vomiting

Much time is spent explaining how to stop vomiting. There *are* times, however, when vomiting must be induced to get noxious waste out of the stomach. When used to start the process of vomiting, a concentrated solution of *blessed thistle* is made. How? Take six teaspoonfuls of crushed thistle leaves. Place the batch in one pint of cold water. Let it soak. Two tablespoonfuls of this tea start the vomiting. Half a teaspoonful is excellent as a tonic.

> **NOTE: There may be some tendency to sweat when blessed thistle is taken as a tea. Expect it. It's all part of the cleansing action.**

BLACK COHOSH . . .
Remedy for Rheumatism

The word "rheumatism" is a general term given to anything and everything causing soreness and stiffness in the muscles and pain and soreness in the joints. It may start with dietary problems as does gout. It may begin with infections such as rheumatic fever. It may be due to any fever or degenerative disease. It may even begin because of "nerves."

Whatever the cause, rheumatism may begin with the person's "feeling lousy." There may or may not be sore throat, tired feeling, chilliness with a joint getting red and tender to touch. The big joints are more commonly involved. Joints may become more tender as the days go by. They may enlarge and even become rigid. Fever may go to 103°F. A person with this problem usually smells sour from his profuse perspiration. His appetite disappears. Urination is not as frequent. His face, first blushing red, becomes pale. His tongue becomes heavily coated. He becomes constipated.

Mike D. came into the office persenting all the typical symptoms and signs. He admitted he'd had a lot of previous treatment and drugs in quantity with no results. After making an exhaustive physical examination, I determined his problem as rheumatism due to autointoxication. In other words, his rheumatism was self-induced. He did it himself. His diet was wrong, very wrong, and he was eating his way to the grave. I told him this and he became angry with me for saying so.

However, after he started using *black cohosh* ("squaw root"), his pains started to disappear. Wherever Mike goes now his *black cohosh* goes with him. Sure, he's had some recurrences, but the pain is nothing now in comparison to what it was. *Black cohosh,* an Indian herbal remedy, is used not just for rheumatism. It's also good for menstrual problems. As a syrup it's good for coughs and colds. As a poultice it may be used on all areas of inflammation. As a tincture (diluted alcoholic solution) five drops of it in sweetened water may be given to a child for whooping cough. To make the tincture pulverize the root. Add two ounces of root to each pint of gin, vodka, or whiskey. Wine may also be used.

BLUE COHOSH. . .
Indian Remedy to Conquer
"Female Complaints"

One of the better Indian remedies using teas is that of *blue cohosh* for female pelvic or uterine problems. *Blue cohosh* was also given to Indian women for predelivery relief from pain. How was the remedy concocted? A tea was made from the roots of the *blue cohosh* plant. This tea, taken for three weeks prior to delivery, was found to make childbirth easier, quicker, and almost painless. There is no restriction on quantity consumed. For rheumatism take two ounces of *blue cohosh* root and one ounce of *blood-root* and soak these crushed roots in whiskey or brandy for a week. Take a shotglass full three times daily. It's quite a remedy!

BUCHU BERRIES
. . . Solution to Problems
of Your Urinary System

Martine L. had had kidney problems for years. She simply couldn't hold her urine. She was constantly going through the embarrassment of knowing she was dribbling and it always happened in the most public places. On a warm day it was especially offensive, as you can well understand. It also burned and kept burning until she started using *buchu berries*. From her drugstore she obtained *buchu* powder and took one tablespoonful of powder three times daily in water, milk, or brandy. Another way she took her dosage of *buchu* was to make a tea from an ounce of crushed *buchu* leaves. Two to four tablespoonfuls of tea were taken twice daily. Martine found that only *buchu* berries were available in her area. She steeped them in hot water overnight. She drank a glassful of the fluid twice daily to cleanse her kidneys and bladder and within weeks her inflammation and hurt went away.

BUCKBEAN . . . the
Treatment Kelly R.
Used for "Shingles"

Buckbean sounds like a strange remedy but it's a good one that has been used successfully for a long time. Railroad man Kelly R. had an eruption of painful little blisters along his lower ribs on his right side. They followed in a line along his ribs and became agonizingly painful to the point where he couldn't do his job as yardmaster. He was instructed on how to make a tea using one ounce of dried *buckbean* leaves (obtained from the health food store) to one pint of boiling water. Four tablespoonfuls of the tea were taken three times daily. Kelly said, "I didn't believe it, but I guess I'm proof-positive that it works. My shingles disappeared just like that!"

NOTE: Buckbean tea may also be used for rheumatism and scurvy where there has been a lack of vitamin C.

BUSH HONEYSUCKLE
. . . Antidote for Poison Ivy

I wasn't aware of *bush honeysuckle* as a remedy for anything until one year on the farm I got a bad case of ivy poisoning. The country doctor instructed me to go home, strip some leaves and twigs from our *bush honeysuckle* and make a tea. He said all I had to do was apply it to my skin and the itching and inflammation would subside. I did and it did. He said I could drink any amount of the tea along with the external appplication.

NOTE: Bush honeysuckle is also good for conquering kidney and bladder stones.

CALIFORNIA LAUREL
. . . and How to Make
Muscle Cramps Disappear

Take ten drops of *laurel* tea in a wineglass of water twice daily. That's what I told Catherine S. who had developed leg cramps as a stock clerk in her father's factory. Like all other herbs, *California laurel* is obtainable at all health food stores or drugstores. Catherine made a fluid extract of the laurel leaves and took ten drops daily in water. Within three days Catherine reported that her leg cramps were gone.

NOTE: For headaches inhale the odor of crushed laurel leaves. Stop inhalation the moment the headache stops. For quelling a toothache or earache saturate cotton with this fluid extract and place it on the area of pain. Chills and fever may also be held in abeyance by taking ten drops in a wineglass of water twice daily.

CAPSICUM . . . As a
Way to Check Vomiting After
an Alcoholic Party

To celebrate his promotion, Tommy T. stopped at every bar on Main Street on his way home. By the time he reached his residence he was no longer happy with good news. He was full of booze and sick. He got out of the car, started vomiting and ran inside. His wife took one look, one sniff and ran for the *capsicum* (cayenne pepper). She mixed a quarter teaspoonful into a half-pint of tomato juice and made him drink it. Within moments the abdominal spasms were gone and that was the only lesson that Tommy needed.

NOTE: Cayenne pepper may be sprinkled on plasters for external application. It may be mixed with liniments for use for rheumatism and areas of neuralgia. For gas, colic or headache take five drops of diluted tincture of capsicum by mouth.

Quick Review
on Additional Valuable
HERBS

NOTE: The following unusual and unorthodox remedies are taken from Indian and pioneer days. They are folk remedies that have withstood time and use . . . and proven valuable. They are briefed for at-a-glance information and quick know-how.

Herb:	DILL
Purpose:	For *gas* and *dyspepsia*, and *after childbirth*.
How to Apply:	Make an infusion (tea) of dill seeds in boiling water (two tablespoonfuls in one pint of water). Drink as desired.

Herb:	ELDER (sweet)
Purpose:	For *bruises, erysipelas, pleurisy, gout* and *rheumatism*.
How to apply:	Make a tea of the flowers and berries *only*. Bark of the roots may be used *only* when berries and flowers are not available.

Herb: EUCALYPTUS
Purpose: For *head colds, stomach ulcers, external ulcers, bladder* and *vaginal problems* and *bad breath*.
How to apply: Place four drops of eucalyptus oil in a steam atomizer, cover your head and breathe in the steam. For odorous ulcers place two tablespoonfuls of oil in one pint of warm water. Rinse external ulcer craters with this fluid three times daily.

Herb: FENNEL
Purpose: For *colic* in children, *dyspepsia*.
How to apply: Pulverize three tablespoonfuls of fennel seeds. Make tea in one pint of hot water. Take half teaspoonful per dose on the hour until relieved.

Herb: GENTIAN
Purpose: For *severe diarrhea, stomach* and *bowel* inactivity.
How to apply: Make tea of roots and tops of the gentian plant in one pint of boiling water. Flowers may be added to this tea. *Dose*: one tablespoonful with brandy.

Herb: GINGER
Purpose: For *diarrhea, colic, dysentery, muscular rheumatism, toothache, headache, neuralgia*.
How to apply: One-third teaspoonful of powdered ginger well-diluted in one pint of water. Take a wineglassful until symptoms depart. May be applied externally as a hot wet application* to relieve muscle pain, toothache and neuralgia.

Herb: JUNIPER
Purpose: Diuretic for *dropsy, skin diseases*.
How to apply: Mash and steep one ounce of juniper berries in a pint of boiling water. Take a cupful on the hour over a period of twenty-four hours.

Herb: LEEK
Purpose: For *inflammation* (external), *burns, ulcers, insect bites*.
How to apply: Mash a fresh plant, apply externally to the ulcer or burn

*Hot wet applications are called *fomentations*. The herbs (entire plant) are boiled in a bag. Wring out the liquid and apply the bag to the aching part.

or area of inflammation. For internal use make a syrup by bruising the greens. Squeeze out the juice. Add an equal weight of sugar. Take one tablespoonful of the liquid every two hours until symptoms stop.

Herb: MARSHMALLOW
Purpose: For *tumors*, treatment for *swelling*, stops *itching* and *burning*.
How to apply: Apply a poultice* externally to the swelling or tumor. The root should be cut into small pieces, mashed and boiled in sweet milk to make this poultice effective. To this mass add a teaspoonful of powdered elm bark to the boiling material until it becomes thick. Apply as hot as is comfortable. Reapply when dry. In ointment form it may be applied on areas of burns and itching. For mouth cankers use a half-ounce of dried roots in two pints of water. Boil down to one pint. Use as a mouth rinse.

Herb: MUSTARD
Purpose: For *pain* (external) as a *foot bath* and as a *plaster*.
How to apply: To make a mustard plaster beat the white of one egg. Add a little flour and ground mustard seed. Apply plaster where needed. To "draw blood from the brain" or start sweating place feet in a hot mustard foot bath (two tablespoonfuls of powder in a half bucket of hot water).

Herb: ONION
Purpose: For *colds* and *croup* (children), as a poultice for *infections* to release *suppressed urine*.
How to apply: To make an onion syrup roast the herb. Cut it up and mash it. Squeeze out the juice. Add sugar. Give a child one tablespoonful for colds or croup (until symptoms are gone). For treatment of boils, carbuncles, or infected areas, place half a baked onion on the area. Fix in position overnight. Eating fresh onions is a good method for releasing urine locked in the bladder.

Herb: PEPPERMINT
Purpose: For *heartburn, nausea, vomiting, gas*.

---

*A poultice, when applied, gives a prolonged moist heat and thereby relieves pain. It brings suppuration to a head.

How to apply: Peppermint may be given as an oil, as a powder or as a tea. To make an infusion (tea) boil one ounce of peppermint leaves in a quart of water. Drink as much as desired. Where there are abdominal problems, mash fresh leaves and apply the mass as is externally to the abdomen.

Mary McK. had had heartburn for years. She complained of acid coming up from her stomach to cause a burning sensation in her throat. She continued to have this discomfort despite all the prescribed anti-acids and other potions. The problem didn't interfere too much with her activity but it did make her feel miserable day after day. She got to the point where she didn't want to eat any more because food made her feel worse. This pyrosis, or burning, simply got worse and when I saw her the burning in her throat was already interfering with her speech. Her throat was inflamed and swollen. I'd never seen a case go so far. In fact, I suspected it was more likely to be a drug allergy than pyrotic in origin. I started her on peppermint tea. The first three days there were no appreciable results. Then a mashed fresh peppermint leaf poultice was placed on her tummy. That's when results made themselves apparent. I started her on soft foods and within days she was her smiling self again. After years of heartburn, the symptoms simply disappeared.

Where every other treatment had failed, peppermint tea and the application of mashed leaves on her tummy caused a cure. Mary watches her diet now. She takes her peppermint tea regularly and there hasn't been a recurrence since.

Herb: **PLEURISY ROOT**
Purpose: For *pleurisy, chest pain, low grade fever* in a teething baby, *acute rheumatism.*
How to apply: Make tea by crushing one ounce of pleurisy root and boil in one and one-half pints of water. Take a half teaspoonful three times daily. This remedy may also be taken as a powder to relieve difficult breathing as well as the pain of pleurisy. It may also be used to start perspiration in breaking a fever.

Pleurisy is no fun. John M. found this out the day after getting cold chills after sitting in a duck blind on a wet miserable fall day.

He had stabbing pains in his left lung. It became worse when he tried to breathe deeply or when he coughed. His fever went up to 103° F. His face was pale. He had a perplexed or anxious look about him and when I walked into the examining room he was lying on the side that hurt him most. He said that he had already been to another doctor and had been given a prescription but the hurt along the margin of his ribs still continued. Sometimes the pain shot into his belly. This area was tender on finger tip pressure. He had difficulty breathing. This was further complicated by the fact that he started to hiccough. In all, John was miserable. He laughed when I told him about *pleurisy root* but he got some anyhow. The next day he returned to the office with an amazed expression on his face. "I can't believe it!" he said. "The pain's gone. I can breathe. My fever's gone. A few cents' worth of pleurisy root did it when all those expensive drugs failed. I simply don't understand it at all!"

Herb:	PRINCE'S PINE
Purpose:	For *sciatica, gout, chronic rheumatism*.
How to apply:	*Prince's pine* is also known as "rheumatism weed" or "ground holly." A tincture is made from this herb by placing a quarter-pound of dried herb into a quart of wine. Seal the container. Keep in a dry place for two weeks. Use as desired to relieve the problem.

Herb:	PUMPKIN
Purpose:	For all *urinary problems* (spasm, scalding urine, etc.).
How to apply:	Boil two ounces of pumpkin seeds in one and one-half pints of water. Take a wineglassful three times daily. This remedy is also said to be good for getting rid of tapeworms but I have never had this experience.

Herb:	RED CLOVER
Purpose:	*Neutralize gastric acidity, purify the blood,* apply on *external ulcers*.
How to apply:	Make an infusion of the roots and drink as desired. Tea may also be applied to ulcers and sores externally. Good for cold sores and sore lips. A syrup may be made by boiling red clover blossoms in water.

Herb:	RED RASPBERRY
Purpose:	For *cankers, proud flesh, sore mouth, burns, scalds*.

How to apply: Crush one ounce of dried leaves and boil in one pint of
                    water. Use as a mouthwash. For poultices, thicken the
                    tea with elm bark and crackers and apply to cankers and
                    proud flesh. For children make a tea of the leaves and
                    sweeten with honey for improved taste.

It was happenstance that Tom K. discovered raspberry leaves as a
treatment for proud flesh. Tom had had a fingernail infection. A
felon developed. Irritated tissues piled up around the nail. It was
sore and festering before he started pruning and clearing away his
red raspberry bushes on the small garden plot behind his house. In
the process of clearing the brambles, chunks of the dried leaves
clung to the moist, festering proud flesh. He didn't think anything
about it until the next morning. The inflammation, redness and
swelling had subsided. The superfluous tissue had begun to shrink.
He stopped me on the street to tell me about his discovery. You can
make this for yourself. A tea made of dry red raspberry leaves to
which has been added elm bark and crushed crackers makes a good
treatment for proud flesh. The angry irritation is quick to depart.

Herb: SAGE
Purpose: For *tonsillitis, tiredness, fever, colds,* and *coughs,
                    thrush, "summer complaint," worms in children.*
How to apply: Make an infusion, or tea. This fluid may be used as a
                    gargle for thrush and tonsillitis or taken internally an
                    ounce at a time.

Herb: SKUNK CABBAGE
Purpose: For *asthma, coughing, catarrh.*
How to apply: Skunk cabbage may be administered as a powder, a
                    syrup or as a tincture. Tinctures and syrups are made
                    from the roots and seeds. Powdered root may be given in
                    five-grain doses.

Herb: SLIPPERY ELM
Purpose: For *wounds, burns, frostbite, felons, ulcers, erysipelas.*
How to apply: For external application *slippery elm* bark is boiled in hot
                    water (one pint) and is applied to the lesion as a hot mass
                    between two pieces of cloth. Slippery elm tea is also
                    good for those who are just recovering from any illness.

Herb: SPEARMINT
Purpose: For *nausea* and *vomiting, piles* (hemorrhoids).
How to apply: Mash a handful of spearmint leaves and drop it into a quart of boiling water. Take tea as necessary to relieve nausea or vomiting. For kidney and bladder stones, make a tincture by mashing the entire green plant and dropping it in gin. Drink as desired. Saturate a wad of cotton with this same tincture and apply to hemorrhoids for quick relief.

Herb: THYME
Purpose: For *headache, to promote perspiration.*
How to apply: Add seven ounces of turpentine to one ounce of thyme oil. (This herb is cut while in bloom.) It may be used as a liniment.

Herb: VIRGINIA SNAKEROOT
Purpose: For *snake bite, fever, colds, bile problems,* to check *vomiting,* to soothe the *stomach.*
How to apply: A third of a teaspoonful of powdered snakeroot may be added to water and boiled. Take four tablespoonfuls of this tea every three hours.

Herb: WILD CHERRY
Purpose: For *colic, dyspepsia, intermittent fevers, diarrhea, dysentery.*
How to apply: Crush a handful of wild cherry bark and soak it in cold water (*not hot water*), for forty-eight hours. Take a wineglassful of this tea three times daily for any or all of the above problems.

Herb: WITCH HAZEL
Purpose: For *hemorrhages, piles, ulcers, external inflammation, tumors* (external).
How to apply: Make a poultice of bark and apply externally to all painful piles, sores and other inflammations. Make a tea from the leaves and apply externally as an astringent.

There's one I'd like to add. It's out of alphabetical sequence but it will interest you as much as it did me.

ALLIGATOR PEAR
. . . Treatment for Neuralgia

Adrienne A. was only twelve years old but she was having parox-
ysms of acute pain in her arms and shoulders. Sometimes the sharp
pain lasted for seconds, sometimes it lasted for minutes. It was the
child's crying that brought her to my office. Many diagnoses of her
problem had been made but none of the tests showed positive for
any ailment and no part of her physical history indicated possible
bone or soft tissue complications. I was inclined to diagnose her
pain as *neuralgia* but since children are seldom affected with it I
doubted that this would be the problem.

One thing was certain, the child was experiencing pain. Nature
was crying out in anguish. So was Adrienne. When exposed to cold
she became worse. When I learned that her mother and grandmother
had had the same thing, this made for a possible hereditary connection.

The child was fatigued most of the time. Simply stroking her skin
made her hurt. Her muscles jumped. There was no tenderness along
the course of her major nerves but there were points of pain enroute.
I remembered a professor at school saying, "When neuralgic pain
occurs, it is the nerve's prayer for healthy blood." Our treatment
began right there: healthy blood. Along with a changed diet,
alligator pear was applied externally on the area of pain. One and a
half ounces of fluid extract rubbed into the skin, which was then
covered with warm flannel. Within days the pain was gone. Within
weeks her skin was no longer hypersensitive. Her muscles no longer
jumped. There were no recurrences. Today Adrienne is a healthy
young woman. She has her own family now, and whenever her
youngsters have the same kind of pain out comes the alligator pear
juice and the pain subsides.

Yes, all of this is said to be unorthodox and unusual, but the herbs
of yesterday still continue to be excellent treatments today.

Chapter 3

Magic Minerals Called "Cell Salts"

and an amazing route to health

NOTE: This chapter is a long one. It contains a mountain of usable information. All of this is given to you at-a-glance for easy reading. Read slowly! Absorb it! Note how it applies to you.

Your body is a concentration of power cells and it remains a dynamo of power until the basic source of energy is cut off.

Each tiny body cell is specialized in its own way. Every organ and body part is made up of these cells, and the structure, the total health of these organs and body parts, is determined by incredibly small particles of minerals or biochemical salts that feed them, and therein lies the very secret of health!

77

Herein also is the story of what happens when health fails and how you can use those unusual and unorthodox remedies called "cell salts" to come back to living better, living longer and being free of aches and pains.

What Does "Biochemical" Mean?

"Bio" means living matter in all its forms and phenomena: its beginning, its growth, its reproduction, its makeup and its structure. In other words, *bio* means *you*! "Chemical," as the word implies, is the makeup of substances that cause certain reactions to take place when minerals or salts are absorbed into the human body . . . *your* body. Each mineral or chemical salt is individually good for each individual organ, tissue or body part. Each has a purpose and a role. Without cell salts or minerals we do not have health. We cannot survive. We are totally dependent on their might. As powerhouses of potential energy, these biochemical substances create Nature's own tiny miracles that take place within us day after day. This dynamo of power flows by the way of the bloodstream.

BLOOD . . . Master Conveyor Belt to Health

The secret to health lies in the lifelines through which your bloodstream flows. It's the chemistry of life flowing nonstop through miles of subways and this network of tubes is the conveyor belt that makes you tick. As a supercharged pipeline it carries magic miracle foods as long as they are being fed into the system. These incredibly amazing health-makers are at work day and night.

Blood circulates through your heart, arteries, capillaries and veins. In the form of liquid plasma and cells it carries nourishment and oxygen from head to toe. It transports daily food needs to their destination and picks up waste to be transported to physiological dumps such as the bowel, the liver, the lungs, kidneys and skin. In twenty seconds it runs the entire vascular route and there's no comparably efficient system that can beat it.

> *Floating in this magic stream are the miracle-makers, the chemistry of cell salts, that control everything about you. In the plasma, as well as in the blood cells, are water, fat, and such minerals as calcium fluoride, iron, lime, magnesium, silicate, soda and potash. All of these are known as "cell salts," each with a particular destination, each with a significant function, each with a controlling interest in the specialized tissues that demand them. The secret of administering these miracle-makers lies in a minimal dose . . . .tiny flotillas of health without which we cannot live.*

**Nature Deals in Atoms
. . . Only Small Amounts
Are Required**

"The use of small doses for the cure of diseases in the biochemical method is a chemico-physiological necessity," according to the father of cell salt therapy, Wilhelm Schussler, M.D.*

Minerals, or cell salts, in the blood cell are in the minutest amounts. For example, in 1,000 grams of blood cells there are only 0.99 grams of iron, 0.13 grams of potassium sulfate, 2.3 grams of potassium phosphate, 3.07 grams of potassium chloride. Plasma, on the other hand, has inorganic materials (minerals) in even lesser amounts with the exception of sodium chloride (common table salt) 5.5 grams of which is found normally in every 1,000 grams of plasma. Milk, said to be the "perfect food," provides only minute traces of all the cell salts vital to body health and physiological normalcy. It is computed that one blood cell contains about a billionth part of a gram of potassium chloride. So you see, when we deal with the human body, we are dealing with fractions of cure and overdosage is something we can't afford.

---

*Schussler, W. *Biochemical Treatment of Disease*. (Philadelphia, PA: Boericke and Tafel, Publishers, 1946, p. 36).

Body Vitality Is Determined
by the Substances That Feed It

Cell salts, as Nature's remedy for building health and body vitality or restoring it, are normally the end products of the digestion of food after it has gone through the process of metabolism. Through metabolism inorganic substances, or minerals, are taken into the body and converted into kinds of materials necessary for this process: specific minerals for building tissues of the kidney, special minerals for the bone, and so on.

Deplete these minute miracle-food substances for any reason, remove or lose them, and poor health begins. What is an example of just this? What follows in the wake of cell-salt shortage?

The end product of calcium deficiency came on with a vengeance in the case of Mary V. It started with what appeared to be rheumatism. She exhibited sleeplessness, nervous exhaustion, body aches and muscle tremor. Each symptom was a signpost pointing to a health problem and a basic calcium imbalance. As a result of a deficiency in these magic, minute minerals, Mary's physical resistance went down. Her dynamic powers were depleted. Her energy was gone and she became a candidate for just about anything that came along.

If this doesn't convince you, let's take the case of John R., accountant. John developed a hard, dry cough. Then came the misery of erysipelas (St. Anthony's Fire), which turned his skin into a burning, itching mass of pain. He had nosebleeds and hemorrhoids. His gums and eyelids were inflamed. He had carbuncles and ulcers in his skin. He was a ready victim for colds and was quick to develop influenza, bronchitis and bronchial catarrh. All of this started with an iron deficiency. In Mary's case, where calcium was added to her diet, and in John's case, where iron phosphate was added, the lives of both changed. These minute additives changed the course of their lives, just as they change the course of the life of a child who is deficient in iron and begins to wet the bed.

Iron salts in solution in the body possess the power to transform sunlight into body energy. This energy is then transported to all body cells via the hemoglobin that is in each blood cell. Nature is the master chemist. Nature wields the mortar and pestle of quantity,

Nature uses them to promote healing, develop internal anti-toxins, precipitins, agglutinins and bacteriolysins, which the bloodstream uses to fight infection.

These magic salts such as iron phosphate must be in balanced control in the hemoglobin of blood cells to prevent *anemia*. They generate the dynamo of life. According to Gilbert, "When these tissue remedies enter the body they become a living force."*

HOW DO YOU ACHIEVE HEALTH?
WHAT CAN YOU DO?

The Power of Cell-Salt
Therapy Is in Your Hands

Under normal circumstances, with proper food control, proper digestion and proper metabolism, mineral salts pass from the intestine into the bloodstream. By way of this master conveyor belt they are transported to the specialized cells that demand them for survival and health. As long as wholesome nutrition is maintained, there is no physical, mental, or infectious conflict and the body remains calm. Health is maintained. Just as the farmer places nutriments in the soil to keep his plants flourishing, so must our bodies be properly fed. If health circumstances are not normal, signs and symptoms of nutritional deficiency are quick to follow. What we are going to do in this chapter is show you how to recognize these signs and symptoms and then how to counter them with those magic minute minerals that can change the course of your life. With the taking of these magic cell salts you become the architect and builder of your own body and life!

Health, therefore, is a state of regulated cellular balance. Health is a physical and mental state in which all cell salts are supplied as living forces to activate structures that make the person and personality you are. These cell salts, as life forces,

*Gilbert, H. "Biotherapy." (Grantham, England: British Biochemic Association Publishers, 1935, p. 15).

help you repair, regenerate and reconstruct. They restore the
well-being that is inalienably yours.

Disease, on the other hand, is what occurs when mineral salts, for any reason, are lacking in the bloodstream. The phenomenon of disease develops due to shortages and cure comes *only* with the restoration of cellular balance. To rebuild health then it is necessary to know which cell salt to use for what. If you would conquer ill health it is necessary to follow the rules of health and the natural laws of biochemistry within you. Only then will the equilibrium of health be accomplished. Only then will disease be cured. Only then will body function be restored so that you can live longer, live happier, and stay young!

Under Normal Circumstances
Cell Salts Are Extracted
from Foods . . . Sometimes

"The normal American diet gives us what we need in the way of vitamins and minerals." That's what authorities tell us. However, despite outraged professional talk that Americans have "good diets," they are among the worst fed in the world because American foods are dangerously inferior and devoid of vitamins and the magic minerals we need. Our eating habits are even worse because nobody remains normal on a diet of hamburgs. french fries, and cola. Foodstuffs, grown in the modern manner, heavily processed with preservatives, are no longer wholesome. American processed foods, with all their additives, are today contributing to disease rather than supplying those mineral needs so desperately needed. There is more illness in the United States than ever before. Adulterated foods are part of this problem. Because American foods have become inadequate our bodies demonstrate this lack immediately by way of one or more signs and symptoms that you are herein going to learn. And as you investigate further into the cell-salt saga, and realize the little miracles it can create for you each day, you will know why you have the aches and pains you have, and which cell salts you can take to chase them. Like magic you will rectify nutritional errors as is being done in the animal laboratories today. And why not? Isn't it health that you and I want?

What Are the Names of These Amazing Cell Salts So Important to Health?

There are twelve major cell salts upon which our brain and body thrive. In fact, our very life is dependent upon them. Without them the garden of life stops growing. Take one or two cell salts away and illness sets in. Take all of them away and we are destined for the end. So let's think about these minute miracle-makers. Let's give exact names to these amazing cell salts that are so vital to health and longer life. Let's use those unusual and unorthodox remedies of yesterday in our search for well-being today.

Those Twelve Amazing Cell Salts That Make Your Life Worth a Fortune

NOTE: Both Latin and common names are given so that it will be easier for you to order them at the drugstore or the health food store.

1. *Kali Muriaticum* (potassium chloride, chloride of potash)
2. *Natrum Muriaticum* (sodium chloride, table salt)
3. *Calcarea Sulphurica* (calcium sulfate or gypsum)
4. *Natrum Sulphuricum* (sodium sulfate or Glauber's salts)
5. *Kali Sulphuricum* (potassium sulfate or potash)
6. *Calcarea Phosphorica* (calcium phosphate, lime)
7. *Ferrum Phosphoricum* (iron phosphate)
8. *Kali Phosphoricum* (potassium phosphate or potash)
9. *Natrum Phosphoricum* (sodium phosphate)
10. *Magnesium Phosphoricum* (magnesium phosphate)
11. *Calcarea Fluorica* (calcium fluoride, fluoride of lime)
12. *Silicea* (silica)

*Here's Your Magic Key
for Self-Treatment*

Phosphates are used as remedies for nervous system problems.
Chlorides (as well as phosphates) are used for treatments of
    muscles.
Sulfates for treatment of bone. (Also see *Additional Treatment
    Tips* that follow.)

*The Treatment Key
for Cell-Salt Therapy
Is Simple to Learn*

Each cell salt has a definite duty. Each is a specific for a particular part of your body or a certain function. To simplify knowing which cell salt to use, the following key is provided. After you have learned the characteristics of the remedies and have determined your own signs and symptoms, you can render self-therapy. For example: If there is *inflammation* in a body part (as in sore throat) the remedy is *Ferrum Phosphoricum.* If there is *soreness,* but no inflammation, then your remedy is *Natrum Phosphoricum.* There is no need to memorize any of this, and no need to be frightened by the technical terms. Just consult the following key.

Additional Treatment Tips

General Symptoms	Cell Salts to Use
Inflammation	iron phosphate
Soreness and acidity	sodium sulfate
Pain	magnesium phosphate
Low temperature making pain worse	calcium phosphate
Fever or soreness after exercise	potassium phosphate and sodium phosphate
Problems worsened by warmth and improved by coldness. All discharges yellow in color	potassium sulfate

General Symptoms	Cell Salts to Use
Muscle spasms, cramps, pain relieved by warmth or pressure	magnesium phosphate, calcium phosphate, and quartz
Croupy cough, dental problems, bulging varicose veins	calcium fluoride
All bilious problems	sodium sulfate
Greyish-white secretions on the tongue	potassium chloride

Where Are Cell Salts Available?

Your local health food store or drugstore may have these "salts" in stock. Also, manufacturers such as Boericke and Tafel of Philadelphia and Luyties of St. Louis, Mo., may be written to on this matter. In any event I am now going to give you a number of common ailments and how they can be treated. Only ailments treatable at home are considered here. In this book of unusual and unorthodox treatments you may find a lot of answers to personal problems. You, too, may restore health by using Nature's own remedies. The little tablets you get from your druggist or health food store come in various potencies. The most generally satisfactory potency or strength is 6X. NOTE OF CAUTION: *When improvement sets in DISCONTINUE the remedy!*

Potassium
Chloride (*Kali Muriaticum*) chloride of potash

The Story: Body chemistry is pretty much an unknown to most folks. In explaining potassium chloride to Marcella and John R. and their family here's what I said: "Potassium chloride is a cell salt found normally in nerve, muscle and blood cells. The time to take this cell salt is when a greyish-white secretion appears on the tongue or when an illness is chronic. Anyone suffering from a deficiency of potassium chloride finds that any or all his symptoms and hurts are *emphasized by motion*, that his belly is easily upset by eating rich or fatty foods." Marcella and John's family was remarkable in its potassium chloride deficiency. What was more remarkable was that each of them was affected differently.

At-a-Glance Chart to Know Whether Your
Symptoms Demand Treatment by
POTASSIUM CHLORIDE

Body Part	Symptoms
Head:	John R. showed snowy shoulders as a result of his potassium chloride deficiency. He had dandruff and eruptions on his scalp. He had sick headaches, stuffy head colds, and his skin was saffron or jaundiced in color. There was a chronic white discharge from his ears. He had earaches and heard strange noises. His mouth was raw, his tongue white and slimy. He coughed up white slime. There was swelling, inflammation and fever when sore throat set in.
Throat:	With Kelly R., male, aged eight, the symptoms were somewhat like his Dad's with his throat a warehouse for bacteria. Pharyngitis and chronic sore throat were constant with deafness in one ear. He had tonsillitis and even lost his voice for a time.
Gastric System:	After eating rich food Marcella R.'s potassium chloride deficiency showed up as white mucus in her throat. Her liver became inactive. Diarrhea followed eating. She had chronic constipation and a tender abdomen, dysentery and general abdominal discomfort.
Pelvis and Sex Organs:	Kathy R., aged fifteen, reacted differently. Her potassium chloride deficiency showed up as an inflamed bladder with sand in her urine. She had a white discharge (leukorrhea) and what appeared to be an ulcer in her uterus. Her breasts were inflamed. Her menstrual period was suppressed and usually overdue.
Respiratory System:	Potassium chloride deficiency made itself known in Jackson R., aged eleven, as croup and pleurisy. As a result of this cell-salt deficiency he was an asthmatic.
Back:	Millie, aged sixteen, had pain in her back when lying in bed. These pains were emphasized by movement. But that was the sum total of her discomfort.

Extremities: Tommy, aged seventeen, on the other hand, had pain in his big toe joints and it wasn't gout. His joints swelled. He experienced rheumatic pain when moving around. His muscles went into spasm.

Skin: With John R., Jr. potassium chloride deficiency showed up in the skin. He had acne, cold sores and pimples. His skin was scaly and dry.

The point here is that the whole family was affected and yet each was affected in a different way. All folks do not react the same way to a potassium chloride deficiency, or for that matter to any other deficiency.

Addition Health Problems
for Which Potassium Chloride Is Helpful

Croup	Bronchitis
Diphtheria	Broncho-pneumonia
Dysentery	Rheumatism
Pneumonia	Asthma
Epilepsy	Pleurisy
Eczema	

Rx: Take two 6X tabs every two hours until symptoms are gone.

Sodium Chloride (*Natrum Muriaticum*) Common table salt

As I explained to Madeline De L., who had been on a salt-free reducing diet for over a year, *sodium chloride*, common as it is, is vital to health. As a part of every liquid and solid in the human body it regulates most of the body's activities and is important to its function. Sodium chloride regulates the passage of minerals through cell walls. It regulates the amount of moisture in tissues and when this regulatory force is lost, swelling and/or dehydration may begin. Sure, removing salt from her diet was a way for Madeline to lose weight, but it also set up a series of complications. Sodium chloride influences all the body's systems, its organs and parts. It especially affects the blood, liver, spleen and mucous membrane of the alimentary canal. Aches of all kinds are benefited by regulating salt balance such as toothache, headaches, aches in the cheek or jaw, or even stomachache. Where vomiting has occurred, salt must be resupplied. Where there has been excessive diarrhea, the water balance has to be rebalanced and salt is vital in this matter as well.

On the other hand, when too much salt is taken with meals it creates a definite influence on the intestinal tract. Those little absorption depots called villi cannot absorb liquids in the intestine and the reverse takes place. Instead of absorbing fluid it pours *into* the intestine, and a watery stool and diarrhea result. Even the stomach wall exudes this bitter fluid, which is often vomited up as "water brash." As with potassium chloride, note that sodium chloride loss doesn't affect everyone the same way.

At-a-Glance Chart to Know Whether Your Symptoms Demand Treatment by SODIUM CHLORIDE

Body Part	Symptoms
Head:	Nelson A. had a sodium chloride deficiency that led to mental depression. His brain was tired. He had sick headaches, hammering headaches that were at their worst in the morning. His eyelids were inflamed. He itched along the hairline at the base of his skull. His vision was impaired. He lost his sense of smell and taste. He had cold sores on his lips. His neck muscles felt weak, his skin was sallow, and he had nasal catarrh. He complained of being dizzy.
Gastric System:	Tom R., on the other hand, had an extreme thirst as a part of his general feeling when he went without salt. He had a feeling of hunger. He vomited up bitter water. His breath was offensive and there was a feeling of heartburn in his chest. His anus burned after his bowels moved and constipation was a constant problem, as were hemorrhoids and fissures (cracks) in his anus.

Urinary System
and
Sex Organs: With Joyce B. it was still another matter. Her sodium chloride deficiency showed up as a bladder problem. Involuntary squirting of urine occurred. It was frequent and embarrassing. Sometimes it occurred at night. Her vagina burned after urinating. It also prolapsed (dropped). A burning white discharge plagued her. She had annoying menstrual difficulties and all of this brought on mental depression.

Back: Richard R.'s reaction to lack of salt was to feel chilly. His back ached even when lying on a soft mattress. His hips were painful when he lay on his side. Backache was pretty much constant.

Extremities: The legs of most folks suffering from salt deficiency feel weak. Their joints creak and snap.

Additional Health Problems
for Which Sodium Chloride Is Helpful

Anemia	Mumps
Coryza	Chronic catarrh
Intermittent fevers	

Rx: Take two 6X tabs twice daily until symptoms are relieved.

Calcium
Sulfate *(Calcarea Sulphurica)* gypsum

This cell salt is found normally in the connective tissues of the body and in the bile. Deprive the connective tissues and skin of *calcium sulfate* and characteristic problems follow in its wake. Pus may form and it is at this stage in an infection that calcium sulfate is at its best for healing. The way to gauge when to take this cell salt is when skin eruptions come to a head. Calcium sulfate plays another role in the human body. It helps eliminate, or get rid of, worn-out blood corpuscles. It is also of value where any body part has been showing discharge for a period of time without healing. This minute mineral is one of the cell salts that does not remain in the biochemical system of the body. When they are taken into the body they are held only long enough to take care of an existing problem. This was the way it happened with the Johnson family.

At-a-Glance Chart to Know Whether Your Symptoms Demand Treatment by CALCIUM SULFATE

Body Part	Symptoms
Head:	Yellow mattery sores and scabs appear on the heads of children when there is a lack of calcium sulfate. Pimples and pustules appear on the face and this is often the cause of teenage acne. Sometimes the scalp looks and feels like it has been scalded. The rims of nasal openings are tender to touch, and a thick discharge comes from a cold in the head. The cornea of the eye may develop an abscess and yellow discharge. The gums bleed easily and may develop boils. There is sore throat. Neck glands may ulcerate. The ears sometimes have a discharge of pus mixed with blood. There may be headaches with pain worse in the front part of the head. This may be accompanied by nausea but not necessarily vomiting.
Respiratory System:	Bronchitis and catarrh develop with thick, lumpy phlegm. Often there is a high fever in the person who is very deficient in calcium sulfate. Such a person has a short, hard cough. Strangely, and I can't account for it, when he coughs eruptions appear on his skin.
Back:	Aches may occur in the entire back. Usually the pain is worse in the low back. Herpetic eruptions (painful blisters) may break out on the back. These occur along the shaft of the ribs or between them.
Extremities	The soles of the feet itch furiously and may burn. Herpes, boils, carbuncles and abscesses may break out. This person gets frostbite very easily. Ulcers develop on his legs. All the sores that develop suppurate. His injuries are hard to heal. Felons may occur around the nails of his toes.
Gastric System:	The stool is often green in color.

Pelvis: Menstrual periods prolonged.

Additional Health Problems
for Which Calcium Sulphate Is Helpful
    Kidney problems
    Neuralgia in the aged or weak
    Colds

Rx: Take two 6X tabs on the hour for one week.

Sodium
Sulfate (*Natrum Sulphuricum*) Glauber's salt

This sodium salt appears only in the intercellular fluids and never in the tissue cells themselves. Its job is to regulate water loss. In this role it is important in the control of bilious conditions, liver diseases and dropsy. Deficiency in this cell salt is marked by a greenish-brown coating on the tongue. For folks who have uric acid problems it is *the* antidote and is of equal value to those who live in damp places and have muscle and joint pain. Fondulac de L. lived in the Louisiana bayou country. I first met him at a Miami Beach doctors' convention. He complained of his aches and pains but refused to move from the place where he was born. I suggested *sodium sulfate* as an antidote to his problems. The next time I saw him at a New Orleans convention he reported that his pains were gone.

There are some interesting facts about sodium sulfate that you should know. It does *not* act like sodium chloride in the body. Sodium sulfate attracts water *only* after water has been created as a waste product by the tissues. Sodium chloride (table salt) *attracts* water that the body's cells will use. Sodium sulfate draws water *away*, especially from white cells (leucocytes) in the blood and kills them. Thus it could be an aid in treating leukemia. Sodium sulfate stimulates the nerves to the bile duct, the gall bladder and liver, the pancreas and intestines. It aids them in their duties of secretion as well as excretion. Any disturbance in sodium sulfate balance in the body may be expressed as chills, fever, vomiting, biliousness, diarrhea, edema and even herpes. Let's take a look now at the symptoms of sodium sulfate deficiency.

At-a-Glance Chart to Know Whether Your
Symptoms Demand Treatment by
SODIUM SULFATE

Body Part	Symptoms
Head:	Bilious diarrhea may bring on sick headaches. Most of the headache pain will be at the base of the skull. There is nausea and vomiting. The white of the eye becomes discolored yellow (bile). The skin becomes sallow and jaundiced. The mouth has a bitter taste and is full of thick catarrhal mucus.
Lungs:	Asthma that is worse in damp weather, difficult breathing, cough with ropy expectoration, bronchial catarrh, purulent expectoration (greenish), bronchitis and soreness in the chest.
Gastric System:	Vomiting up of bile, gassy colic, dark stool, diarrhea, biliousness is worse in the morning and is especially bad during wet weather. Stool is clay-colored and there is painful distress in the liver.
Urinary System:	Sand in the urine.
Skin:	Abscesses and fistulae appear. Skin is jaundiced.
Back:	Neck muscles pull. Entire spinal column aches.
Extremities:	Swelling may occur in the extremities complicated by sciatic pain and gout in the joints. The extremities twitch during sleep and there is often pain just beneath the nails of the fingers and toes.

Additional Health Problems
for Which Sodium Sulphate Is Helpful

Gout	Sciatica
Dropsy	Cholecystitis
Diabetes	Leukemia
Intermittent fevers from any cause	

Rx: Take two 6X tabs every two hours for a week, thereafter only as symptoms appear.

Potassium
Sulfate *(Kali Sulphuricum)* **potash**

Potassium sulfate is found in all body cells where iron is found. Acting with iron it aids in the transfer of oxygen from the lungs to the red corpuscles. Folks deficient in potassium sulfate always feel chilly. Such a person experiences vertigo (dizziness), toothaches, headaches and pain in the extremities. Because potassium sulfate helps regulate healing via the red blood cells it is very helpful in problems of the skin. It throws off or exfoliates external segments of the skin damaged by scarlet fever, scarletina, measles, etc., and even does the same for the bronchial tubes.

In most part the skin and mucous membrane are strongly influenced by potassium sulfate. In the later stages of inflammation it is the cell salt you can take to get maximum results when treating yourself for symptoms that occur as the result of deficiency. Remarkable about folks who need this minute mineral is that their problems are worse toward evening. They are worse during warm weather or when subjected to heat. They are relieved by coolness or going out into the open air. Another factor to remember is that those who need potassium sulfate added to their diet usually have a yellow mucous discharge from organs or parts involved by illness or damage. Deficiencies in this cell salt leave a person with the problems described in the following table.

At-a-Glance Chart to Know Whether Your
Symptoms Demand Treatment by
POTASSIUM SULFATE

Body Part	Symptoms
Head:	Headaches and dizziness are par for the course in potassium sulfate deficiency. Warmth makes the problem worse, especially toward evening. The person with this problem loses his sense of smell. His nose is obstructed and the discharge released is usually yellow in color. He has dandruff. Eruptions occur in his scalp. All such eruptions have an offen-

sive odor. Burning thirst develops. So does a yellow-coated tongue. This person dislikes hot food or liquid.

Chest: Catarrh and bronchial asthma are often offenders in this deficiency. The person with this involvement feels as though he's suffocating during hot weather. Coughing is worse at night. There are mucous rattles with the cough.

Abdomen: There is a feeling of pressure in the abdomen, a yellow slimy diarrhea alternately with chronic constipation.

Sexual Organs: A yellow discharge comes from the urethra and vagina of the female.

Extremities: Rheumatic pains in the low back and legs. Pain shifts from place to place.

Skin: Itchy eruptions break out. The skin gets scaly. A person with potassium sulfate deficiency is highly susceptible to poison ivy, poison oak, etc. His nails are quick to become diseased. Eczema or erysipelas break out.

Rx: Take two 6X tabs every two hours until symptoms are relieved.

Calcium
Phosphate (*Calcarea Phosphoricum*) lime

Calcium phosphate is found normally in all body tissues. It is called "the great tissue restorer." As the remedy for proper body growth and nutrition it provides the building blocks for new cell construction. It repairs and generates bone. As the answer to imperfect growth and decay calcium phosphate hastens repair of fractures and the development of sound teeth. It affects soft tissues such as those that line the bursa sacs. Its absence causes bursa sacs to become inflamed and painful. Excess fluid gathers within them. Such a swelling on the knee is known as "housemaid's knee." Simply by taking calcium phosphate orally the fluid in the bursal sac is absorbed because cellular balance has been restored. The minute minerals are at work.

In the absence of calcium phosphate in the bloodstream and failure of cell salts to get to their proper destination an illness called *anemia* may begin. If this lime salt is not present to do its physiological job for which it is predestined, the body's muscles begin to go into spasm. This happened to go-go dancer Casey J. It started with pains shooting through her curvaceous body. Her skin began to itch. She said her skin felt numb and cold. Crusty secretions formed on her skin and any young woman who is deficient in calcium phosphate usually has a very waxy-looking skin. Such young ladies usually feel depressed and have frontal headaches. They may have white vaginal discharges and be pestered by painful menstrual periods.

Absence of calcium phosphate in the body leads to other troubles. When lacking this cell salt, folks get dyspeptic. They have digestive problems and calcium phosphate is an excellent method for relieving gas. Anyone deficient in calcium phosphate usually sweats heavily around the head and neck. Urine is scant. Teeth are quick to show decay. When the cold damp weather comes on, rheumatic pain is quick to follow. I got Casey started on calcium phosphate and within a week her aches and pains were gone.

At-a-Glance Chart to Know Whether Your Symptoms Demand Treatment by CALCIUM PHOSPHATE

Body Part	Symptoms
Head:	In a calcium phosphate deficiency the head feels cold. Memory is impaired and there is vertigo (dizziness). A person with this problem is irritable, fretful and peevish. His scalp doesn't just itch, it is tender to the touch. There is pain around the ears. Such a person is bothered by headaches. A baby with this deficiency is marked by fontanels that fail to close (the soft spot on top of the baby's head).
Face:	The skin is sallow and waxy. It is greasy and marked by pimples and other blemishes. The face aches at times.
Eyes/ Ears:	Lids twitch, eyes are red, ears feel cold. During puberty a youngster with a calcium phosphate deficiency has difficulty seeing clearly.
Mouth/ Throat:	A baby with this deficiency develops teeth slowly. Teething

is painful. The throat is sore with swollen glands. The child is constantly coughing up phlegm.

Bowels: There may be rectal pain in this deficiency. This may be due to a fistula or due to the watery stool that burns the soft tissues of the opening. There is noisy gas passage and the odor is offensive.

Stomach: Heartburn and gas, pain from eating, craving for salt is present in this deficiency. Babies with a lack of calcium phosphate constantly crave nursing.

Bladder: In youngsters there is bed-wetting. In the aged there is incontinence.

Sex Organs: Women demonstrating this deficiency often have a displaced uterus, heavy menstrual period, and leukorrhea (white vaginal discharge).

Lungs: There is constant coughing. The chest is sore.

Extremities: In the absence of calcium phosphate in the diet the limbs are cold and sometimes even numb. They may ache. Weather changes (coldness, dampness) aggravate a rheumatic-like pain. Housemaid's knee may follow with swollen joints and twitching. Youngsters may develop bowlegs and muscle flabbiness.

Back: Lumbago.

Additional Health Problems
for Which Calcium Phosphate Is Helpful

Anemia	Chlorosis
Rickets	The process of aging
Bone disease	Night sweats
Heartburn	Aching shoulders
Pain in kidneys	Lung problems
Pain and numbness	

Rx: Take two 6X tabs every two hours until distress is relieved.

Iron
Phosphate (*Ferrum Phosphoricum*)

Iron is concentrated in the blood cells. Its purpose, along with that of sulfur, is to pick up and carry oxygen to all body parts. As a

result all human tissues contain iron. Therefore, anything affecting
the iron balance in your body leads inevitably to congestion and
hemorrhage. In Jimmy D's case it led to loss of muscle tone and loss
of circulation to all parts of his body. When Jimmy's muscle cells
were deprived of iron they became flabby and weak. As a result
even the muscle walls of his blood vessels collapsed. He developed
varicose veins and hemorrhoids. The giant artery in his chest developed a weak spot and expanded. Because all these bulged areas
contain unusual masses of blood, circulation slows down. The heart
strains to do its job. In turn, when there is an absence of iron in the
diet inflammation may start in any organ or part. It may begin in the
villi of the intestine. In the absence of *iron phosphate* the villi
cannot perform their function of absorbing liquids. In fact, the process reverses itself and water is expelled. This converts to watery
stool or diarrhea, and in just this way does an illness begin. The
large bowel may lose its capacity to function because of iron deficiency, and constipation begins. This was how it happened with
Jimmy D. Ferrum Phosphoricum (iron cell salts) was his antidote to
inflammation, hemorrhages, contusions discoloration and sprains.
Iron salts hasten healing, and this miracle of healing all begins with
iron found in the red blood corpuscles.

At-a-Glance Chart to Know Whether Your
Symptoms Demand Treatment by
IRON PHOSPHATE

Body
Part   Symptoms

Head: Throbbing sick headaches are quite often due to iron defi-
               ciency. The scalp becomes sore to the touch. Strange noises
               may be heard. There may even be deafness as a result. The
               eyes are bloodshot and inflamed. The face is red, hot, achy
               and the cheeks feel sore and feverish. The nose may bleed
               easily. Babies have teething problems with this deficiency
               and cry constantly. The child is feverish, his gums hot. He
               is thirsty. His throat is dry, inflamed and may show a thick
               membrane across the inside of the throat.

Bowel:	There is gastric pain, vomiting of food that may be accompained by blood. Food passes through undigested and diarrhea and hemorrhoids may be complications.
Urinary System and Sex Organs:	Bed-wetting is a complication of this deficiency in children. In older folks there is frequent urination, profuse and early menstrual periods and pelvic pain.
Respiratory System:	Painful coughing and chest pain may be accompanied by fever. When coughing the urine can't be controlled. Bloody phlegm is expectorated. There is hoarseness and loss of voice, heart palpitation, colds, influenza and whooping cough as complications.
Back:	Lumbago is one of the back problems in this deficiency. There may be rheumatic-type pain that *feels better when warmth is applied* but hurts more when the body is in motion. The vertebral joints ache and the neck gets stiff.

Adolescent girls sometimes develop a form of anemia called *chlorosis*. This is sometimes referred to as "greensickness" and is often due to faulty eating habits during puberty when there is a tremendous need for iron salts. It happened this way with Rhonda D. A hamburg/french fries/cola diet brought on a host of problems. She was tired and achy and had difficulty breathing. Her ankles swelled. She had headches. Sometimes she had diarrhea. Sometimes she had periods of vomiting. Her tongue was red, sore and dry. She was a sick girl and within days after cell-salt therapy was begun she showed improvement. Within weeks she was back to her own cheerful hardworking self. Iron cell salts, the powerhouses in each red blood corpuscle, restored her health.

Additional Health Problems for Which Iron Phosphate Is Helpful

Listlessness and apathy in children	Bronchitis
Colds	Erysipelas (with fever)
Coughs	Lumbago
Inflammation of eyes ears, nose, skin, wounds, ulcers	Anemia
	Pneumonia
	Tonsillitis

Rx: Take two 6X tabs every two hours until symptoms dissipate.

Potassium
Phosphate (*Kali Phosphoricum*) potash

I've watched this cell salt work what may be called little miracles in some very delicate areas. Men, crying like babies under stress, were restored to normal and their self-respect restored, as well as their nerves settled, under the cellular influence of *potassium phosphate*. *Kali Phosphoricum* or potassium phosphate is the remedy of choice for brain cells, nerve cells and the bloodstream. As a cell salt it is a constituent of all body tissues and fluids. It neutralizes nervous distress and neurasthenia. It acts as an antiseptic in the body and halts decay. When there is a lack of potassium phosphate in the bloodstream and body tissues, there is prostration, depression, brain fatigue and loss of personal drive. Even the blood itself deteriorates and all of this lays the groundwork for hemorrhages, stinking diarrhea, dizziness, nervous exhaustion and many other complications as you will note in the At-a-Glance Chart. An interesting factor about potassium phosphate deficiency is that anything the person has is aggravated by noise, drafts, and air conditioning.

Potassium phosphate is found normally in abundance in the nerves, blood corpuscles, muscles and cells of the brain. The chemist finds it also in the blood plasma and lymph fluid. When anything changes the normal balance of the cell-salt system the body is immediately affected. For example: When there is a loss of potash the *sensory nerves* may become paralyzed. When the *motor nerves* are affected by deficiency the muscles become weak. They may degenerate into paralysis. When the brain is deprived of potassium phosphate the person becomes anxious, suspicious, and forgetful. He is despondent and is inclined to weep over anything. He is depressed. Now stop and think about the folks you've know with those very symptoms. Think of the complex treatments they've had when maybe all it took was a few cents' worth of the right cell salts, those amazing minute mineral miracles, to restore them to health.

As your doctor will tell you, potassium phosphate is not just a good treatment for depression, it is excellent for muscle spasms, cramps, scurvy, carbuncles and stomach ulcers. Sound impossible? Try working a few little miracles of your own. You will become a believer as I have.

**At-a-Glance Chart to Know Whether Your
Symptoms Demand Treatment by
POTASSIUM PHOSPHATE**

Body Part	Symptoms
Head:	During a deficiency of this cell salt there may be nervous prostration or "nervous breakdown." There may be delirium, sleeplessness, depression, and forgetfulness. The person may be snappy, irritable, and can't control himself. He has constant headaches, is drowsy, suspicious and always anxious about something. The person is fearful, dull, nervous, lacks energy and feels weak.
Face:	Nosebleeds may be common occurrences, facial muscles may become paralyzed as may the vocal cords. The skin is greasy and has an offensive odor. Pustules may form on the face for no apparent reason.
Mouth:	The tongue becomes dry in potassium phosphate deficiency and has a dark brown coating. Along the sides of the tongue are sore areas of redness. The gums may bleed. There is a great deal of odorous phlegm and the breath is horribly offensive. The mouth may be cankerous and sore and the throat hoarse.
Ears:	Fetid discharge.
Stomach and Bowels:	The person with a potassium phosphate deficiency may suffer from constant agony in the pit of his stomach. He usually has gas, diarrhea and a sore rectum. His stool is dark brown in color and highly fetid. The bowel sometimes tends to prolapse. This person has constant hunger pangs and is in a state of total discomfort.
Chest:	Asthma and hay fever seem to accompany this problem. The person is short of breath and complains of a feeling of pressure in his chest.
Extremities:	Where this cell-salt deficiency has led to mental depression I have noticed that there is a concurrent problem of neuralgic pains in the extremities. The feet burn and sometimes feel numb. The legs may feel weak and sciatic pain shoots down from the low back to the heels. All of these complica-

tions are accentuated by cold damp weather. Legs may ache during menstrual periods where potassium phosphate deficiency exists.

Urinary System
and
Sex Organs: Bed-wetting by children or incontinence in the aged is one of the consequences of potassium phosphate imbalance. Women may have profuse and premature menstrual periods. There may be pains in the ovaries and across the low back. A scalding, blistering leukorrhea (yellow-white discharge) may develop. During the menstrual period the woman with this deficiency is sleepy and mentally dull.

Connie McL. was twenty. She hadn't had a menstrual period in two years and pregnancy was not the cause. She complained of feeling drowsy all the time, headachy, nasty-tempered, and flying into uncontrolled tantrums. Her eyes bothered her but her opthalmologist said she didn't have an eye problem. Her psychiatrist said she was not "losing her mind." After using *potassium phosphate* for one week Connie did a complete about-face in personality. She was happy, cheerful and organized once again. Her vigor returned. Her headaches were gone and it was potassium phosphate that did the trick.

Additional Health Problems
for Which Potassium Phosphate Is Helpful

Epilepsy	All menstrual problems
Pulse irregularity	Bright's disease
Diabetes	Muscle spasms
Cramps	Scurvy
Carbuncles	Stomach ulcers

Rx: Take two 6X tabs twice daily.

Sodium Phosphate (*Natrum Phosphoricum*)

Like other body salts, this cell salt is found in the blood, the muscles and nerve cells. In addition it is in all cells and their inter-spaces. When present it neutralizes the formation of waste lactic acid. It regulates digestion. When there is excess gastric acidity *sodium phosphate* is the treatment of choice. As a neutralizing agent it assists the normal function of all the abdominal organs as well as the function of the lungs. It quells sour stomach, stops sour-smelling diarrhea and colic. The keynote here is that sodium phosphate is the antidote to acidity and sourness.

Sodium phosphate normally dissolves uric acid around joints and relieves acute arthritis. Because sodium phosphate is good for saponifying (turning to digestible fluids) fatty foods it is excellent for the treatment of dyspepsia.

At-a-Glance Chart to Know Whether Your Symptoms Demand Treatment by SODIUM PHOSPHATE

Body Part	Symptoms
Head:	In a deficiency of sodium phosphate sick headaches may be followed by vomiting. Creamy yellow secretions exude from the eyes. There may be a yellowish nasal discharge and a yellowish coating on the tongue. One of the amazing things in this deficiency is that some folks grind their teeth.
Gastric System:	Sour eruptions, nausea, vomiting, flatulence, colic, heart-burn, diarrhea and a sore, raw and itching anus may develop. The feces smell sour. After fatty foods are eaten there is pain in the belly. There may be intermittent fever along with vomiting as a consequence.
Respiratory System:	Pain in the chest from no known cause.
Back:	Feeling of weakness.
Extremities:	The person with this deficiency may report that his legs give way when walking. His knees and ankles hurt. His wrists ache. He has rheumatic pain in his joints.
Skin:	The skin in such persons demonstrates itching, hives and rash. It is chafed and characterized by sour-smelling sweat.
Sex Organs:	(male) Frequent emissions but loss of sex drive.

Additional Health Problems
for Which Sodium Phosphate Is Helpful

Gout	Rheumatism
Catarrh	Spermatorrhea
Dyspepsia	Colic in children

Rx: Take two 6X tabs every two hours until relieved.

Magnesium Phosphate (*Magnesium Phosphoricum*)

This cell salt is a fundamental part of all muscles and nerves. Because it plays a role in the contraction of muscles and their proper metabolism, if there is a deficiency of *Magnesium phosphate* in the diet, cramps and even convulsions will follow. Because of this magnesium phosphate is an excellent remedy for folks having charley horses in their arms or legs. It is most effective when taken in hot water. As a remedy for the muscles of the heart it is of value in the treatment of angina pectoris or even muscles of the bowel wall. This was brought into focus for me by Marteen M., a small, thin intense woman, dark complexioned and aged twenty-five. When I saw her she was doubled up with abdominal pain. Her face, normally dark, was beefy red. She said she felt like a knife was stabbing her in the gut. She seemed like she was ready to scream in her agony but she didn't let it out. The available physical evidence pointed to magnesium phosphate as a probable cure. This was used in hot water. Within moments she relaxed. Her pain was gone.

At-a-Glance Chart to Know Whether Your Symptoms Demand Treatment by MAGNESIUM PHOSPHATE

Body Part	Symptoms
Head:	In the absence of magnesium phosphate in the diet there

may be pain around the eyes, which is often worse on the right side for reasons unknown. There may be neuralgia in the scalp especially after hard use of the eyes or intensive studying. Swimming in cold water or being exposed to draft may cause a quick earache. Application of heat and magnesium phosphate relieves it. Facial muscles may twitch with this deficiency, the eyelids twitch and there may be deafness. When pain occurs in the face it has a darting or tearing nature that is acute and sudden. There may be hay fever and a clear watery discharge as a complication. Coughing may follow.

Joints: Gouty joints with intense pain. (Take 6X dosage of magnesium phosphate with hot water for quick relief.)

Gastric
System: There may be hiccoughing as well as gastralgia (pain in the stomach). There may be heartburn, gassy dyspepsia, bloated abdomen, cramping and watery stool. Constipation. There may be diarrhea with intense cutting pain.

Pelvis
(female):   As a result of this deficiency there may be premenstrual pain. Pain may be intermittent. The ovaries may be painful. Menstrual period may be earlier than usual.

Chest: Coughing is worse at night or when lying down. A feeling of oppressive weight is on the chest, and a feeling of constriction around the throat and down the chest. Asthma is a complication. There may be anginal pains in the chest and the heart palpitates. There may be pain between the ribs or intercostal neuralgia. Bronchitis, chronic winter cough and running colds are continuous complications.

Back: Intense shooting pains may occur in the back. Sometimes the sensation is tingling and prickling.

Extremities: The feet get very tender when there is a magnesium phosphate deficiency. Sometimes the feet tingle. Cramping may occur in the calf of the leg. Alcohol and other stimulants when consumed make the legs feel leaden, heavy and exhausted. Legs and toes may move uncontrollably.

Additional Health Problems
for Which Magnesium Phosphate Is Helpful

St. Vitus's Dance	Chorea
Hiccough	Gout

NOTE: This may take months to alleviate. Take dosage three times daily (St. Vitus's Dance and chorea)

Rx: Take two 6X tabs hourly until symptoms are gone.

Calcium
Fluoride (*Calcarea Fluorica*) Fluoride of lime

Calcium Fluoride is found in the outer surface of bones, the enamel of teeth, the skin and in the elastic fibers of the body. Change the molecular chemical balance of these cell salts and tissue changes begin immediately. For example, when muscles and other elastic tissues are deprived of calcium fluoride they become flabby. Muscle walls of blood vessels dilate (varicose veins). Hemorrhoids result. Glands harden. Because the elastic fibers holding the uterus in position are affected, they loosen and the uterus changes position or becomes displaced. The bowel sags. Bony joints enlarge. The remedy for much of this is calcium fluoride. What to look for in determining whether you need calcium fluoride added to your diet is noted in the following.

At-a-Glance Chart to Know Whether Your
Symptoms Demand Treatment by
CALCIUM FLUORIDE

Body Part	Symptoms
Head:	In Randy B's case I noted that deficiency in calcium fluoride was marked by significant head problems. Randy had a stuffed-up nose and head colds. The constantly draining phlegm in his head was thick, lumpy and odorous. And it wouldn't let loose. His scalp had hard swellings in it. There were boils on his jaw, cold sores and cracks on his lips. His soft palate was swollen, and pain and tickling were in his throat. He complained of little lights flickering in his eyes and wax in his ears that was hard to remove.
Gastric System:	Folks who have a lack of calcium fluoride in their system usually have constipation and hemorrhoids. Their piles itch and are swollen and hard. These hemorrhoids may be internal as well as external. Randy had both. Vomiting is a symptom of this deficiency, as is hiccoughing.

Back:	Gnawing low backaches.
Pelvis (female):	Where there is a calcium fluoride deficiency the uterus tends to get displaced. There are "dragging pains" or feelings of heaviness in the uterus and profuse menstruation.
Extremities:	The lower extremities are involved by varicosities, gouty thickening of joints and joints that pop. Knee joints become inflamed and develop knots when there is a deficiency in this amazing cell salt.
Respiratory System:	The person who is deficient in calcium fluoride often has a hoarse voice and coarse cough. His throat tickles and there is a thick mucus in his throat. His lungs are not involved.
Skin:	The skin gets easily chapped. Lips may split. Little sores form at the corners of the mouth. Boils may form on the gums and swelling appear along the jaw. Blood tumors (hematomas) may appear under the skin after trauma (harsh blow).

Additional Health Problems
for Which Calcium Fluoride Is Helpful

Croup	Varicose veins
Hiccoughing	Bad teeth
Bone problems	

Rx: Take two 6X tabs every two hours until symptoms are gone.

Silica (*Silicea*)

Silica is related to calcium fluoride. It works with it in the body As a cell salt greatly needed in the human body it is located in the hair, fingernails, toenails and the skin. Yet, when it comes to conquering infections, silica salts are an excellent remedy. It influences the activity of bone growth, stimulates glands, and improves nourishment. As an anti-infection agent it controls suppuration and helps bring it to a head. Silica is of special value in helping the absorption of blood at sites of trauma (ankle sprain, etc.). When taken alternately with *Calcarea Phosphoricum* it promotes absorption of blood deposits after injury (ex: black eye). Silica is used to relieve arthritic pain and in turn helps get rid of kidney or bladder stones. Silica was given in the past in treatment of cataracts and amblyopia. It helps muscles to relax. It restores perspiration in the hands and feet of those who have dry skin and sweat glands that have been suppressed because of faulty nerve function. For folks who are always chilly it helps restore a feeling of warmth as these tissues return to normal once more.

At-a-Glance Chart to Know Whether Your Symptoms Demand Treatment by SILICA

Body Part	Symptoms
Head:	Pain at the base of the skull is not uncommon where there is a deficiency of this magic cell salt. A person deficient in silica is often irritable, dizzy, and hypersensitive to everything including noise. His headache becomes worse if overexerting or from studying or reading too much, when confronted with bright lights, or even straining at stool. He gets sties on his eyelids. When he keeps his head warm he feels better. His middle ear tends to get infected. Catarrh forms in his nose and becomes very odorous.
Gastric System:	This deficiency is marked by being hungry all the time, but the person with the problem can't stand warm food or meat A baby with this deficiency vomits after nursing. The bowels of the adult become somewhat paralyzed in their function and bulge with constipated waste. The rectum has no ability to open and expel.
Pelvis and Sex Organs:	Tumors are sometimes present, glands enlarge, hemorrhoids become painful and protruding, fistulas may occur in the anus. Women with silica deficiency usually feel icy cold during their menstrual period. They may have a white vaginal discharge.

Respiratory
System: A sore, tickly throat brings on a constant cough. Odorous,
               gravelly phlegm is coughed up. A person with this defi-
               ciency often has a hoarse voice and is marked by persistent
               night sweats. There's pain deep in his chest and his heart
               does not function at par. He has high fevers for no apparent
               reason.

Back: The back aches and there is pain between the shoulder
               blades. Chronic sciatica extends from the low back to the
               heels.

Extremities: The feet are odorous. They hurt. The toenails of persons
               with this deficiency are rough, brittle, ingrown and break
               easily. They become infected easily. Glands in the groin
               enlarge to handle the infection but healing is difficult.
               Rheumatism may be a complication and it's chronic.

Skin: Abscesses, felons, ulcers, boils, carbuncles, swellings con-
               tinue as long as the silica deficiency exists.

Additional Health Problems
for Which Silica Is Helpful
                    Catarrh
                    Sciatica (chronic)
                    Bone problems
                    All skin problems

Rx: Take two 6X tabs per day if problem is chronic.

FOODS TO SUPPLY
CELL-SALT NEED
WHERE COMMERCIAL SALTS ARE NOT AVAILABLE

Calcium (sources):
    Green vegetables, eggs, oranges, buttermilk, nuts, carrots,
    beans, hard water.
    (Note: Fish, meat, fruits, and white bread are poor sources
    of calcium)

Phosphorus (sources):
    Fish, milk, meat, eggs, cheese, beans, lentils, whole meal,
    oatmeal and rye meal.

Iron (sources):
   Meat, potatoes, bread, kidney, liver, egg yolk, green peas, carrots, cereals, cabbage, watercress.

Sodium chloride((sources):
   Present in most foods.

Magnesium (sources):
   Green vegetables, bread, meat.

SPECIAL NOTE

Once more, what do these cell salts do? Their purpose, and their magic, lies in the fact that they fill a physiological need. They repair deficiencies. They overcome chemical deficiencies. They regulate bio-electric and hormonal defects. They repair hurts and avert disease. As synergists they work with other chemicals in the body. As catalysts they step up the action of food metabolism and ingestion. They reconstruct, revitalize, and in so doing convert the minute minerals in biotic power! All in all these cellular salts are powerful agents in the healing and prevention of human disease. Unorthodox and unusual as they may seem to be they continue to be a vital part of your life. For acute conditions take your dosage one or two hours apart. When there is a great deal of pain they may be taken fifteen minutes apart. For chronic problems take two to four doses daily.

Chapter 4

Raw Vegetable Juices
. . . a Route to Better Health

The *rule of resupply* is constant in your body. The body demands food. If you do not resupply its daily losses, if you do not replenish the elements of which you are made up, if you do not bring back to normalcy that which the body requires, you become ill. The rule of resupply demands that we eat right, that we have a balanced diet, that we must eat immediately assimilable foods so that body cells can continue to regenerate, rebuild and revitalize each day. This supply may come through the magic stream of raw vegetable juices.

Our bodies are made up of sixteen major elements*and a number of lesser or ''trace'' elements. As indicated in the previous chapter on cell salts, these elements are in the bloodstream. To maintain health balance these food-dynamos are transported via the bloodstream to all body parts including the brain. Without these elements at par we become ill.

---

*Carbon, calcium, chlorine, fluorine, hydrogen, iodine, iron, magnesium, manganese, nitrogen, oxygen, phosphorus, potassium, silicon, sodium, and sulfur.

In the Land of Plenty
We Starve

In the plenteous United States today we live the strange paradox of dietary deficiency. We eat great amounts of the best food and yet our bodies starve. This means dietary imbalance. It means proper food supply is not being replenished. As a result degeneration begins in one or more body parts.

In establishing the rule of resupply with vegetable juices, fruit makes an excellent additive. The fruit must be ripe. Fruits contain all the sugars that the body needs. *Fruit juices are the body's cleansers but the builders of the body lie in the vegetable juices you consume each day.* They resupply and regenerate. They contain the magic minerals, salts, amino acids, vitamins, enzymes, etc., so vital to life. To obtain juices at their best, have the vegetables at their freshest. The vegetables must be raw and not laden with inorganic chemicals or preservatives! The very life of the vegetable goes into the human digestive system as tiny dynamos of power and herein lies the secret to living longer, staying younger, and being full of the vigor you desire.

Raw Vegetable Juices
Provide Instant Goodness

Fresh vegetable juice converts into body energy in less than a quarter-hour after ingestion. In slightly more than ten minutes nourishment pours into the body's cells and tissues. As a source of quick energy raw vegetable juice is not to be considered as a concentrated food. It is not concentrated like sugar. Sugar is 4600% more concentrated than celery juice, which is not an acid maker as is sugar or popcorn or soybean.

Do Not Place Milk in
the Juice Category

Although the chemistry of cow's milk has the same volume of water as does carrot juice, the resemblance ends there. *Milk is NOT a health food.* In fact, in some folks it is a direct contributor to ill health. Think back. Visualize some of those friends and relatives who drink lots of milk. Usually they are the ones with runny noses, colds, tonsillitis, bronchitis, odorous breath, and all problems with mucus and catarrh. Carrot juice, on the other hand, eliminates mucus, and children who drink vegetable juices and eat vegetables are brighter, more active and happier. Their resistance to illness is high.

Children living on devitalized foods, milk, and soft drinks are listless, without energy or drive. They are more concerned about riding then walking. They have pimply faces, give up easily, and are attacked by every illness that comes along. They, or their parents, have not controlled diet and provided for the rule of resupply. When milk is used instead of vegetable juices, human cells break down. Resistance goes down. Illness begins. To prevent this, systematically cleanse the body with juices and regeneration, reconstruction, and health begins.

What Controls the Amount of Juice to Be Consumed?

Moderation is always the rule. Nature regulates you automatically by telling you when enough's enough. You drink what you can and still be comfortable.

What Is the Minimum Amount That Can Be Taken for Best Results?

Although two to six pints of juices may be taken daily without discomfort, one pint is the minimum that can be consumed and still get good results. In the rule of resupply the body recovers its losses in direct proportion to the amount of juices taken by mouth. Remember that vegetable juices are *the* power source. The greater the amount of juice, the greater the amount of repairing vitamins, minerals, hormones and other food values to do the job of health-making.

Are Hand-Juicers
of Any Value?

Locked deep in the fibers of vegetables are its truest and best values. A vegetable or a fruit is water for the most part. But there is more than water in their cellular structure. Vegetables and fruit fibers have to be broken down. The true values have to be extracted from these fibers. In the fluid that is extracted are organic elements that are the health-makers so vital to life.

A hand-juicer cannot free these elements from the fibrous structures of the plant. All it is capable of doing is express the water content. Heavier electric juicers are better equipped for this purpose. Specific curative powers locked deep in the vegetable or fruit are released. Potent forces that combat disease are released.

Vegetable juices are subtle powers, persuasive and therapeutic. It is true they work slowly. It is also true they are effective and many a disease has been eliminated through raw juice therapy. Many a body has been detoxified so that glands can function once more. Blood begins to flow normally once more. Muscles and joints begin to function and it all comes about when you release the powers of vegetable juice into your body. You'll start feeling better once more. Toxic waste locked within you will be released and with the release is re-established your go-power. So buy an electric juicer. It may be the best investment you ever make.

Are YOU Interested in
Living Longer and Living
Better?

Folks who live on pastries as well as on lots of meat, candy and heavy starches, whose food comes mostly out of cans, bottles and the frozen food department, and who "simply can't stomach vegetables and fruit" are those who are constantly ailing, whose lives are shorter, whose faces and bodies age fast, who are bloated, fat or scrawny, whose energy level is constantly low, who are fearful and filled with tension. Even more than that, *they are the people who have a reaction to raw vegetable juices in the very beginning* as the rule of resupply takes place.

With release of toxic waste there is temporary discomfort until the waste clears out through the skin, the bowel, the liver, the lungs and kidneys. Some of that waste may make itself known as a nasty breath. The very fact that this is happening is an indication of improvement. The new energy supply is forcing toxins out of the body's vital tissues into the bloodstream and recuperation can begin *only* when this waste is cast off!

How Effective This Can Be Was Noted in the Case of Jennie D.

Everyone agreed that Jennie D. had bronchitis. After she ran the gamut of many treatments and medication, no one agreed as to the cause of her problem or why it continued. What had begun with poor diet and concurrent exposure to cold resulted in coughing, expectoration, low-grade fever, pain under the breastbone and rattling in her chest. The cough became persistent. When exerting herself she found it difficult to breathe, and because she didn't have the money to travel to the prescribed warm climate she had to fight it out at home. As a mail carrier she couldn't avoid inclement weather. She simply couldn't afford to live in vacationland so I put her on fruit juices to cleanse her and raw vegetables to replenish her ailing system.

What happened? The first thing was that all Jennie's coughing and spitting stopped. Her constipation disappeared. The rattling in her chest went and so did the substernal pain. In a matter of weeks Jennie was back in her U.S. mail truck. It took persistence and guts on her part but she did it and the rule of resupply worked in her favor. It can do the very same for you. The following tells exactly what you can do.

VEGETABLE JUICES
YOU CAN USE TO HELP YOURSELF
BACK TO HEALTH

Vegetable juices contain vitamins and all the magic minerals and cell salts vital to living the healthy way of life. If juices are to be derived from raw vegetables, the vegetable fibers must be totally shredded and squeezed to deliver all their wonder-making foodstuffs. Alphabetically listed now are the vegetables from which you can derive the juices that can change the course of your life. For quick reading the nonhealth problems they effectively treat are added.

ALFALFA JUICE and the
Mysterious Chlorophyl Element

The green chlorophyl element in plant life is comparable to the hemoglobin of our red blood cells. One of the richest sources of chlorophyl is *alfalfa*. One of the best ways to assure more vigorous old age is a farm plant that is so potent it should never be taken internally as a juice by itself. Alfalfa should preferably be combined with carrot juice. In such combination these raw juices provide new life for the heart, the arteries, veins and lymph vessels. When taken with cleansing enemas it clears the bowels out. Gas disappears. Lung problems clear up. Even sinusitis disappears.

The mysteries of chlorophyl became even more intriguing when Jack L. reported that after taking alfalfa juice, with carrot and lettuce juice added, for a period of three months hair started to grow on his bald head. I didn't believe that one pint of these raw juices a day could do it but it did! And that's what counts in this matter of unorthodox and unusual therapies that folks may use on themselves each day. Jack grew a crop of hair when everyone said it couldn't be done!

ASPARAGUS Juice
and the Health-Giving Alkaloid Element

An alkaloid known as *asparagine* is the wonder element in asparagus. It is a health-maker that is lost when asparagus is cooked, canned or otherwise prepared. In the treatment of anemia and kidney ailments asparagine is the agent that brings about cure. It gets into the bloodstream immediately and breaks up oxalic crystals that have collected in the muscle system and in and around joints. Therefore it is good for rheumatism, neuritis and prostate trouble, too. Asparagus juice is best combined with beet, carrot and cucumber juice for full health effect.

BEET Juice
as a Blood Builder

Never take more than a wineglassful of beet juice at a time. It is potent and may even make you feel uncomfortable after you drink it. Therefore, in building the blood (treatment for anemia), combine beet juice with carrot juice at the rate of four ounces of beet juice to one pint of carrot juice. Beet juice is excellent for menstrual problems and should be taken at the rate of two ounces per day. Beet juice contains a high quantity of sodium (50%) as well as iron and calcium (5%), potassium and chlorine. When beet juice is mixed with carrot juice it becomes a natural blood builder because it is also rich in phosphorus, sulfur, vitamin A and many trace elements. Beet juice may be added to carrot and cucumber juice as a remedy for gall and kidney stones and as a gallbladder and liver cleanser. For a gallstone problem, carrot, beet and cucumber juices should be supplemented with the juice of one lemon in a glassful of hot water.

How Jane M. Rid
Herself of Gallstones

Jane M. had been having digestive problems for some years. There was a tenderness over her gallbladder area and a pain radiated up into her right shoulder and back. Along with the pain there was sometimes vomiting and sweating. She had the colic when her stomach was empty and pains occurred an hour after she ate rich food.

Jane was one of those people who are anti-surgery and anti-drugs, and nobody could convince her otherwise. She believed in Nature's remedies and started taking carrot, beet and cucumber juice daily. In addition to the one pint of juices, she drank ten glassfuls of hot water with fresh lemon juice added. On the third day she had intense pain in her abdomen. She said she thought she was going to explode. Each day for five more days she had pains that lasted almost a quarter of an hour. On the fifth day she passed her stones. Her pain vanished. There has been no recurrence since.

CABBAGE Juice
for Reducing as Well as Cleansing

Cabbage juice in its raw state is high in sulfur, chlorine and iodine. It cleanses the intestinal tract because of this. The formation of gas after cabbage juice is drunk indicates the presence of abnormal conditions in the bowel and because of this the taking of cabbage juice actually becomes a test for the condition of the abdomen. To obviate unnecessary discomfort, however, it is wise to cleanse the bowel with enemas or colonic irrigations before starting the cabbage juice regime. Of further assistance in getting acclimated you can take carrot and spinach juice or just plain carrot juice (a wineglassful). Because raw cabbage juice is high in Vitamin C it is good for pyorrhea or infected gums, skin blemishes as well as constipation. *Do not add salt or vinegar*. Because of its cleansing capacity cabbage juice is excellent for reducing. Weight is brought under control with the rebalancing of foodstuffs.

CARROT Juice
. . . the Normalizing Agent

High in vitamins B, C, D, E, G, and K, carrot juice may be consumed without harm from one to five pints daily. One pint of carrot juice contains more mineral value than twenty-five pounds of calcium tablets. Because of this it is invaluable to the nervous system and creates vigor. It helps resist infection, cleanses ulcerated areas as well as cleanses the liver and intestines. A rather interesting misinterpretation of facts leads some people to believe that the yellow skin resulting from drinking large quantities of carrot juice occurs because of the color of the vegetable. However, carotene in the juice has no more tendency to make the skin yellow or orange than does chlorophyl to make the skin green or beet juice to turn the skin red. The problem lies in the liver that the carrot juice is detoxifying. When that load of bile lets loose, the skin as well as the feces turn yellow. In addition to cleaning the liver and gallbladder, carrot juice is excellent for eye problems and skin problems. It helps to lengthen life. It is a general body cleanser that aids healing and lowers the number of diseases a person may get.

CELERY Juice
. . . Rich in Calcium

Celery is an excellent source of organic calcium so vital to body rehabilitation and growth. In providing sodium it assures fewer involvements of the lungs. Celery is high in iron and magnesium. It is of value to the nerves and blood and counteracts such problems as hemorrhoids, varicose veins and rheumatism.

CUCUMBER Juice
. . . the Natural Diuretic

As well as being an excellent cleanser for the kidneys and bladder, cucumber juice, when added to carrot, spinach and lettuce juice, aids hair and fingernail growth, cleans up skin conditions, and counters rheumatic disorders as well.

DANDELION Juice
. . .the Valuable Tonic
for Everyone

Dandelion juice is rich in magnesium, iron, calcium and sulfur, all of which are builders of the body. This juice also acts as a nervous system control because of the presence of these magic minute minerals. It is therefore an excellent remedy for problems of the teeth and bones.

ENDIVE Juice
. . . Counter-Agent Against Cataracts

Endive is often called chicory. It is a vitamin-rich vegetable that, when consumed as a juice, is an antidote to eye troubles. When combined with carrot and celery juice it is valuable for neutralizing asthma and hay fever. When combined with parsley and celery juice in equal parts it is good for the heart.

LETTUCE Juice
. . . a Restorer of Hair

Like alfalfa lettuce is high in iron and magnesium and thus valuable to the development of red blood cells for those who have sustained a high blood loss (from surgery, wounds, menstrual period, etc.). Lettuce juice is a source of vitality for the brain and its nervous system. It aids as a muscle developer, and as a hair restorer it is excellent. Leaf lettuce, rather than head lettuce, is best for this purpose.

PARSLEY Juice
. . . the Kidney Cleanser

In addition to being a kidney cleanser, parsley supplies properties that maintain the proper function of the thyroid and adrenal glands. It maintains the well-being of the smaller blood vessels (venuoles, arterioles, capillaries). Of particular note is its effectiveness in the treatment of weak eyes and other diseases of the eye. When mixed with carrot juice and endive juice, parsley juice becomes a powerful physical aid. For women with menstrual irregularity it is a treatment of choice.

GREEN PEPPER Juice
. . . Aid for Improved Nails and Hair

Because green pepper juice provides a large quantity of silicon it is of value, when combined effectively with carrot and spinach juice and taken one pint per day, in improving hair and nail growth. It helps get rid of abdominal gases and should be drunk *before* eating.

POTATO Juice
. . . the Skin Blemish Remover

Potato juice, combined with carrot and celery juices, is excellent for folks with gout and sciatica. It is excellent for those with muscle, nerve and gastric complications, and is especially effective when all meats are eliminated from the diet.

SPINACH Juice
. . . Ideal Cleanser for the Intestinal Tract

As an alimentary tract cleanser spinach juice also regenerates the stomach, duodenum and small bowel lining. It is also used in the treatment of neuritis, abscesses and boils, loss of vigor, impaired heart function, headaches and blood pressure changes. Spinach juice, added to raw carrot juice, provides one of the most effective and potent health drinks available. Spinach also contains Vitamin E and thus becomes a factor in preventing miscarriage in women who are susceptible to this problem, impotence and sterility. Spinach should *never* be cooked or heat processed! *Cooking converts its oxalic acid content into dangerous inorganic crystals* that cause kidney pain and trouble. Oxalic acid, as long as it remains inorganic (uncooked) is a valuable stimulant for peristalsis in the stomach and bowel.

TOMATO Juice
. . . Good Only When Fresh!

Processed and canned tomato juice is almost devoid of food values. Folks who drink a lot of canned juices come up with kidney and bladder problems. But when tomato juice is fresh it is high in calcium, potassium and magnesium. *Tomato juice should be consumed only if there is no starch or sugar on the menu!*

TURNIP Juice
. . . the Tooth Hardener

The juice of turnip leaves provides more calcium than any other vegetable. Because of this it is of great value when bones have softened or when teeth have not hardened. When combined with celery and carrot juice, it is of value in quelling hyperacidity. Calcium, valuable to bone formation, is also vital to metabolism in the nervous system and the musculature of the body. Because calcium feeds muscles and nerves it is of particular importance in the treatment of hemorrhoids and varicose veins. It strengthens the walls. The venous walls tighten. The hemorrhoids begin to disappear. This is especially true when turnip juice is combined with equal amounts of spinach, watercress and carrot juice and all foods except vegetables and fruit are eliminated from the diet.

REMINDERS
About Juice Therapy

(a) *Whatever equipment you use to get your juice, keep it sterile and clean.* A dirty apparatus may contaminate and spoil an entire batch in a short time.

(b) *Don't expect immediate miracles!* Whatever your problem is, it has taken years to get that way so never expect an overnight cure. Remember that when the juices start cleansing your body a number of aches and pains will show up as toxic waste in the body lets loose. Stay with it. Consume additional juices, knowing full well that this reaction has to take place and that after the waste is removed healing begins.

(c) *Drink a large glassful of fresh citrus fruit juice the first thing each morning.* While you are going through this process use no other foodstuff.

(d) *Detoxify with an enema.* To "get the plug out" each morning use a warm saline solution (one tablespoonful of salt in an enema bag of warm water). Repeat for three or four days at the beginning of your juice control program. After the fourth day go to more solid foods. Salads are suggested. These may be made up of fruits as well as vegetables.

Chapter 5

Fasting:
The Miracle Method
to Achieve
a Longer and Healthier Life

In the fascinating story of fasting let's take some examples from real life.

JANICE C. was forty-two years old. She had four children and all of them came hard. Raising them was even harder because she was a war widow, and the kids, plus holding down two jobs, were enough to break anyone down. The inevitable happened. She became ill. She coughed constantly. Her muscles ached. Her throat was sore. She coughed up mucus. Her fever went to 102° F. Her lungs rattled at the base and one physician diagnosed her problem as bronchitis. Another debated over the complications that were setting in and said a heart problem could possibly be the original cause and suggested expensive therapy. She couldn't afford it. She heard about *fasting* and said, "What have I got to lose?" She fasted for three and a half weeks and lost eighteen pounds but she also lost her cough. She no longer hacked up phlegm. Her chest no longer hurt. She felt strong. On the twenty-first day natural hunger returned and that was her cue to terminate the fast. The job was done. Mrs. C. stayed on liquids for the following week and then returned to solids and her two jobs and children. She was able to face the world once more. Now she could stand up to her responsibilities and it was all done with fasting. It was a "miracle cure" in her own words but it was actually an everyday occurrence in Nature. All she had to do was let Nature do the job.

LOIS Von F. was twenty-eight years old. She was five foot five, weighed 208 pounds and had a list of complaints nonstop. Her big problems were her headaches, her backaches, her joint aches and her feelings of depression. She said she couldn't go on. She said she was through with all the expensive drugs her husband couldn't afford. She even contemplated suicide. This obese woman was a candidate for the psychiatric ward when, in a more rational moment, she made a decision. She was going to fast! Her love of life was stronger than her love of food and she did it! Four weeks went by. The first week was the hardest. Hurts were magnified. The second week she awoke one morning able to get out of bed without a groan. The third week her chronic tears dried up. The fourth week she weighed herself and found she was down to 180. In the mirror she saw a more shapely woman. With the disappearance of hurts in mind and body, a whole new world awakened for Lois. Her normal hunger returned but now she was totally convinced of the values of fasting and food control and went on a sensible diet. Her old symptoms simply disappeared. Her husband looked at her once again with desirous eyes and as far as Lois was concerned this was all she wanted in the first place.

Jack T. was a professional football player. He was tough, rough, and a backfield hatchet man. He played until the years caught up with him. No one would even take him on a trade so in a splash of national publicity he retired, and sudden obscurity threw a block into his body and soul. He hit the saloons up and down Main Street. He drank nonstop. This former great athlete became a slob, a frustrated personality, with nothing but mean words to say about the press, the public, and professional football. He became mentally and physically sick and landed in a sanitarium. This sanitarium advocated fasting as a rest cure. The detergent of fasting cleansed both his body and mind. He began physical workouts after the third week of fasting, slowly, surely, reporting that he was feeling great, that there was no loss of energy, no depressive moods. While working out physically he hit on an idea. Why couldn't he represent an athletic goods concern to the athletic goods trade? Salesman? Ambassador of goodwill? Why not! So he projected the idea to a national manufacturer of athletic goods and the concern, pleased with what they saw in this rehabilitated star, hired him on the spot . . . and it was fasting that made all this possible.

TOM L. was a retiree. He had spent thirty-five years as a foreman in a large automotive plant but was still hale and hearty when company policy put him out to pasture. Suddenly he had nothing to do after a lifetime of activity. A vast emptiness engulfed him. He converted his wife into a nervous wreck with his aggravating presence. Constantly nagging, constantly fussing, constantly giving her orders, he drove her up the wall. Worse than that he drove himself up the wall. He became constipated. Suddenly he was tired all over and a vast feeling of weakness engulfed him. He got strange tingly sensations in his arms and feet and thought that he was going to have a stroke. One side of his head hurt. He made the inevitable round of doctors, and tranquilizers seemed to be the therapy of their choice. He bumbled around under drugs like a sodden vegetable until one day his wife took matters into hand and changed all this. Her father had been a Naturopathic doctor and suddenly she was remembering all that he had said about the wonder of fasting. It worked! Tom L. went out of retirement. He developed a mobile welding shop and turned a lifelong job into a new career. At age sixty he was still wanted, still needed. But it was Mrs. L.'s memories of fasting that opened up the door to a whole new life.

MABEL B. was fat, fecund and forty. During pregnancy she developed biliary colic but didn't think too much about it because she

had had the same thing every time she had her menstrual period
previously. The symptoms weren't strong at first. They started as a
little cramping in the belly after she ate a heavy meal. Then, with
increasing severity, the pain radiated up under the right shoulder
blade and clavicle. Her upper right abdomen became rigid and
tense. She had nausea and vomiting and attributed all these to her
pregnancy. But she had other complications, fever and clay-colored
stool. Her skin took on a yellowish tinge and this continued even
after her pregnancy was over. Each year it got worse. So did her
teeth. She suffered from leg pains and backaches. Her right arm
hurt. She was told that she had *cholelithiasis* (gallbladder stones)
and that an operation was necessary. A doctor of other than medical
persuasion advised a *fast*. She went along with it. At the beginning
of fasting her aches and pains became more magnified. They became so bad she was almost convinced that surgery was necessary.
Then suddenly the pains stopped. Her headaches went away. She
had more good days than bad days. On the seventeenth day she
passed the stones and from then on her recovery was remarkable.
She has had no trouble since.

> **NOTE: For these five people Nature played the same role.**
> **The body was cleansed. The body was rested. Self-caused**
> **illness was eliminated and a health miracle took place.**

Sickness Begins With One
Common Denominator . . . Toxemia

All illness begins with poisonous waste in the human body. Healing and health can follow only when these poisons are eliminated.
When waste is eliminated, warning signals such as pains and aches
stop. And how is this best accomplished? Through *fasting*. Fasting
is an answer to personal contributions to willful negligence, but you
have to know what you're doing to correct the problem. This chapter tells you how.

Understand Fasting Thoroughly
Before Starting on Your Way

Let's make one thing plain: *There is no help for you through fasting unless you want to do it.* There is no help for you if your demand to eat is greater than your desire *not* to eat. Maximum benefits are not obtainable when you abuse your body by eating too much each day.

Remember that the average person loses about a pound a day when he is not eating. Most people eat twice this amount or more and as a result fat continues to store itself up in the tissues. The bowels clog. Constipation or diarrhea, or even both, sets in. There's no pep or energy. Nerves are on end. Circulation stands still. A general breakdown may occur and none of the body's systems are at "Go!" This overloaded, overworked body reacts. It develops and demonstrates tattletale signs and symptoms that tell you that acute or chronic disease is about to begin. And as the "Father of Medicine" Hippocrates once said, "The more you nourish a diseased body, the worse you make it." And the whole point in fasting is that you are bound to get well long before you starve to death.

Because all body parts are equally helped by fasting and purification, a lot of unrelated signs and symptoms disappear: tonsillitis, high blood pressure, pleurisy, jaundice, etc., all go away. As the cleansing takes place they depart.

In self-confession here's what James M. had to say about his contribution to health delinquency:

> "Instead of keeping the routes of elimination open, I closed them with lack of proper diet, lack of exercise and improper breathing. I didn't breathe right. I couldn't stand the thought of drinking water. I stuffed myself with food day and night and my joints got to aching so bad I couldn't get out of a chair. Every movement was hell. The doctor said there was nothing wrong with me, just a little constipation. Well, that's when I decided on fasting. My body was clogged and I did it myself. I

was simply poisoning myself day after day and it was up to me
to fight my way clear.''

James M.'s story is the story of millions of Americans. Possibly it
is your story as well. Maybe *your* kidneys, bowels, skin, liver and
lungs need help. Maybe you have been contributing to health delinquency by clogging the avenues of elimination. Maybe you are
consuming foods that decompose and convert to poisons that make
you ache all over, toxic waste responsible for headaches and joint
pain making you feel low. Maybe *you* need to fast. Maybe *you* need
to use Nature's most simple remedy for illness. Remember, when
Nature takes your appetite away it is saying something very important to you. It's *making you fast!*
  With this in mind, let's answer some of the questions that folks
bring up:

1. "Will fasting make me weak?"

You've probably heard folks say to those who are ill, "You've
got to eat to keep up your strength." Or, "You've got to feed a
cold." All of this is false. In fact, such irresponsible statements
have contributed to disease and death. It's a statement made by
those who know nothing, or care nothing, about the amazing work-
ings of human physiology. Such statements are made by people who
are themselves stimulated by food and believe that to go without a
few meals is to have the bottom of the world drop out. Fasting will
not make you weak. In fact, as the waste clears away you will
become stronger each day.

2. "How do I know when fasting should stop?"

It is true that during the first stages of fasting you will feel hunger
pains. However, a mere glass of water allays all this. Hunger disappears and fasting can go on for days and in some folks even months.
Professional fasters, to the amazement of health investigators, have
gone months without eating. When weakness occurs during a period
of fasting it is due only to disease within the body. Hunger returns
only when the body has eliminated all waste. Nature sets the time

schedule. It tells you when. When hunger arrives it means that Nature's job is done. Fasting stops. It's that simple.

3. "Does strength actually increase with fasting?"

Here's a letter I had from a patient:

> "At the very beginning of fasting there was a great feeling of exhaustion. I began to expel a lot of waste and it was like magic. My body strength improved. My get-up-and-go came back and now I can attest to just how wonderful fasting can be. It's the best thing that ever happened to me and I'm living proof that it happened.

4. "When I'm sick should I force myself to eat?"

The jaded appetite of the ill should never be tempted. No one, including you, should ever be forced to eat. For example, have you ever had an illness where every smell of food made you feel sick? Was there ever a time when the very thought of food made you feel worse? Have you ever had a cat or dog who refused to eat or lap water? That's Nature's way. It's Nature at work! Whether it's household pets, children, or you, *never force anyone to eat*. When the body's devitalizers and appetite detractors are gone, the desire for food will return. When the body is physiologically clean, health returns. Remember that illness is the body's effort to purify the system, a reparative process in the beginning that is not helped by continued eating. Illness is actually a process of self-help if you just stop and observe what is going on. It is actually the cure, and fever, skin eruptions, headaches, chills, etc., are just manifestations of this curative phase at work. The sicker the person is, the greater the necessity for fasting. There is also a greater need for sleep because *it is rest and sleep, and not food, that re-establishes energy!* It is Nature at work!

5. "Should I eat breakfast?"

Breakfast is best . . . when *not* eaten! Begin each day with a short fast. Go without breakfast in normal life. Eat later in the day only when you are hungry. Do not glut yourself or consume coffee and cola for stimulation. After you've gone through the fasting cure, stick with bland diets and reap positive benefits instead.

6. "What IS fasting? What does it really do?"

Fasting is a deliberate rest-cure, a premeditated stoppage of food consumption to permit the removal of previously consumed food that failed to digest or that has decomposed in the intestinal tract. Fasting gives the digestive tract a rest and period of repair. Physiological chemistry reorganizes and recuperates. As all this improves so does the mind. Alertness returns and you're ready for your job in life once more!

7. "A lot of strange things have been said about fasting. Just exactly what am I supposed to believe?"

Those who know no better have said many adverse things about fasting, most of which is patently untrue. For example, fasting does not paralyze the bowel as has been declared, nor does it produce acidosis or cause acids to eat through the stomach wall. At no time does fasting cause the heart to weaken or contribute to collapse. The stomach does not shrink nor do its walls grow together. At no time does fasting contribute to lowered body resistance or injure the nervous system. It does not bring harm to the body's many important glands, bones or teeth. It never made anyone mentally unbalanced, caused fits or bad dreams. Fasting is a method cure. Where such matters as the previous problems exist, they exist only because disease is already there. On the other hand, fasting clears all this up and helps chase disease away.

8. "When is it best to fast?"

Any time of the year is good for fasting but summer is best. It's best because people who fast usually feel a little chilly and must be kept warm. For those who are ill fasting should begin immediately. Winter or not, there's no time to waste.

9. "How long should my fasting last?"

There is no rule or criterion for the number of days required to fast. Nature determines all this for you. In some cases going without breakfast is the only fasting necessary. In chronic problems it means going without eating until Nature breaks the fast by bringing on the desire to eat. This may take five days. It may take ten or forty. It may take only two. The rule of the road in fasting is that when Nature signals the end of fasting with hunger pains, stop fasting right then and there! Babies and animals all do this intuitively.

10. "Must I go completely without eating?"

If you are not going to fast completely, don't start in the first place! Arguing that you have to have at least a little food to survive on is a self-admission that you are not truly interested in fasting, that you love food more than you love life. Eating food to supposedly maintain strength is a halfway procrastination that succeeds in doing nothing more than worsening the situation that already exists. In the first place, after the second or third day of fasting you will have no desire to eat. Food may even seem repulsive. You'll even be surprised, as your fast continues, that you have even more energy than before! Learning to control your food intake is the biggest step you'll ever make in your life. It will be the first time that you really have self-control.

11. "Should children fast?"

Youngsters, other than newborns, may fast with equally good results. This does not hold true of the highly emaciated child with a malignant disease or one who has been deprived of food. Physician-controlled fasting in children holds special values and not only gets rid of disease but also adds years to a sickly child's life.

12. "What if I get a headache from fasting? Should I eat?"

When you are fasting, *fast*! Permit yourself no excuses or alibis. *Do* expect reactions as toxic waste in your body lets loose. You may have a headache when this occurs. Your joints may ache. The very fact you are having a headache indicates how badly you are in need of fasting. Your headache is only a warning, a clue, that you have to stick to the rules. As quickly as the eliminative organs release their accumulated poisonous debris, that's when your headaches and other signs and symptoms will vanish and you will start feeling better once more.

13. "Once my hunger starts how much should I eat?"

Eat sparingly once your hunger returns after fasting. Eat regularly in small quantities. Stick to fruits and vegetables. Avoid fats, proteins, starches and sugar. Avoid meat. It's the worst luxury you can afford.

14. "If I fast do I become deficient in vitamins and minerals?"

People have yet to develop scurvy or beri-beri as the result of fasting. There are no known cases because there is a reserve of vitamins and minerals waiting in the body until such time as needed. In fact, such problems as nervous conditions clear up during the fasting period. In true scurvy and beri-beri the nerve problem gets worse. Remember to keep in mind that there is a big difference between therapeutic fasting and starvation! No one advocates that you starve, only that you eliminate food for a while to cleanse your body of accumulated waste. When Nature calls, through hunger, *then* eat . . . and eat sparingly.

15. "Should I do anything manual during fasting? Should I rest?"

Folks who work less should eat less. People who fast should labor less and rest more. There should be no heavy labor or exercise.

There should be plenty of relaxation, plenty of sleep, and relief from tensions and worry. Walking is the best suggested exercise. In the first few days of fasting there will be a feeling of weakness, a feeling of discouragement, of aches and pains, but once you're over the hump strength will come flowing in. As waste is eliminated the natural dynamos within you will begin to work. As this happens you will find yourself doing more and more.

16. "What should I do about clothing while fasting?"

At all times keep warm. Wear warm clothing when up and around. Be well covered when in bed. Do not wear tight clothing. Make sure that even your shoes, stockings and gloves fit loosely.

17. "How much water should I drink?"

Drink whenever you are thirsty or whenever your stomach is growling during those first few days of the fast. Drink at least a quart of water or vegetable juice per day. Add lemon juices for taste if you desire.

18. "Should I take a bath when fasting? How often?"

Take warm baths daily. In the summertime follow your warm bath with a cool shower and rub your body down with a coarse towel until you are glowing. Do not use cold applications in spring, winter or fall when the temperature is down. Keep warm at all times. Keep active.

19. "What about exposure to air and breathing deeply?"

Get plenty of fresh air day and night. Breathe deeply and as easily as possible. Relax. As your fasting continues you will find relaxation easier and easier to accomplish. Many of the signs of clogged sinuses, stuffed noses, etc., will clear up. Admittedly fasting is no panacea. It does take courage and fortitude on your part. It takes guts to get well, but if your desire is strong enough, if you really want to get well, fasting is a method of choice. Remember, it took you a long time to get in your present condition. Nothing is going to make your problem disappear overnight, not even good clean air. Fasting is a rest cure, so as you rest breathe deeply and help yourself along.

20. "Should I take an enema to help things along?"

If you have been constipated, and your bowels refuse to move, it is absolutely necessary that this avenue of waste removal be opened. You will find that even with prolonged fasts (the absence of food) a daily enema will often continue to expel unbelievable amounts of waste, some of it hard, some of it tarry, some of it like stone. Use saltwater enemas (one tablespoonful of salt to one enema bag of warm water) whether you have been constipated or have been having diarrhea.

21. "How should I prepare for fasting?"

You may prepare for the purpose of internal cleansing by nudging Nature with a laxative. Ground senna leaves, prunes, etc., help loosen the fecal mass and prepare it to move out. An enema may also be used once daily for a week before the fasting begins. Retain the enema water as long as you can without discomfort. One additional point is necessary to remember: in preparing for fasting you must be mentally as well as physically prepared for it. You must *want* to fast! And then not just want it but *do it*!

22. "What can I expect from fasting?"

A lot of changes will take place. Some you will least expect. Most of them are good changes. While fasting, in the early stages, you will notice that your breath becomes most foul, that your tongue gets a very heavy coating, and it's wise to look at your tongue each morning. As the tongue comes back to its normal color and the coating disappears, it is indicative of the amount of improvement that is taking place in your alimentary canal. Usually the clearing of the tongue is concurrent with a feeling of hunger and it's your cue that fasting has come to an end!

Your pulse may become a little rapid as you fast. In some persons it slows down. Variations exist in everyone. In most part the pulse remains normal. In the event it appears fast you will notice a fantastic thing occur. The moment your hunger for food returns your pulse will normalize. The heart is strong. There will be no vestiges of fever.

Your courage level will be your most trying problem. The first three days of fasting are the hardest. The biggest problem will be that of breaking old habits, especially the habit of eating morning, noon and night. You may become anxious, nervous, irritable, feel nauseated and queasy inside. By the fourth day the poisonous waste in your body will have begun to move out. Your organs will be at rest as they become cleansed. Revitalization will have begun. Your comeback to health is assured.

Body temperature often becomes subnormal when entering a fasting period unless a fever is already present. In either case, as the body progressively cleanses and rests, the temperature of the body adjusts to normal.

Weight loss is something else you can expect. This quite often is at the rate of approximately one pound per day. This amount usually reduces with each day of fasting until everything is back to equilibrium once more. The moment hunger comes on establish a regulated eating program. Stick to fruit and vegetable juices (see chapter 4) in the beginning stages of postfasting care.

Internal organs take weeks for total cleansing. The lymph vessels and bloodstream have to be filtered. Waste has to be removed. In the beginning there may be some loss of sexual desire but this returns sharply and strongly when fasting terminates. The nervous system and general senses improve and with this comes mental as well as physical peace.

23. "Is there anything else I can expect from fasting?"

There's no doubt that fasting is not simple. It takes courage. It takes a person with stick-to-itiveness to get past those first few days

when fasting is at its worst. Yes, there may be some fever. There
may be some chills. There may even be some nausea, dizziness and
headaches, too. Some folks complain of insomnia in the first stages
of fasting and that they can't void their urine. Others may complain
of muscle cramps, belly cramps and even diarrhea. But don't stop at
this crucial moment! Maintain your fast! Open up your bowels with
enemas. Drink lots of water and/or vegetable and fruit juices. Apply
hot compresses to your abdomen and an ice bag at the nape of your
neck. Place cold cloths on your face and head for a delightful feeling
of relaxation. Do all this knowing that Nature is healing you. Do
this knowing that keeping food from your body is not starving you.
Rather it is starving the disease that made you ill in the first place! In
fasting lies an answer to health.

An unusual and unorthodox method for achieving health? You bet
it is and it's one of the best. Jesus Christ fasted for forty days and
nights. When he returned to his flock he came back cleansed, rested
and whole. You can do the same!

Section C

(The section that teaches you to control pain)

Unusual and Unorthodox
How-to-do-its in
PHYSICAL THERAPY
FOR IMPROVING YOUR HEALTH

Chapter 6
Somatherapy and the magic of soft-tissue manipulation
   for pain relief

Chapter 7
Cupping and Skin Rolling to relieve those aches

Chapter 8
Spinal Concussion, Percussion and Vibration
   to rid yourself of hurts

Chapter 9
Clay Packs and the mystery of how they heal

Chapter 10
Aquatonics—the waterway to health and how to do it

CHAPTER 6

Somatherapy . . .
The Magic of Soft-Tissue
Manipulation for
Pain Relief

When pain comes, pain relief is something that everyone desires. An old-fashioned remedy, now considered unorthodox, offers you a way to do it. It is called *somatherapy*. Somatherapy is as old as time and yet as brand new as each day you use it for personal health. It is as close as your finger tips and immediately available without inconvenience or cost. It is yours to use whenever desired.

In your hands I place a technique that you can use on yourself and your family. It's simple. Anyone can do it. All you have to do is follow directions as did Gwendolyn R. and her husband who used somatherapy to change the course of her life.

Gwen had that all-American problem called neurasthenia. It started out with persistent headaches at the base of her skull. She

was depressed, couldn't concentrate, couldn't sleep. She reported
that her head felt like it had a tight band around it. Her back felt
weak and she had a feeling like little bugs were crawling on her
skin. Sometimes she felt dizzy. Her sex life had ground to a halt.
Her heart palpitated. Even her sense of smell became perverted and
things went from bad to worse at home. I started her on somatherapy
and showed her husband how to continue the procedure. In two
weeks the problem she had had for years disappeared. She no longer
felt miserable. Family life returned to normal and it all came about
through somatherapy and the magic of soft-tissue manipulation.

What Is Somatherapy?

Somatherapy is a technique of nerve or muscle stimulation or
inhibition by physical means. *Soma* means the body. Here is an
easy-to-do procedure using your hands on the body in a form of
massage or soft-tissue manipulation. So easy to do! So effectively
fast!

What Does It Do?
How Does It Bring Relief?

Somatherapy (1) stimulates spinal and other nerves, (2) inhibits
or slows down these same nerve centers when needed, (3) releases
muscle contractions, and (4) neutralizes or regulates excessive
blood supply, or lack of blood supply, around the spinal colum and
cord.

Key Nerve Centers
Control Pain

Each and every one of your body parts is controlled by a spinal
nerve. Pairs of these nerves exit from the spinal column. To
suppress nerve and blood flow, pressure is applied gently to control
pain. To *excite* nerve or blood flow, heavier pressure is applied. All

of it done with nothing more than your finger tips. Key nerves control your state of health and you have the master touch that holds them in abeyance.

Think about it. When nerves fail to receive their normal quota of blood supply, the organs and parts they feed go hungry. Like a garden without water these organs die a little bit each day. Lack of nerve and blood supply is called *anemia*. When there is a highly excitable change going on and the area is glutted with too much nerve and blood supply it is called *hyperemia*. All of this leads to malfunction and all can be prevented simply by locating and placing your finger tips on the right nerve centers.

There's nothing to memorize. Just check the diagrams. Identify the pressure points you want. Then apply massage action. Let's take a look at those spinal bones and nerves and give them names and numbers. The spinal column is composed of thirty-three vertebrae. Seven are in the neck. There are twelve thoracic vertebrae in the middle and upper back, five in the lower back called lumbars and the rest of them in the sacral and coccygeal (tailbone) areas.

How to Identify Landmarks
Where These Nerve Centers Are

The second cervical vertebra is the first one that can be felt from the rear at the base of the skull. Find that hollow at the base of your skull. Move your finger down slowly. The first bump you come to is called a spinal process. It belongs to cervical two. Continue down the neck to the biggest bump of all. This is cervical seven. Continue your count down. Count down the twelve thoracic vertebrae. Then the lumbars. Using these bumps as your landmarks, and Figure 20 as your guide, you have bone and nerve immediately on target.

Nerves Are the Vital Keys
in Making a Comeback to Health

Let's take some examples. Say that you have a pain in your arm. Check the first and second thoracic vertebrae on the illustration.

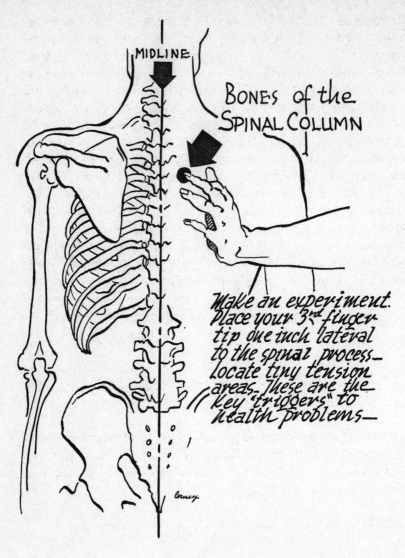

MIDLINE

BONES of the
SPINAL COLUMN

Make an experiment.
Place your 3rd finger
tip one inch lateral
to the spinal process.
Locate tiny tension
areas. These are the
key "triggers" to
health problems—

Figure 20

144

Note how nerves from this area go to the arm. That's your key treatment point. Nerves from the ninth to eleventh thoracic vertebrae go to the bowels. The ninth thoracic feeds the gallbladder. Nerves from the eleventh thoracic to the second lumbar go to the legs. See how simple it is? You identify, locate, and then use somatherapy on your nerves. To somatherapy you may add hot or cold applications as are described in the techniques that follow. The roadmap is there! Immediately at your finger tips is relief. With your own personal touch you stimulate or inhibit nerves, aid elimination of waste in local soft tissues and improve circulation. Consult the following illustrations and their accompanying explanations. Stick to the rules by simply following directions. Practice the technique until your hand goes out automatically to do what has to be done. *Somatherapy* is at your finger tips whether you're on a plane headed for Europe or working in the basement of the five and dime. Just apply it! Anytime! Anyplace!

**Homestyle Somatherapy Techniques
to Relieve Discomfort and Pain**

The SPINAL COLUMN

Pressure Point Procedures

Pressure points on the spinal column may be treated by leaning against a door frame, lying with two fists or golf balls in position. Maintain pressure to inhibit the angered nerve supply causing pain (Figure 21). (Also refer to Figure 6.)

Local Fingertip Traction

Nerve centers all along the spinal column may be inhibited by finger tip pressure by pulling gently on their anchorage. This is done, as soft tissue traction, beside each spinal process involved. The finger tips must not be permitted to slip on the skin (Figure 22).

Single Pressure Point Technique

Place the tips of your third finger on the single treatment point desired.

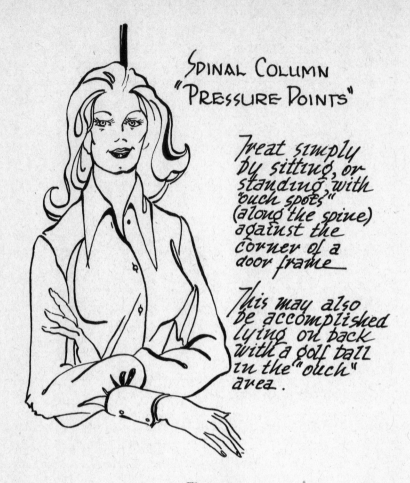

Spinal Column "Pressure Points"

Treat simply by sitting, or standing, with "ouch spots," (along the spine) against the corner of a door frame

This may also be accomplished lying on back with a golf ball in the "ouch" area.

Figure 21

146

LOCAL FINGERTIP TRACTION

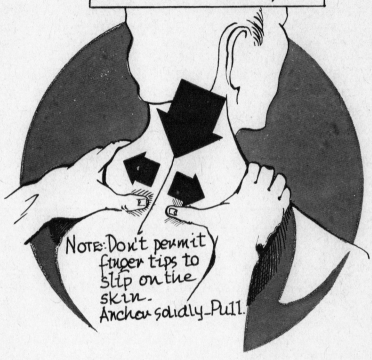

Figure 22

If you are doing it to someone else, bring that person's shoulder toward you with slight pressure. A finger placed on a key point will elicit pain. Maintain pressure to inhibit or quiet the involved nerve of organ (Figure 23).

Spinal Muscle Stretch

With all finger tips parallel to the spinal processes, anchor them in the muscle and pull toward you. Stretch them gently but firmly. Note, as they relax, how the little knots and ropelike tensions disappear. Keep fingers anchored as you pull (Figure 24).

Muscle Stretch with Torso in Half-Twist

The added half-twist gives just enough added pressure to the involved muscles. A general application from neck to low back may be administered, or it may be applied just on the specific area of concern (Figure 25).

Thumb Pressure Glide Technique

Patient is face down. While standing at his head place your hands on each shoulder. Place your thumbs on each side of the spinal processes. With even pressure glide your thumbs down to the base of the spinal column (Figure 26). Repeat. Feel the muscle tension release beneath your finger tips. Applying lotion on the skin preceding this move facilitates the action.

Palmar Thrust

With one hand over the other, place the outside of the underneath hand over the spinal process of the nerve involved. Give a sharp quick thrust with both hands. Hit like a little hammer (Figure 27).

Palmar Circle Rub

Place hands as in the palmar thrust. Instead of making a sharp impact, use the side of the underneath hand to make small circular actions on each side of the spinal processes involved (Figure 28).

Single Pressure Point

Technique
(with muscle stretch)

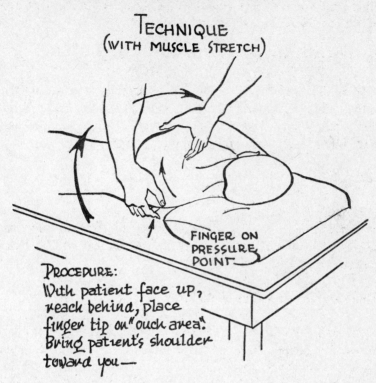

FINGER ON
PRESSURE
POINT

PROCEDURE:
With patient face up,
reach behind, place
finger tip on "ouch area".
Bring patient's shoulder
toward you—

Figure 23

SPINAL MUSCLE STRETCH
(WITH PATIENT FACE DOWN)

PROCEDURE:
Place finger tips parallel to spinal processes. Anchor finger tips. Press. Then gently pull.

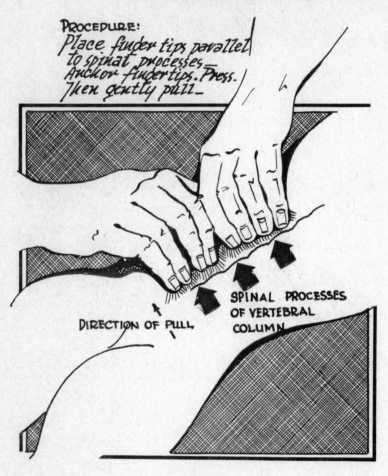

DIRECTION OF PULL

SPINAL PROCESSES
OF VERTEBRAL
COLUMN

Figure 24

150

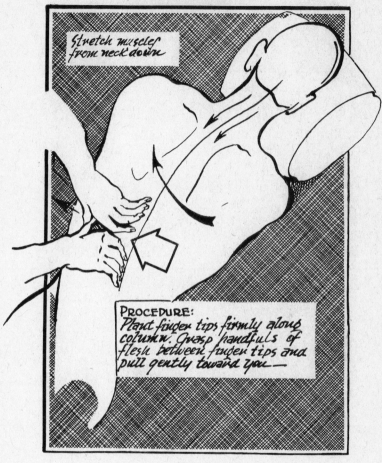

Figure 25

151

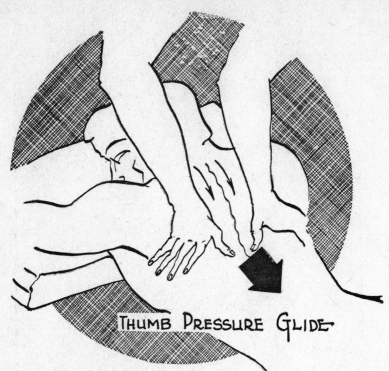

THUMB PRESSURE GLIDE

PROCEDURE:
From position at patient's head, place
thumbs on each side of spinal
process. Press. Lean weight forward.
Release. Repeat from neck to pelvis.

Figure 26

PALMAR THRUST
(PATIENT FACE DOWN)

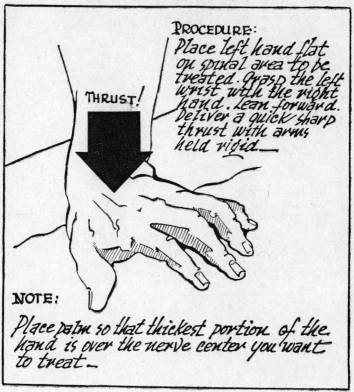

PROCEDURE:
Place left hand flat on spinal area to be treated. Grasp the left wrist with the right hand. Lean forward. Deliver a quick sharp thrust with arms held rigid.

THRUST!

NOTE:
Place palm so that thickest portion of the hand is over the nerve center you want to treat.

Figure 27

153

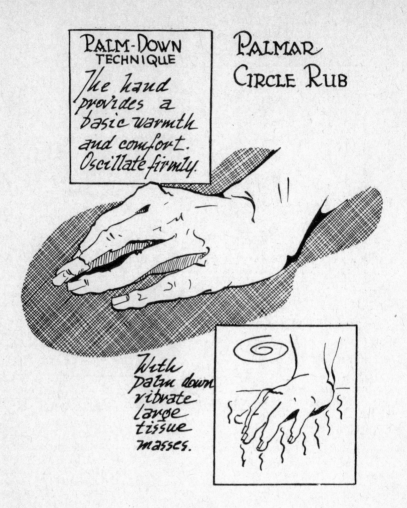

PALM-DOWN TECHNIQUE

The hand provides a basic warmth and comfort. Oscillate firmly.

PALMAR CIRCLE RUB

With palm down vibrate large tissue masses.

Figure 28

Spinal Roll

With the patient on his side and you facing him, place your right
hand on his hip and your left hand on his shoulder. With reverse
pressures bring the shoulder forward and the hip back (Figure 29).
Stretch the muscles gently. Hold. Relax back to position. Rest.
Repeat three times.

The NECK

Head Circle-and-Stroke Relaxation

With the patient on his back, lock his head in your two hands by
placing them under his neck. Move the head gently from side to
side, then in a circle. Then stroke the outstanding muscles of the
neck from the skull down (Figure 30). Ease the tensions. Note the
knots. Now stroke the forehead. You may do the same on yourself.
On yourself: Reach up and place finger tips at the base of the
skull. Make a gliding excursion down the muscles of the back of the
neck to the shoulders. Note the hard knots. Pause on each knot and
apply gentle pressure (Figure 31). Note how the muscle twitches,
moves, and then relaxes. Repeat same on the front of the neck and
sides. This will often remove a headache. In all cases massage
deeply at the base of the skull.

The SHOULDERS

On someone else: Stand behind the patient seated on a straight-
backed chair or ottoman. Systematically go over the scapula and
find each painful trigger point. Apply pressure on each. Feel the
knots twitch and then release (Figure 32).

The ABDOMEN

Abdominal Massage

While lying on your back apply the butt of each hand into the area
below the ribs. Press deeply (Figure 33). One hand may be placed
over the other in doing this if your arms are not particularly strong.

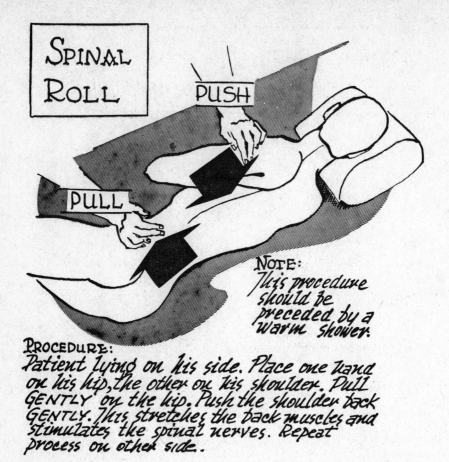

Figure 29

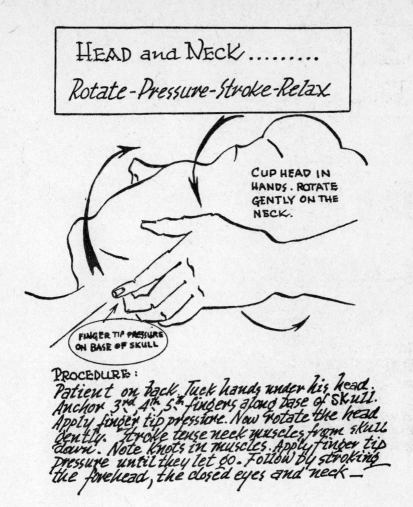

HEAD and NECK..........
Rotate-Pressure-Stroke-Relax

CUP HEAD IN
HANDS. ROTATE
GENTLY ON THE
NECK.

FINGER TIP PRESSURE
ON BASE OF SKULL

PROCEDURE:
Patient on back. Tuck hands under his head.
Anchor 3rd 4th 5th fingers along base of skull.
Apply finger tip pressure. Now rotate the head
gently. Stroke tense neck muscles from skull
down. Note knots in muscles. Apply finger tip
pressure until they let go. Follow by stroking
the forehead, the closed eyes and neck —

Figure 30

157

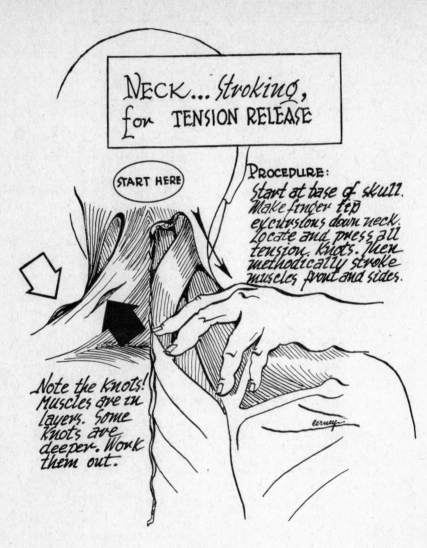

Figure 31

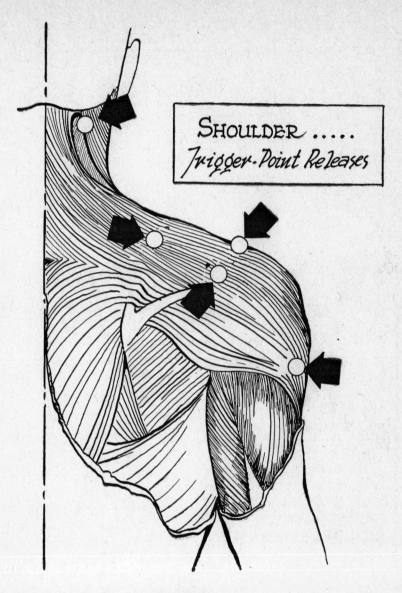

Figure 32

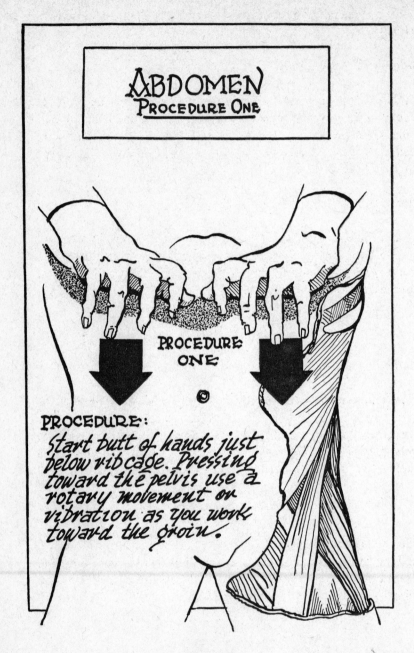

ABDOMEN
PROCEDURE ONE

PROCEDURE ONE

PROCEDURE:
Start butt of hands just below ribcage. Pressing toward the pelvis use a rotary movement or vibration as you work toward the groin.

Figure 33

160

To this may be added a rotary movement as you traverse the abdominal wall.

Abdominal Muscle Pull

While lying on your back place your finger tips deep in the muscles of the lower abdomen. Pull up toward the chest (Figure 34). Come up in progressive steps. There will be points of pain until tensions relax. Actually you are lifting the belly's contents and invigorating them.

Solar Plexus Pressure Point

Bury your finger tips in the area just below the tip of the breastbone. Press deeply making rotary motions from the umbilicus up to the tip of the sternum (Figure 35). Press deep. Find that area of extreme tenderness on pressure.

The SKULL

Thumb Pressure on Crest of Head

In working on yourself place your finger tips at the midline on the top of your skull. You will note tender areas you didn't know were there. Use a rotary massage motion along the midline from the forehead backward (Figure 36). An alternate to the rotary motion is simply deep pressure on each trigger point of pain in the scalp.

The FACE

Stroke the temples from the forehead back to the ears (Figure 37). Use both hands. Note the pinpoint trigger points of pain. Continue massage until the pain is gone. Sit back. Relax. Go to sleep if you desire.

The EYES

Place one finger tip flat on one eyeball. With the index finger tip of the other hand tap the underlying fingernail (Figure 38).

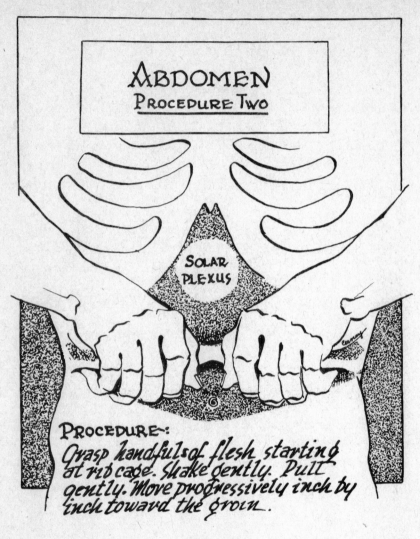

ABDOMEN
PROCEDURE TWO

SOLAR PLEXUS

PROCEDURE:
Grasp handfuls of flesh starting at rib cage. Shake gently. Pull gently. Move progressively inch by inch toward the groin.

Figure 34

162

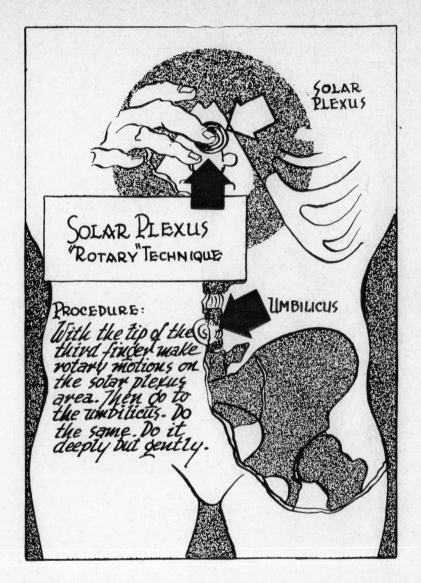

Figure 35

163

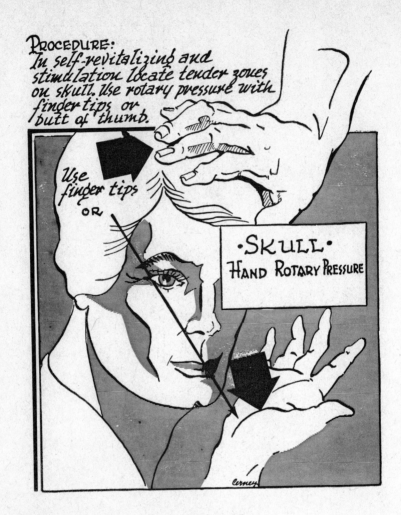

Figure 36

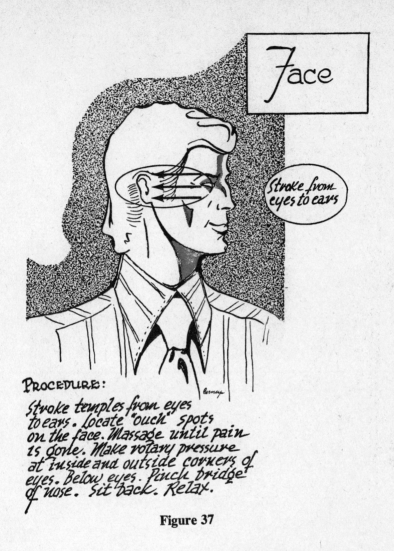

Figure 37

The purpose is to stimulate nerve and blood supply to that eye gently. This act improves eyesight and you see it happen.

Physical Therapy Follow-up

How to Use COLD Applications
After Soft-Tissue Manipulation

For additional personal care of your health problem, cold applications may be placed on areas of distress or pain. Once you learn how this adjunct to somapathic massage and pressure brings you results you won't want to do without it. Consult your chart of the spinal column and the nervous system (see Figure 7). Note the organs or body parts being fed by this system. If, for example, you want to treat cramps in your legs, you place a cold pack or ice bag over the nerve origins at the base of your spine. (*Note:* Never place ice bags over the eyes, breasts or scrotum.) If the skin becomes mottled blue under this therapy, massage the skin back to its normal color and repeat the procedure. This rub may be done with a cloth glove (gardener's glove) soaked in cold water. Remember that cold is always used when there is hyperemia around the spinal column. Use that key test, that million-dollar *spinal vasomotor reaction test,* to check this out. This hyperemia has to be inhibited and cold packs may follow finger pressure.

How to Use HOT Applications
After Soft-Tissue Manipulation

Heat is used when your vasomotor test elicits two white lines up and down the spinal column. Stimulation is necessary and hot water bags or compresses of wet toweling may be used. Bags of hot salt or sand may also be used.

How well and how efficiently hot and cold applications may be is noted in the following alphabetical listing of seventeen common nonhealth problems.

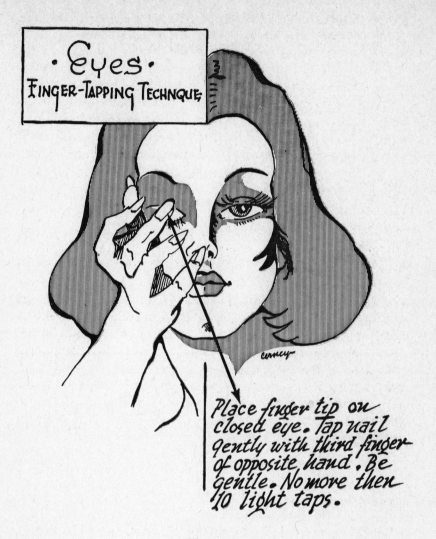

Figure 38

167

SEVENTEEN NONHEALTH PROBLEMS
TREATABLE BY SOMATHERAPY AT HOME

Asthma

Procedure: Apply heat to the entire thoracic and cervical areas of the spinal column. One day of the treatment week apply cold first and follow with heat. *Treatment time:* twenty minutes cold, one hour heat. This method quickly relieves the asthma attack. Follow with massage of the muscles of the neck and back (see Figures 21-29, 31, 32). Eat no heavy meals. Consume no pastries or sweets or gas-forming foods. Walk away from excitement, anger, fright, etc. Refuse to get involved.

Bed-Wetting

Procedure: Apply cold packs on the lower thoracic and lumbar areas of the spinal column. *Treatment time:* thirty minutes. Repeat twice weekly. A cold footbath is also helpful. Take a cool sponge bath each morning. Rub briskly until you glow. Drinking water is permitted during the day but not for three hours prior to bedtime. Relax the low back muscles (see Figures 14 and 24).

Bronchitis

Procedure: A constant hacking cough makes this problem undesirable and annoying. Chest pain and difficulty in breathing call for a hot pack from the fourth cervical to the seventh thoracic vertebra. Massage both the back and the abdomen (see Figures 22-29, 33-35). The cough usually abates. Breathing becomes easier under this method of treatment. Fever, if present, tends to drop. Take an enema or a laxative to keep the bowels open. Drink hot lemonade before going to bed. Administer a hot mustard footbath before bedtime. Treat on alternate evenings.

Catarrh

Procedure: Treat the upper thoracic or cervical areas with a cold wet towel pack or ice bag. *Treatment time*: Thirty minutes twice daily. Gradually extend the treatment time up to one hour per treatment. Sniff saltwater up into the nose, throw the head back and let it drain into the mouth (two tablespoonfuls of salt to a quart of water). Massage the back, chest and abdomen. Use deep abdominal massage.

Colds (general)

Procedure: Apply hot water pack to the entire spinal column (toweling saturated in hot water and wrung out). Follow with neck and back massage (see Figures 21-29, 31, 32). Also massage the solar plexus area (Figure 35). Follow with a hot footbath, drink hot lemonade and get into bed. Remain in bed if fever is present. Treat daily until the cold is gone. Be sure your bedroom is well-ventilated at night. Take a cool sponge bath daily and follow with a brisk rub with toweling.

Constipation

Procedure: Twice a day, for an hour each session, apply a hot water bottle or hot wet toweling from the seventh thoracic vertebra down to the sacrum. Follow with deep massage of the abdomen and solar plexus. Massage the back muscles. Use a warm saltwater enema (one tablespoonful per hot water bag of water) at the beginning to "get the plug out." After that rely on abdominal massage to get action. Watch your diet. Add bran bread and vegetables with heavy residue (cabbage, squash, cauliflower, pumpkin, etc.).

Cramps (extremities)

Procedure: If the cramps are in the *upper extremities* use heat on the lower cervical and upper thoracic area of the spinal column. *Treatment time:* twenty minutes daily. Massage the neck and upper back (see Figures 22, 25, 26, 30, 31). Massage the extremity on the side of the cramping (if there are no varicose veins present). Where the *lower extremities* are concerned, place a hot pack from the eleventh thoracic vertebra to the second lumbar.

Diarrhea

Procedure: To check diarrhea, inhibit the lower thoracic and upper lumbar areas with cold packs and/or an ice bag. Administer warm saltwater enemas. Massage the back, neck and abdomen gently and eliminate the cause of the diarrhea (food, water change, poison, weather change, emotional distress, etc.). Stick to boiled milk diet until the problem clears up.

Earache

Procedure: Place hot water bag on pillow. Cover it with warm, moist toweling. Place affected ear on toweling. Massage neck and upper back muscles until relaxed.

Gastritis

Procedure: Gastritis is a problem that plagues a lot of people living in a tense world. To treat it place a heat pack over the solar plexus and over the area of the vagus nerve exiting from the spine. Cold packs should be applied simultaneously over the thoracic area. Treat daily for one hour. Massage the solar plexus and abdominal areas (see Figures 33-35).

Headache

Procedure: Most headaches begin with tension. The muscles of the neck and back should be the first to be massaged after applying cold packs for twenty minutes and inserting the hands in a bucket of cold water. Use deep massage on the abdomen and solar plexus. Place an ice cap on top of the head and a hot pack at the base of the skull. Follow with massage of these areas as well as down over the temporals from forehead to ear. *Treatment time:* thirty minutes on alternate days. Use warm saltwater enema to clear the bowels. Avoid all drugs when using this method with the exception of a cup of hot black coffee!

Hemorrhoids

Procedure: Use deep massage over the lumbar and sacral areas of the low back (see Figures 14 and 24). Treat for constipation (see Constipation, this chapter) or other causative factors. If there are no organic complications this treatment will get results. Take long walks. Avoid overexertion. Do not sit in cold, damp places. Do not partake of alcoholic beverages or highly spiced foods.

Insomnia

Procedure: Follow hot/cold packs on the spinal column with deep massage of the neck and back muscles. Massage deeply into the abdomen. When cold is applied on the back use a hot pack on the abdomen and vice versa after every fifteen minutes. Take a hot shower and go to bed. Place a cold pack on the belly and sleep peacefully. Where constipation exists get the bowel cleared out.

Laryngitis

Procedure: Treat the neck for twenty minutes with a cold water pack on the back of the neck and a hot pack on the front. Do not use ice! This may be preceded with a warm saltwater rectal enema. Follow hydrotherapy with deep massage of all neck muscles and those of the back and upper chest.

Lumbago

Procedure: The low back is usually involved in lumbago and the place to start treatment with alternate hot/cold therapy is over the lower thoracic and lumbar areas. Apply cold water pack for a quarter hour. Follow with a hot pack for the same length of time. Then begin low back deep massage of the musculature as indicated in Figure 24. Use heavy thrust (Figure 27) over the spinal column in the lumbar area.

Sciatica

Procedure: All tissues over the course of the sciatic nerve have to be released of tension. This covers the area from the low back to the feet. To heat this much territory all you have to do is sit in a tub of hot water (104°F.). Follow this with gentle but deep massage over the lower dorsal vertebral area, the lumbar area, the buttocks, hip, thigh, calf, heel and plantar areas of the foot. Note the painful spots along the way. Apply pressure on these ''Z'' or trigger zones until the pain recedes. When separate hot packs are used on the buttocks and thigh, place an ice bag on the lumbar or low back area.

Sprains and Strains

Procedure: Apply ice promptly for a period of twenty-four hours. Every twenty minutes massage the involved area. Treat twice daily for the best results. After the first twenty-four hours start heat therapy. This technique will eliminate discomfort if you wrap a cotton elastic roller bandage around the affected area after treatment.

These somapathic treatments are simple to use. Keep them simple. Don't add. Don't subtract. Of the many unorthodox and unusual treatments available, somatherapy is one of the most efficient and practical to use.

CHAPTER 7

Cupping and Skin-Rolling for Pain Relief

Of the many useful therapies that have come to us from yester-day, *cupping and skin rolling* for the relief of pain continues to be a practical method of self-help. The procedure goes back 3,000 years in Chinese medical history and it still persists today even though it has become classified as unusual and unorthodox as related with modern care.

What Is Cupping and Skin-Rolling?

Cupping and skin-rolling is a method in which the skin over an area of sensitivity is grasped with the finger tips and lifted upward from its base. Its purpose is to stimulate blood vessels and nerves in a local area. It is a local soft-tissue tonic with far-reaching results. The thumb and index finger are all you need. However, some folks go a step further and use a vacuum cup. A vacuum cup is a small glass container with a central aperture and a rubber ball attached. Squeezing the air out of the ball creates a vacuum within the glass. The skin against which it has been placed is sucked upward. Such a glass or cup is available at any drugstore under the name of "breast pump" or "Bier's Cupping Glass" (Figure 39).

Materials Needed:

> *Bier's cupping glass* (breast pump) 1½" diameter
> *Olive oil*

Technique:

Liberally apply olive oil to the area involved. Place the cup. Squeeze the suction bulb so that the skin is drawn gently up inside the glass. Treatment has now begun. Release the rubber bulb. Grasp the glass cup and lift it evenly up and away from the skin surface. Do not elevate or depress any one part of the rim of the glass. Now gently re-place the glass on the skin. Squeeze the bulb once more and you're ready to continue the process. Here's what you do: simply and gently push the cup along the oiled surface even while maintaining traction on the skin. If air leaks in suction will be lost. The vacuum will be gone so start again. Keep the cup moving over the surface of the skin until the skin is uniformly pink in color. NOTE: Over joints and bony prominences the cup may become detached. Simply re-apply. Start again. Experience quickly teaches you to counter this problem. Under all circumstances be *gentle*! If the application is rough little capillaries beneath the skin break and black-and-blue marks result. This is not dangerous but it is unsightly. WARNING NOTE: There *is* a factor about this black-and-blueness of which you should be aware. If you have a chronic dietary deficiency and lack vitamin C you will bruise easily in this manner. When this occurs simply take vitamin C (with bioflavonoids) to rid yourself of this problem.

CUPPING TECHNIQUE
BIER CUPPING
GLASS
or "BREAST PUMP"

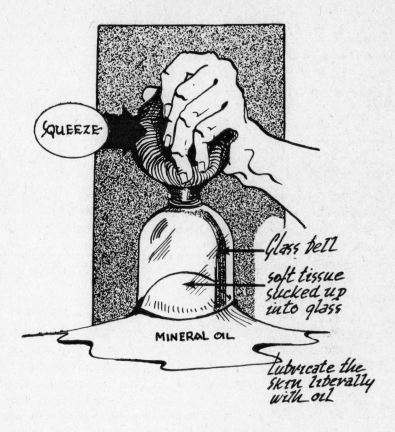

SQUEEZE

Glass bell

soft tissue
sucked up
into glass

MINERAL OIL

Lubricate the
skin liberally
with oil

Figure 39

The IRISH and CHINESE TECHNIQUES
for CUPPING and SKIN-ROLLING

The Irish Method

In the Emerald Isle, the Irish, to rid themselves of evil, were known to place a penny on the belly button. On the penny was placed a lighted candle. Over the lighted candle was placed a glass. By the time the candle went out a vacuum had occurred. The skin was sucked up. In so doing evil was lifted up and out of the pit of hell.

Although I was not concerned with evil in saintly little Janice D., I was concerned with her imperfect digestion and the allergies to medication that were playing havoc with her body and soul. A method had to be used that would relieve her abdominal pain and still fascinate her sufficiently to get her over her fear of doctors. We played a game with the penny, cup and candle, and it worked. Cupping was exacted on her abdomen. Her bowels began to move the next day. Can I explain it? I can't. It just worked. Unorthodox, unusual, but it worked! The child is back to being her vivacious self once more.

The Chinese Method

Long before there were vacuum cups, the Chinese with their different variations of acupuncture techniques were grasping the skin over areas of tenderness and achieving health results. As Stephen Palos said in his excellent text:

> Man's original medical tool is his hand, which he has always instinctively used in order to alleviate pain. Whenever he is struck, stung, or seized with a cramp, he involuntarily puts his hand to the painful spot in order to protect it or to rub, knead, or massage it . . . in China it was realized very early that massage not only helped to relieve pain, that is to say, that its effects were merely local; it was also seen that stimulation of certain area of the skin could affect the internal organs.*

---

*Palos, S. *The Chinese Art of Healing,* (N.Y.: McGraw-Hill Book Company, 1221 Avenue of the Americas, New York).

In the course of Oriental medical history the Chinese developed eight different forms of remedial massage that even today are taught in Chinese medical schools. In one of those methods, like *cupping*, the skin is grasped and lifted from its dermal attachments. How to do this is described as follows:

(1) *Grasping* (Chinese term—*"Na"*). Na is used for toning the muscles, joints and underlying tissues. To execute it grasp the skin between index finger and thumb. Vibrate, shake, or roll the skin between these two fingers. Do it gently at first. Gradually increase the action. Increase it until you are actually shaking it. *Shaking* (Yao-fa) may progress deeper into the underlying tissues. Muscles may be grasped and shaken vigorously. This method may be used on the neck for whiplash injuries.

(2) *Skin-rolling* is often used where the epidermis is too tender for cupping or other procedures. It may also be used to follow the cupping procedure. The skin is picked up between the thumb and index finger with both hands creating a wave of skin and subcutaneous tissues. Keep this wave moving like a wave rolling on the ocean by grasping, moving, releasing, from one side of the body part to the other.

It will take a while to become adept at this method. It's not easy. Until the skin is free from the underlying tissues these tissues will hurt. But keep doing it. The disappearance of discomfort is your criterion of growing success in rendering this excellent treatment on yourself or on others. If you have arthritis *do not move the joint* where you are treating the overlying skin. A half hour of skin-rolling and you will be an expert. Do not continue too long over any one spot. Terminate the procedure by gently stroking or massaging the skin. Where hurt or tenderness appears to be in deep, use a heavier friction or pressure.

As you become more adept at *cupping and skin-rolling*, you will become conscious of the fact that there are numerous little tensions in the skin and underlying tissues. These areas need special attention. They are collections of waste. They may also be adhesions. And as long as they are present there will be discomfort or pain. Back in 1918 Dr. Radcliff wrote on page 103 of the *Lancet* (British) medical journal: "After some weeks of practice I was able to localize the tender areas . . . after three weeks treatment the deposits break up, disappear and the pain vanishes.''

Said John McL., a patient of mine, ''I used that *skin-cupping* and *rolling* method you taught me on my neck after my automobile accident. The stiffness gradually disappeared. I didn't believe it would happen. But it did!''

CHAPTER 8

Concussion, Percussion, Vibration: Unusual Treatment Techniques

how to use them to bring you health

Of the many unusual and unorthodox healing methods known to mankind over the years those physical procedures applied to the spinal column have persisted the longest and strongest. The intimacy of the nerve structures exiting and entering the spinal column makes treatment of each specific nerve possible. Some of this is accomplished by actually moving a spinal bone to influence the nervous system, but this belongs in the hands of a specialist. However, in your hands is the ability to influence that same nerve with *concussion, percussion* or *vibration* over the same area. How to do each in home therapy is discussed briefly in this chapter. Study each method. Learn it. Practice. Be conservative in your application and never overtreat or treat too hard. Learn how Mrs. Maude M. treated her daughter Julie's asthma, how Howard R. treated his emphysema and John K. stopped the sciatica that had plagued him for years. By diplomatic effort you can help yourself, or your family, back to health using the same methods. There's no cost, very little time spent, and all it takes is a little practical diligence on your part. Let's take them alphabetically.

CONCUSSION
AND HOW IT WORKS ITS WONDERS

At first Maude M. refused to believe that anything like *concussion* could do anyone any good healthwise and she had every right to believe that way. She just didn't know about it. She was skeptical. She was doubtful about its values when it was explained to her and she simply couldn't see how it could be used to restore her daughter's health. So I re-explained how *concussion* is a gently forceful blow, a hammerlike pitter-patter, to one or both sides of the spinal processes of the spinal column for the purpose of relieving pain, relieving symptoms and sending reflex stimulation to other body parts.

How Is Concussion Applied?

Here's what I instructed Mrs. M. to do: Place a one-eighth-inch thickness of piano felt or other type felt over the spinal process to be concussed. At the rate of 100 strokes per minute use a little rubber hammer, or the knuckle of the index finger, on target. This takes only one minute. The blows should be only as strong as the patient will tolerate. The blows should be about as hard as it takes to drive a tack into soft wood. Under the patter of blows underlying blood vessels dilate. They will contract if the speed of the blows delivered are hastened. Nerves exiting or entering the spinal column at this point are also affected. They carry this stimulation to the very organs and parts they feed. In Julie's case it was to the organs of respiration. She just couldn't breathe.

Treatment time: five minutes.

Add a Special Additive and Double the Results

In addition to concussion, *digital pressure* may be applied on each side of the involved vertebra. This point is about one inch lateral to the projection of the spinal process. The thumbs are best used to provide this pressure.

Naturally you can't use spinal concussion on yourself, but you can certainly use it on your family as did Maude M. when she applied it to her daughter's back for bronchial asthma. Julie's asthma had come on suddenly and was worse at night. The child was constantly depressed, tired and chilly. Her nose itched and her chest felt full. She said she felt like she was suffocating all the time. When I checked her over, her lungs were rattling like castanets. She was having difficulty trying to exhale as well as get rid of the sticky sputum that filled her throat.

Whether it is asthma or some other problem, turn to Figure 40. Study the illustration. Locate the vertebra recommended for treatment by concussion. In Julie's case it was the fourth and fifth cervical vertebrae involved. While Julie sat backward on an upright kitchen chair her head was bent forward. A piece of felt was placed over the spinal process involved. Then Mrs. M. counted down to the third and fourth thoracic vertebrae and repeated the process. This was followed by one minute of thumb pressure on either side of these same vertebrae.

"There's nothing to it!" exclaimed Mrs. M. From the standpoint of home remedies that's all that has to be done. But from the standpoint of what is going on inside, that's something else. Within weeks the results were remarkable. Julie was no longer depressed. No more tiredness. She could breathe again. She was alive and

Concussion
Hand or Hammer Technique

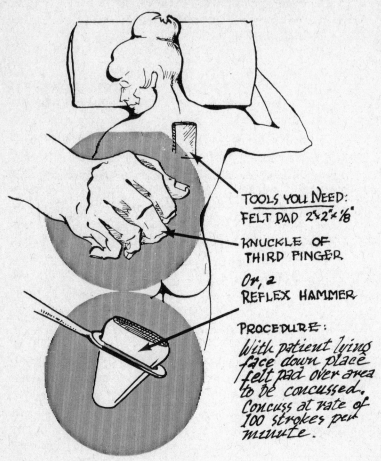

TOOLS YOU NEED:
FELT PAD 2"×2"×⅛"

KNUCKLE OF
THIRD FINGER

Or, a
REFLEX HAMMER

PROCEDURE:
With patient lying
face down place
felt pad over area
to be concussed.
Concuss at rate of
100 strokes per
minute.

Figure 40

going like any young person. The chills and itching disappeared, and Mrs. M. was elated with Julie's progress. The proof was in the pudding. Mrs. M. had watched with her own eyes how concussion worked. Under the magic of her own hands it happened. With spinal stimulation the girl's breathing apparatus began to be restored to normalcy once more.

Special Chart Gives You Instant Directions

To help you with some of the more common ailments treatable at home, I have given, on the next page, an At-a-Glance Chart of the more common nonhealth problems. Use the concussion points wisely. At no time force the action. Nature will handle the whole problem for you.

PERCUSSION and How It Is an Unusual Method for Achieving Healthy Results

How Do You Do It? What's the Procedure?

Percussion for general health purposes is delivered in various easy-to-do ways. It may be done by *tapping, clapping, spatting, hacking* or *beating.*

Tapping is a form of finger tip beating of the target area. This technique is used mostly on the head and chest.

Clapping should be done over a greater expanse with the hand cupped to hit the skin, producing a loud sound on impact. It is used where strong stimulation is desirable.

Spatting, on the other hand, is the slapping of the tissues with a stiff flat hand. It renders a prompt reaction when used on cold body parts. They warm immediately under this persuasion.

SPINAL-CONCUSSION-FOR-HEALTH CHART

(Pressure Points Added Feature)

Nonhealth Problem	Spinal Process for Concussion*	Pressure Point
Abdomen (pain in)	4 to 8 T	none
Abdominal pain (menstruation)	3 and 4 T	none
Arm (numbness in)	7 C	none
Arm (pain in)	4 and 5 C	none
Asthma (bronchial)...............	4 and 5 C 3 and 4 T	3 and 4 T
Bed-wetting	5 L	none
Bladder (pain in)	7,8,9, and 12 T	none
Blood pressure (high)	3 and 4 and 10 T	none
Foot (pain in)	12 T	none
Forearm (pain in)	5 and 6 C	none
Hand (pain in)	5 and 6 C	none
Headache	2 C	in hollow at base of skull
Hiccough	4 and 5 C	none
Nosebleed	7 C	none
Nose (cold in)	7 C	none
Piles (hemorrhoids)	1 and 2 S	none
Rectum (pain in)	12 T	none
Shoulder (pain in area of)	2, 3 and 4 C	none
Shoulder (joint pain)	6, 7 and 1 T	trigger points ("ouch" spots) around shoulder

* "C" stands for cervical vertebra
"T" stands for thoracic
"S" for sacrals (tailbone)

Hacking is a chopping motion with the sides of the hands. Fingers are held apart. This technique is used most often on the head, chest and back.

Beating, as its name implies, is striking the target with the half-closed fist. Used on the thighs and low back it is a powerful stimulant to the kidneys and the organs of the pelvis.

What Does Percussion Do?
Where Is the Reaction?

Percussion is a strong excitant on the skin and underlying tissues. As with spinal concussion, direct percussion to the spinal column stimulates the vasomotor nervous system. All internal organs and parts are immediately affected. New life is brought to them through the nerves stimulated by the action.

Percussion is the most powerful of all the manual stimulating procedures, and in addition to applying it on the spinal column it can be applied to the abdomen with intent to treat the organs within.

Percussion has many uses. The great English physical therapy specialist Cyriax uses percussion even to relieve the strange symptoms of "phantom limb" in which the amputee thinks he still has the injured limb attached and is going through all the agony that seems to still be there.

I still remember Howard R.'s problem. Howard was superintendent of sewers in a nearby large town. Earlier he had played in the Navy band and was then transferred to a war zone where he was hit in the chest with shrapnel. He developed emphysema. His rib cage distended as his chest enlarged. The little airsacks in the lungs called alveoli ruptured. The elasticity of his lungs was lost after the war wounds in his respiratory tract healed. He coughed a lot, expectorated a lot, and found it hard to breathe. He took lots of little breaths and was long on exhalation. He was instructed to stop smoking but he wouldn't. He was told to rest but he didn't. Tonics and oral stimulants given him by another physician were of no avail. Nothing helped until he started using the simple little process of percussion. Within weeks Howard was breathing easier. He didn't get rid of his problem. He didn't get rid of his bulging chest but he was able to continue on his job and that's all he asked for in the first place. Said Howard, "The specialists said there was no cure so who could ask for anything more!"

VIBRATION
and How to Do It

Vibration is a shaking motion conveyed to the underlying tissues with one or both hands through: (a) *lateral vibration*, (b) *deep vibration*, (c) *superficial vibration*, (d) *knuckle vibration*, (e) *shaking* and (f) *digital vibration* for the purpose of stimulation.

Rapid vibration with the hands is similar in effect to electricity. It may cause muscles to contract as well as give a pleasurable tingling to the local part. Blood vessels dilate and circulation improves. Local temperature elevates. Cold extremities are relieved. So are numbness and tingling.

> *Lateral vibration* is done by placing the hand flat on the skin without slipping and moving the hand laterally to and fro. It is best used on joints, abdomen and head.

> *Deep vibration* is accomplished by placing the closed fist on the part to be treated and with the arms held straight a shaking or quivering motion is delivered.

> *Superficial vibration* is a shallow version of deep vibration.

> *Knuckle vibration* is executed by placing the knuckles on target, moving them slowly over the target to impart a trembling or shaking motion.

> *Shaking* is the grasping of the part in both hands and literally shaking it. (To be used on the head and extremities.)

> *Digital vibration* is accomplished by the thumb or other finger tips anchored in position while the arm is set into vibratory motion. By way of the hands vibration becomes a powerful means of stimulating circulation, glandular activity, nerve reflex and abdominal peristalsis.

Smoothing vibrations are achieved through the palm of the hand placed flat on the body part. Stimulating vibration is conveyed through the finger tips and knuckles.

The Purpose of Vibration and What It Can Do for You

Vibration relieves pain and tension. It reduces edema, loosens stiff joints, stretches adhesions, loosens scars, stimulates nerves and relieves gas in the abdomen.

John K. was a housepainter. Like a lot of painters going up and down ladders he developed pains in the low back, buttocks and thigh. Sometimes the pain shot all the way down to his foot. Cold, wet days made it worse. The pain was hot and stabbing and usually worse at night. He could put his finger on points of pain down his leg. I pointed out to John that these points of pain were Nature's signal systems to show exactly where to render treatment. Finger tip vibration and pressure on these points were his keys to loss of pain. He used this method. In three weeks he had an almost complete cessation of sciatic hurt. To further supplement the vibration technique, I had him apply alternately hot and cold compresses on his low back and on his thighs. This was followed by the digital vibration.

All body parts are treated in the same manner. For example, Francine K. used shaking and vibration on her nose, larynx and lungs to loosen the adhering mucus inside. Said Cyriax, "Vibration performed on the thorax, together with postural drainage, is of particular value in treating certain pulmonary conditions."*

*Cyriax, J. Textbook of Orthopaedic Medicine, Vol. II: Treatment by Manipulation and Massage. (London: Bailliere Tindal and Cassell, 1959, p. 70).

CHAPTER 9

Healing with the Mystery
of the White Clay Packs

Adrienne De L. had eczema. It wasn't contagious but it was unsightly, uncomfortable and chronic. She had had it for years. It was the weepy kind on her legs, with varicose veins beneath. Her legs were one big walking sore until she started using white clay packs and found healing in the mystery of mud.

Why Is White Clay So Healing?

Exactly why white clay is beneficial, why it heals, why it cools and causes waste matter beneath the skin to be eliminated, I don't know. What I *do* know is that the white clay pack, the modern version of the old mud bath, proved to be a godsend to Adrienne De L.

After the application of white clay on her legs, the first thing Adrienne reported was the cooling effect. The second was the even distribution of compression as it began to dry. She said it felt like a pair of lisle hosiery but without the itch. She said, "You may not believe it, but I could actually feel the heat and inflammation leaving my legs."

On examination I found that the weepy excretion, which previously had run down into her shoes, had now stopped. Such a difference! Previously her legs had been lumpy with varicose veins following multiple pregnancies. Small lengths of veins had converted into tortuous sacks of blood standing still. Each leg was a septic tank holding about a quart of standing blood. As the result of this stasis the external skin and underlying soft tissues broke down. Local tissues swelled. There was acidosis, anoxemia, and a general collection of waste. It was inevitable that this cesspool would break open in many places and the contents of varicose destruction leak out.

I told Adrienne about the possible necessity for surgery and she snapped that she had already had two "stripping" operations in which sections of her saphenous (external veins) system had been removed, that she had been to famous clinics specializing in circulatory diseases for injections in her veins, that she'd had mechanical boots on her legs and that twice she'd had skin grafts. I looked at those fat stumps of legs oozing fluid and I felt sick inside. What could I do? More in desperation than anything else I suggested *white clay packs*.

You may or may not have heard about the healing ability of white clay and other virgin earths, but clay, down through the centuries, has been the mysterious substance used for treatment of congestion, growths, wounds, and skin problems of one kind or another. For Adrienne this appeared to be the final resort because she'd had everything else including tender loving care from her husband who footed the bill.

How Is White Clay Applied?

After wrapping the affected part carefully with layers of cloth or sterile gauze, mix the white clay preferably with rain water. Thin it down until it is the consistency of thick paint. Then apply this puttylike material liberally over the gauze wrap. It may be applied with a paintbrush or with the hands. The latter is very sloppy indeed and not to be recommended. Add two or three coats and permit it to dry.

When there has been fever the entire body may be wrapped and immersed in clay to the neck. The clay is to remain on for at least six hours.

What Happens to the Skin?

The clay apparently acts like a blotter. As it dries it begins to draw out, pull, or absorb the liquid waste collected in and under the skin. Some folks refer to this as "drawing out the poison," and actually that's what it is. Toxic waste exits through the pores of the skin. This drawing power is noted immediately as the clay begins to dry.

Boils, carbuncles and other sores that have refused to come to a head open up and spill their ugly contents into the bandaging material. After the treatment everything is thrown away. The skin is cleansed. This may be done with soap and water, under a shower, or with alcohol. The shower is preferable.

In Adrienne's case, when the clay pack came away, it left a silky soft pink skin in its wake. Ugly corrupt sores were beginning to heal. Little islands of granulation (healing) tissue were showing. She said it felt as if a giant pressure had been removed from her legs. With the removal of the clay pack I was interested to see that the varicose veins had retreated. On standing they didn't fill up grossly as they had before. What was best of all, with continued clay pack therapy her varicose veins got progressively smaller. The angry inflammation departed. The weeping stopped. Healing was complete and her legs were no longer ugly.

Clay Packs Have Many Uses

Bernarr McFadden, in writing his *Encyclopedia of Physical*

Culture, tells about a certain school of hydropathic doctors in Europe that advocated mud as the "Nature Cure" for overcoming disease and eliminating body waste, that the same effects could be achieved by burying the patient in warm sand, that the resulting perspiration would act as a body cleanser. Rheumatism, strains and bruises would thus be given relief. He also warned that there should be no prolonged burial in cold, damp earth because of its chilling effect. He stressed particularly that unsterile mud should not be slapped on open wounds or sores because of possible infective complications, that hot wet dressings or fomentations were satisfactory alternatives.

How to Get Rid of Headaches with White Clay Packs

A compress of white clay may be applied to the forehead and behind the nape of the neck to alleviate a headache. Chest and abdominal distress may be relieved by applying clay packs over these areas. Leg cramps, backache and inflammation are all relieved in the same manner. All you do is apply and permit the pack to dry. Insect stings may be treated the same way. Swelling is reduced, pain allayed.

Today Adrienne De L. gets around like other folks. Her legs are no longer swollen. They no longer weep. The sores are gone. She's back to taking care of her family without any of the burdens of those ugly varicose veins and the eczema that accompanied them. There are scars to show where the ulcers were but other than that her legs are healed. Why? Was it due to the absorptive power of the clay? Did this unusual and unorthodox treatment method merely create a compression boot on her legs to alleviate the problem? As I said, I don't know how it works, but it does!

Where May White Clay Be Obtained?

My last known supplier was the Stanley Phillips Company at 305 Garfield Avenue, Trenton, New Jersey.

CHAPTER 10

Aquatonics
. . . the Water Way
to Health

Yours is the hand that rocks the cradle of personal health. Yours is the ability to use *aquatonic therapy* not only for conquering ailments but preventing them. You can use it in the privacy of your own home with little or no expense simply by using tools that are already at hand. When diplomatically handled, all aquatonic procedures are completely safe so that you can use them to make health vibrantly yours.

Remember that only Nature cures. Nature alone restores health through the magic of the body's own processes. It does this by assisting, stimulating or sedating the body into healing itself. Because of all this *aquatonics* is the indeed the waterway to health! What is *aquatonic therapy*? What does it do? Why is it so successful? Let's take a look.

NINE MAGIC ACCOMPLISHMENTS
OF NATURAL HEALING

(1) *Aquatonic therapy* stimulates those wonder-working endocrine glands (thyroid, pituitary, adrenals, testes, ovaries, etc.), those powerhouses and dynamos and helps them to function normally once more.

(2) *Aquatonic therapy* helps release local obstructions and pressures on blood vessels, nerves, lymph vessels and the organs of the body with which they communicate and control. It relieves the burden of swelling, stiffness, strain, tension, growths, temperature changes, soreness, and collections of corruption that bring about discomfort and pain.

(3) *Aquatonic therapy* activates organs of purification and elimination (liver, kidneys, bowels, lungs, skin, etc.) so that cleansing takes place.

(4) *Aquatonic therapy* enriches the chemistry of the body with the very fluids of life that maintain immunity against disease and aging.

(5) *Aquatonic therapy* regulates the circulation of blood and tunes up the body's intricate system of nerves. It influences that master gland called the *medulla oblongata* at the base of the brain.

(6) *Aquatonic therapy* reduces excess gastric acidity and excess alkalinity in achieving that acid-base balance so important to health.

(7) *Aquatonic therapy* helps clear away any foci of infection.

(8) *Aquatonic therapy* helps bring about peace of mind and body as the body tissues are regulated and restored to normalcy once more.

(9) *Aquatonic therapy* is a tangible "something to do" to help release tensions. Through water therapy you not only relieve aches, pains and hurts, but you also take the edge off emotional stress. Through *aquatonic therapy*, when used by the person who wants and needs help, comes optimum human performance and improved sexual capacity.

Because aquatonic therapy may be somewhat new to you, you may at first question its true effectiveness. You will tend to question that which is in this book about unusual and unorthodox therapies.

And you have every right to do so. Take nothing for granted. *Do* it! Utilize the magic of water and assist Nature. Experience that which happens to you. You will be amazed at the results you get. You will be astounded by your own successes. You will create your own little miracles of health and this you have every right to do.

**Housewife Turns to Water
Therapy When All Else Fails**

Mrs. Kevin R's husband said she was a hypochondriac, that she loved to be ill, that she caused her own troubles. To Mrs. R, however, her aches and pains were very real. She was most sincere in telling about how her heart caused her to be breathless, tired and giddy. She complained of pain in her chest and pointed exactly to the place from where it stemmed. She said the pain came on during stress (anger, worry, anxiety, etc.). She said her face flushed, that her hands trembled and she felt faint. Her breathing hastened so that she could hardly catch her breath. She said she was always sighing.

Dealing with Nature's remedies as I do as a doctor, I started her on cold sitz baths and within weeks her problem was gone. She was *not* a hypochondriac! She simply responded to aquatonic therapy and Nature made her whole again! How did it achieve this? How does aquatonic therapy work?

*Effects of Water Therapy
on the Spinal Cord and
Total Nervous System*

When hot or cold water is applied to the skin and spinal column area, the spinal cord and its interconnecting nervous systems, as well as the brain, are immediately affected. Such an ingenious human electronic device as the *sympathetic nervous system* is affected immediately where the watery influence is applied with gossamer touch, a harsh stingy spray, or with a friction rub. What is the sympathetic nervous system? It is a special set of nerves running down the back on either side of the spinal column. This system supplies and controls nerves to each organ and body part. Stimulate this system and you automatically stimulate everything it controls. Action and reaction sets in. Sedate it and everything it feeds is soothed. Irritate it and reaction is immediate. It's an amazing device and all you have to do is learn to use it.

Specifically, Here's What
Hot and Cold Water Does

For example, cold water (or an ice pack) applied to the back of the neck and the base of the skull immediately increases the blood supply to the brain. It increases circulation to the arms and hands. It elevates blood pressure in those whose blood pressure is low. An ice pack applied to the lower back increases circulation to the lower extremities. Cold hands and cold feet can be made to become warm again through such treatment. That deep coldness felt in the spine itself may be chased away. Heat acts in reverse. Apply heat to the low back and the temperature of the extremities cools off. The hot burning feeling goes away. All of this is a nerve reflex action. The sympathetic nervous system is at work. Learn these plain and simple facts and you are on your way to health and longer life!

Tantalizing Facts That
Help You Restore Health

The secret of water therapy lies in the fact that its temperature affects the nervous system. In stimulating the peripheral nerves and acting reflexively on the brain and sympathetic system it acts as a tonic, increases vitality, increases all forms of elimination and can actually be used to relieve a fever by healthful means!

Alternate hot and cold water treatments are excellent spinal stimulants if you keep in mind that *short applications of cold stimulate! Long applications of cold depress!* A short application of cold on the back of the neck stimulates sex life. Prolong that therapy and sex life is inhibited, or slowed down. In just this simple manner, you do not only control the standard equipment with which you were born, but you control health! You *do* control longer life. You *are* in the driver's seat for better health!

Let's take a look now at some of the nervous system problems that may be treated at home with hot and cold water therapy. Use these modalities efficiently and your life will change as did mine through their use. Covered, in brief, will be *depression, neuralgia, neurasthenia, neuritis* and *nerve injury* to the spine.

**Using the Uplifting Power of Water
to Cure
DEPRESSION**

Sooner or later every family has someone who becomes depressed and melancholic. With the advent of tranquilizers a lot of this has been suppressed. But suppression by drugs, as you are already well aware, is no solution to anything. Drugs mask the already existing problem and lead to further complications. As a result, more and more doctors as well as folks at home are turning back to natural remedies and the kind of water therapy my grandfather used back in Europe. They are returning to "the good old days" when hydrotherapy was the treatment of choice.

What is the treatment for *depression*? I'm going to give you the European approach because it uses water for its relaxing effects, for its tonic stimulation, for its ability to normalize metabolism and stimulate circulation and improve elimination, for its effect on the organs of the abdomen, pelvis and brain. Because of these effects, water therapy is excellent for coping with anxiety and depression when the mechanisms of the brain and body bog down due to mental congestion. Water creates a little miracle in coping with mental depression. I saw it happen at our house when I was a little kid. I'd like to tell you about how my grandfather, in all his old-fashioned European ways, brought my grandmother through a very trying time.

Aquatonic Therapy Regulated
Grandma's "Change of Life"
and Made Her Feel Well Again

Grandmother was going through a strange period. She was hot
one minute, cold the next, red of face and irritable. Most of all she
saw things that weren't there. I heard the grownups whisper that she
was going through the "change of life" and at that time all this was
very mysterious. I didn't know what "change of life" was but I did
see what Granddad did to help her. Each day he washed her down
with cold water and made her walk in the open air. After each cold
tub bath and walk session she had to go to bed for a nap. Before
bedtime he sat patiently beside the big wooden tub where he made
her lie immersed chin deep in hot water. Cold tub in the morning,
hot tub at night, and patience paid off. One day she called me by
name again. There was a beautiful smile on that wrinkled old face.
She was no longer irritable, no longer irrational. The water treatments continued. Her depression departed. Her apathy disappeared.
She was no longer melancholic. The hallucinations were no more.
Granddad's water cures had worked once more!

How to Take the Hurt Out of
NEURALGIA

Neuralgia simply means pain in a nerve. Kenny K. told me that
when his hurts first started his skin over the painful area got red.
Sometimes the part would become numb but the pain remained
pretty much local. Sometimes, however, these pains radiated.
Neuralgic pains, as in Kenny's case, are found most frequently in
nerves of the face, teeth, neck, shoulder, ribs, abdomen, low back
and thighs. Whether to treat with hot or cold water is determined by
the body part involved and the duration of the involvement. To
simplify what to do for yourself on this score, here's a method in
brief

Facial Neuralgia

Steps to take

Your schedule for the day is as follows:

Morning

Hot air bath (Turkish bath) on the face is accomplished at home with an infrared lamp. The lamp should be at least eighteen inches away from the face for ten to fifteen minutes of treatment time. This may also be accomplished under direct sunlight or by sitting in front of the fireplace. Follow this with an invigorating shower on the entire body including the face.

NOTE: *Do not rub the skin after radiant heat has been used!*

> **Special note: Do not use radiant heat on the entire body. This is especially true for folks with heart, kidney, lung or high blood pressure problems. Why? Radical and some- times dangerous reactions take place. This fact has been borne out by the number of deaths in Turkish baths each year.**

Afternoon

Hot wet compresses on the face for a period of ten minutes. Once again follow with a quick cold shower. *This time use a mild friction rub over the painful area.*

Evening

Hot wet compresses for one hour. Follow with a cold shower *with* friction over the area of discomfort. Rub briskly with a coarse towel or mitten.

There Are Other
Kinds of Neuralgia

In addition to facial neuralgia there is *brachial* neuralgia (shoulder and arm), *intercostal* neuralgia (between the ribs), *lumbo* (low back), *abdominal* and *sciatic* nerve neuralgia. To treat each of them effectively, use the alternating hot/cold scotch douche. Even sciatica will respond.

How to Cope with Sciatica
with the Scotch Douche

Steps to take

1. *Hot water spray,* or scotch douche, on that painful low back, buttock, thigh or leg, is one of the more effective procedures you can use. Water should be as hot as you can tolerate without burning yourself. Don't pause in the application. Keep the spray moving to prevent excessive heat from collecting at any one point. Treat yourself from the hips down for two to five minutes *only*! Follow immediately with a quick cold shower on the entire body of no more than five to ten seconds duration. No more! Repeat the process at least three times per session: hot/cold, hot/cold, hot/cold. Then go to bed. Excellent results may also be accomplished by sitting under a blanket tent or umbrella with a teapot or kettle directing steam at the area of sciatic hurt. Follow the steam process (five minutes) immediately with a cold shower or a cold sponging of the sore area with ice water or have a friend spray ice water or rubbing alchohol on the part.

Other Excellent Methods
for Treating Sciatica

Steps to take

2. *Hot half baths* take approximately thirty minutes of treatment

time. Water temperature is 110-115° F. Depth of water in the tub is belly button high. Complete the hot half bath with a cold shower and a brisk rubdown with a coarse towel. The point here is that *when improvement begins to show, and nerve pain subsides, do not stop the treatment*! Continue therapy for at least a week. The half bath may be used alternately with the scotch douche.

3. *Hot retention enemas* often quell sciatic pain immediately. To accomplish the best results fill an enema bag with water (no hotter than 120°F.). Apply the solution slowly (via the anus) as you lie on your back or side on the bathroom floor. If abdominal spasms occur squeeze the cut-off valve. Rest. Relax. Use a flexible rectal syringe. Don't put the enema bag up too high (just about a foot above body level on the floor). This slows the gravitational force. (To the water add a tablespoonful of table salt.)

> Note: In the application of the retention enema LIE ON THE SIDE WHERE THE PAIN IS. Hold the solution as long as you can. This treatment not only lessens the pain but improves digestion and eliminates waste.

Conquering
NEURASTHENIA
with Nature's Water Remedies

There are many causes, some of them very complex, for *neurasthenia* and your doctor is the best one to determine this matter. Let me give you a few of the reasons why some people get it. Overwork, stress and worry are among the major causes. The person with neurasthenia is the one who is overtaxed mentally and physically. One film star I know had neurasthenia that began just that way. Diseased organs of the body, on the other hand, may cause it. This is especially true of organs within the pelvis. The most effective home procedure I know of for this problem is *rest and aquatonic therapy*. To help yourself in this matter here is my special clinic routine schedule to follow.

**Cerney Technique for
Treating Neurasthenia**

Steps to take

> **Early
> Morning**

1. *Tepid full bath* (90-95°F.) has a treatment time of one quarter hour. Submerge yourself to the chin. Relax! Follow with a quick cold shower and brisk rubdown. The key factor to remember here is that *each morning you lower the temperature of the water*. By the end of a week it should be down to 65° F. When water is at this temperature there is no longer any need for a cold follow-up shower. Just rub down with a coarse towel. Then walk around in the nude for a few moments before dressing. Your breakfast should consist of cereals and fruits, toasted bread, all of which should be well chewed before swallowing. Drink milk. Exercise each morning. Do some manual work as well as walk in the open air. Walk in your bare feet in the dewy grass each morning. Five minutes are sufficient. Rub feet briskly and don your stockings and shoes.

> **Midmorning**

2. *Half hip sitz bath* (90°F.) is used for five minutes while you or someone else apply cold affusions (cold water sponged or rubbed up and down the spine). The midmorning half bath may be alternated with cold water treading. Both should be followed with a quick cold shower, a brisk rubdown, and a half-hour rest.

> **Note: Your main meal of the day should be eaten at noon. Use no spices. Do not eat soup, fish and/or meat. Concentrate on fruit and vegetables. Follow the noon meal with an hour's rest.**

Midafternoon

3. *Cold water treading* for five minutes. Follow with active exercise for thirty minutes. Have a snack of fruit and milk immediately afterward.

> Note: Your evening meal should be your lightest meal. It should consist of whole wheat toast, eggs, milk, and a small portion of cold meat.

Night

4. *Wet cold compresses* are placed on the abdomen while lying in bed. Go to bed early (8:30-9:00 PM). Stay under covers in a well-ventilated room. As this day-by-day schedule proceeds, you will note the discomfort in your chest and solar plexus departing. Your hastened heart will begin to slow down. You will be suddenly conscious of the fact that you are more at ease with the world and the people in it. You will be feeling better in mind as well as in body. You will sleep better. I know! I've watched this procedure work wonders with patient after patient for over a quarter-century and it will probably do the same for you. Just stick to the rules.

The Magic of Water for Treating
NEURITIS

Treatment for *neuritis* (inflammation of a nerve) affects different people differently. In other words, what's good for the goose is not good for the gander! Some folks respond best to cold therapy, some to heat. John M. found that hot compresses were the best approach to his neuritis. John is a sheet metal worker. He works a lot of overtime and does a lot of lifting and carrying. Before he started to use the magic of water therapy John said he had tingling in his extremities (pins and needles), sometimes the pain was stabbing and boring. He reported that his pain was usually worse at night, that changes of weather aggravated it, that sometimes his muscles would twitch. Sometimes they'd be sensitive to touch. He said he had areas of redness and sweating over the areas of hurt and once he had herpes (shingles or blisters) around his rib cage. He said that he lost weight and sometimes felt very weak. It all started in his fingers and toes and that's when we started the magic of water therapy. After the third treatment John showed results. To determine whether the hot or cold approach is better for you do a little experimenting. Getting results depends on what you find.

Steps to take

1. *Hot sectional ablutions* (doing one body part at a time while the balance of the body and extremities remain covered). Have a friend sponge one part at a time. Sponge and then cover each part treated. When the body and extremities are completed, follow with a quick cold shower and a brisk rubdown with coarse toweling. In conjunction with this external bath take an internal enema. Keep in mind that results in neuritis are remarkably slow. However, some folks respond almost simultaneously and immediately to this treatment and I hope you are one who does.

2. *Cold compresses* must be applied directly to the area of the inflamed nerve. If you find that cold irritates the existing problem use the Hot Sectional Ablution procedure.

In Johnny M's case the tingling and prickling disappeared under this procedure. He followed through on all instructions about easy exercises and kept in mind that joints should be put through a full range of motions, that muscles have to be stretched, that along with additional protein in the diet (amino acid capsules or pills that you can get at your health food store) there should be diet supplementation of vitamin B (thiamin), vitamin C and brewer's yeast three times daily, that to prevent permanent muscle damage as the result of nerve inflammation this routine should be followed day after day.

Today Johnny no longer suffers neuritis pain. The secret to water therapy for neuritis lies in remembering that exudates (tissue liquids) collecting around an inflamed nerve may be increased by the application of cold. Pain in some people will increase. For some people, on the other hand, heat absorbs these exudates and reduces the hydrostatic pressure causing pain. Where *multiple neuritis* (pain in many places) is present, use prolonged hot baths (with epsom salts). Maintain water temperature at 120°F. for one to two hours. Follow this bath with a quick cold shower and brisk rubdown with coarse toweling. Rest as much as is possible.

NERVOUS SYSTEM TRAUMA

Doctors Said Child Was Destined to a Wheelchair . . . Instead, He Walked Again

After little Michael K. fell out of the apple tree in his backyard and landed on his back, his parents were warned by the attending physicians that the balance of the child's life was more than likely to be spent in a wheelchair. Their anguish was great, as you can imagine. The doctors said there was no possibility of return to normal, that the spinal and sympathetic nerves had been irreparably damaged, that Michael's neck had been injured permanently. Function in both extremities was gone. Pain, however, wasn't. In fact, the pain increased despite all the new forms of medication. The little muscles shrank. The child's eyes retreated in his head because of the lack of sleep and malnutrition. He wouldn't eat. His parents became desperate as they watched him fade. They tried the rounds of more hospitals, more tests, more doctors. When I saw that little boy I told the parents that only God could create the miracle they wanted, that perhaps part of that miracle might come through aquatonic therapy and that with the grace of God he might walk again.

What started as a pitiful little heap of motionless skin and bones was destined for better days. After x-rays and other tests, I ruled out the possibility of complications, manipulated a few bones in the child's neck and started my aquatonic procedures to get the little guy back on his feet. First, I placed him in a tub full of tepid water (90-95°F.) and slowly dropped the water temperature down to 60°F., let most of the water out of the tub and slowly brought the temperature back up to 105° F. The child just lay there motionless, his eyes closed, his pale face startlingly white against the background of the blue enameled bathtub.

I reached down and lifted him out of the tub, turned him over one arm and sprayed his spine with the stinging sharpness of ice water. His body didn't even jump on impact of the cold. His skin, however, did react and that was my first encouraging sign. The child's nervous system *was not dead*! A pleasant redness began to show. I rubbed him briskly, wrapped him warmly, and put him to bed as his parents watched. So did a hawknosed aunt. She was one of the harbingers-of-doom type and looked on with great disapproval. After all, the great specialists had said he would not walk again and she knew absolutely that little Michael K. would not walk again. She had predicted it from the start.

Somehow doom never took place. Just the opposite happened. There *was* a miracle in that water! The next morning, when I made my early morning house call, I touched Michael's forehead. His temperature was normal. His eyes opened and focused. He grinned. I made some reflex tests, asked him to wiggle his fingers and toes. They wiggled. He looked up at his mother. His hands and arms slowly lifted. With tears rolling down her cheeks she gathered her little boy up in her arms. Because of another miracle in aquatonics a whole new world opened for those folks and I was there when it happened.

I explained to the family about the necessity of following the same aquatonic technique to awaken and re-awaken, to set up action to get reaction. I told them that they shouldn't expect total change overnight, but that Michael *would* walk again with God at his elbow, that water therapy and a little bone manipulation quite often, when everything else has been used and failed, contain a miracle system all their own.

The Ice-Water Spray and How to Apply It

Ice water, or even fast-evaporating rubbing alcohol, may be applied with an atomizer. Spray up and down both sides of the spinal column (not over). Keep the major force of the spray about one inch on each side of the column. Then make a parallel excursion about three inches out from the spinal column.

At-a-Glance
Information

Additional Ailments You Can Treat
with
ICE WATER SPRAY

Facial neuralgia
Headaches
"Shingles" (herpes zoster)
Neuritis
Whiplash injury
Colds

Persistent coughing
(inside and outside
the throat)
Migraine headaches
(on the side of the
pain)

Note: Whenever there has been nervous system damage I always advocate going a step further in water therapy. It's a vital step in the re-awakening and re-establishing of all the body's normal processes that have been temporarily stopped. This supplementary process is called the "Friction Rub" or the Swedish Salt Glow. These procedures not only quiet the patient but cleanse the body as well. They awaken those processes so vital to health. They develop go-power, and this is something that all of us need. Right?

INDEX

A

Abdomen:
  nerve to, 28
  pain in, 184
  pulse test, 18, 29-30
  somatherapy for, 155, 160-162
  tension release points, 52, 53
Abscess, 90, 108, 121
Acidity, antidote, 102
Acidosis, 29
Acne, 29
Acupuncture points, 30
Adenoids, 29
Adrenal glands, nerve to, 28, 32
Adrue, for dyspepsia, 61
Aging, 96
  to prevent, 194
"Alarm points":
  diagram of, 33
  guidelines for testing, 34
  how to use them, 34
  tests, 18, 34
  use in treatment, 35
  what they do, 31
  where they are, 31
Alfalfa juice, 116
Allergies:
  hayfever, 29
  hives, 29
Alligator pear, 75
Anemia, 81
  cell salt therapy for, 89, 96, 98
Angina pectoris, 26, 103
Ankle:
  nerve to, 28
  tension release points, 44
  treatment for, 43

Anus:
  burning, 88
  fistula in, 107
  nerve to, 28
Anxiety, aquatonic therapy for, 197
Appendix, inflammation of, 28-29
Aquatonics, 193-207
Arm:
  numbness in, 184
  pain in, 29
  tension release points, 48, 51
Arteries, hardening of, 29
Arthritis, cell salt therapy for, 102
Asparagus, 117
Asthma:
  alarm point test, 35
  cell salt therapy for, 87, 92, 100, 102
  endive juice for, 120
  somatherapy for, 168
  spinal concussion for, 184
Autonomic system, 21

B

Back:
  ache, 192
  cell salt therapy for, 90
  muscle stretch, 150-153
  tension release points, 47
  treatment, low back, 43
Bad breath, 70, 100
Bed-wetting, 96, 98, 101, 168, 184
Beet juice, 117
Belly:
  "button," 27
  pain in, 27-30
Bier's cupping glass, 174
Bile problem, 75

Biliousness, 91, 92
Biochemical, 78
Black cohosh:
   how to take, 66
   rheumatism care, 65
Black eye, 107
Bladder, alarm points for, 33
   herb therapy, 69
   nerve to, 28, 32
   pain in, 184
   problems of, 38, 89
   stones, 68, 71
Blindness, 29
Blood:
   health conveyor, 78
   pressure (high), 129, 184
   supply to head, 28
   vessel maintenance, 120
Blood root, for female complaints, 66
Boericke and Tafel Co., 85
Boils, 29, 71, 90, 105, 108, 121
Bone growth:
   dandelion juice for, 120
   turnip juice for, 122
Bowel cleanser, spinach juice, 121
Breasts:
   nerve to, 28
   pump, 174-175
Breath (short), 100
Bronchial tubes, nerve to, 28
Bronchitis, 29, 90, 92
   balsam of Peru therapy, 64
   cell salt therapy, 87, 98
   somatherapy for, 168
Bruises, herb therapy, 69
Buckbean, treatment for shingles, 67
Burn:
   feet, 100
   therapy for, 70, 73, 74
Bursitis, 29
Bush honeysuckle, 68
Buttocks, nerve to, 28

C

Cabbage juice, 118
Cankers, mouth, 23, 100
Capsicum, to check vomiting, 69
Carbuncles, 71, 90, 99, 101, 108
Carrot juice, 119

Cataracts, 107
Catarrh, 29, 87, 90, 92, 103, 108, 168-169
Cathartic, 62
Celery juice, 119
Cell salts, 77-109
   composition of, 79
   key to self-therapy, 84
   names of:
      potassium chloride, 83, 85
      sodium chloride, 83, 87
      calcium sulfate, 83, 89
      sodium sulfate, 83, 91-92
      iron phosphate, 83, 97-98
      potassium phosphate, 83, 99-101
      sodium phosphate, 83, 101-102
      magnesium phosphate, 83, 103-104
      calcium fluoride, 83, 105-107
      silicon, 83, 107-108
"Change of life," aquatonic therapy for,
   198
"Charley horse," 103
Cheek, nerve to, 28, 98
Chest:
   alarm point, 35
   clay pack therapy, 192
   nerve to, 28
   pain in, 71, 92, 96
   pressure in, 100
   tension release, 52, 54
Childbirth discomfort, blue cohosh therapy
   for, 66
Chills, 68, 91
Chilly feeling, 107
Chlorophyl, 116
Cholecystitis, cell salt therapy for, 92
Circulation, alarm point, 33
Clay packs, 189-192
Cleansing the body, 194
Colds, 29
   cell salt therapy for, 91, 98, 104, 105
   herb therapy for, 71, 73, 75
   ice water spray for, 207
   somatherapy for, 169
Coldness, 29
   extremities, 196
Cold sore, 73
Colic, 69, 70, 75, 103
Colitis, 29
Compresses (wet), 199
Concussion, 179-182

Constipation, 29, 97, 104, 105, 169
Coryza, 87
Cough:
  asthma, 29
  cell salt therapy for, 92, 94, 96, 98, 104
  herb treatment for, 61, 74
  ice water spray for, 207
Cramps, 29, 68, 85, 99, 101, 104, 169, 192
Croup therapy, 29, 71, 87
Cucumber juice, diuretic, 119
Cupping, 173-178
Cyriax, 185

D

Dandelion juice, 120
Dandruff, 93
Deafness, 29
Decoction, how to make, 62
Depression:
  aquatonic therapy for, 197
  cell salt therapy for, 95, 99
Diabetes, 29
  cell salt therapy for, 92
Diarrhea, 29, 91
  cell salt therapy for, 99, 100
  diet with, 63
  herb therapy, 63, 70, 75
  somatherapy for, 171
Diphtheria, 87
Disease, why it develops, 82
Dizziness, 88, 93, 95, 99, 107
Dropsy:
  cell salt therapy for, 92
  herb therapy for, 70
Duodenum, nerve to, 28
Dysentery, 64, 70, 75, 87
Dyspepsia, 29, 69, 70, 75, 95, 103, 104

E

Earache, 29, 104, 170
Ears, 28, 100, 105
Eczema, 29
  balsam of Peru therapy, 64
  cell salt therapy for, 87, 94
  clay-pack therapy, 192
Edema (swelling), vibration to relieve, 187
Elbow, 28

Elder, for:
  bruise therapy, 69
  erysipelas therapy, 69
  gout therapy, 69
  pleurisy therapy, 69
  rheumatism, 69
Endive juice, 120
Enema, retention of, 201
Energy, how to generate it, 39, 40
Emphysema, alarm point test for, 35
Epilepsy, 85
Erysipelas (also see "St. Anthony's Fire"):
  cell salt therapy, 94
  herb therapy, 69, 74
Esophagus, 28
Eucalyptus, 70
Eustachian tube, 28
Eyelids, inflamed, 88
Eyes, 28, 32
  finger tapping therapy, 167
  parsley juice for, 121
  red, 95
  somatherapy for, 161

F

Face:
  achy, 97
  ice water spray for, 207
  nerve to, 28
  neuralgia, 199
Fallopian tubes (nerve to), 28
Fasting, how to, 129
Fatigue:
  how to treat it, 39, 40, 42, 99
  somatherapy for, 161, 165
Feet:
  illustration of, 42
  nerve to, 28
  odorous, 108
  tender, 104
  tingling, 104
  treatment of, to relieve fatigue, 40
Felons, 74, 90
Female complaints, blue cohosh therapy for,
    66
Fever:
  cell salt therapy for, 92, 97, 108
  herb therapy for, 68, 75, 90, 91
Fomentations (how to make), 70

Foot bath, 71
Forearm:
    nerve to, 28
    pain in, 29
Forehead, 28
Fracture, repair of, 94
Frostbite, 74

G

Gallbladder, 29
    alarm point for, 33
    beet juice therapy for, 47
    carrot juice therapy for, 119
    treatment point on feet, 42
Gallstones, beet juice therapy for, 117-118
Gas (in bowel), 29, 69
    cell salt therapy for, 100, 104
    juice diet for, 116, 121
    peppermint for, 71
    vibration therapy for, 187
Gastritis, 29, 170
Gentian, 70
Gilbert, H., 81
Glands, stimulation for, 194
Goiter, 29
Gout:
    cell salt therapy for, 92, 103-104
    herb therapy for, 69, 73
    potato juice for, 121
Ground holly, 73
Growth, celery juice for, 119
Gums, bleeding, 100

H

Hair growth, 116, 119
    green pepper juice for, 121
    lettuce juice for, 120
Half baths, 200
Halitosis, 100
Hand, tension release points, 48, 51
Hayfever, 100
    endive juice for, 120
Headache, 29
    cell salt therapy for, 89, 93, 95, 97, 102,
        107
    clay pack therapy for, 192
    herb therapy, 62, 65, 68, 69, 70, 75, 92
    ice-water spray therapy, 207

Headache, (cont.)
    somatherapy for, 170-171
    spinal concussion for, 184
Health, what to do, 81
Heart:
    alarm points for, 33
    angina pectoris, 26
    endive juice for, 120
    nerves to, 28, 32
    problems of, 29
    spinach juice for, 121
Heartburn, 72, 88, 96
Hemorrhages, 75
Hemorrhoids, 29
    celery juice therapy, 119
    cell salt therapy, 105, 107
    herb therapy for, 75
    somatherapy for, 171
    spinal concussion, 184
    turnip juice for, 122
Herbs, 61-75
    kinds:
        adrue, 61
        agrimony, 61
        alligator pear, 76
        American senna, 62
        angelica, 62
        aspen, 63
        balsam of Peru, 64
        blackberry, 64
        blessed thistle, 65
        black cohosh, 65
        blue cohosh, 66
        buchu berries, 67
        bush honeysuckle, 68
        California laurel, 68
        capsicum, 69
        dill, 69
        elder, 69
        eucalyptus, 70
        fennel, 70
        gentian, 70
        ginger, 70
        juniper, 70
        leek, 71
        marshmallow, 71
        mustard, 71
        onion, 71
        peppermint, 71
        pleurisy root, 72

Herbs, *(cont.)*
    prince's pine, 73
    pumpkin, 73
    red clover, 73
    red raspberry, 73
    sage, 74
    skunk cabbage, 74
    slippery elm, 74
    spearmint, 75
    thyme, 75
    Virginia snake root, 75
    wild cherry, 75
    witch hazel, 75
  remedies you can use, 61-75
  value of, 60
  where purchasable, 60
Herniation, 29
Herpes zoster (*see* "Shingles")
Hiccough, 29, 104, 105, 184
High blood pressure, 29, 121
Hip:
  nerve to, 28
  tension release for, 43
Hives, 102
Hoarseness, 29, 98, 100, 108
"Housemaids knee," 94
Hunger pangs, 100

I

Ice therapy, on trigger points, 41
Ice-water therapy, 200, 206-207
Impotence, spinach juice for, 121
Indigestion, blackberry therapy, 64
Infection, therapy for, 71, 119
Inflammation:
  cell salt therapy for, 84, 98
  clay pack therapy, 192
  leek therapy, 70
  wild cherry, 75
Influenza, 29
Infusions, 69
  how to make, 63
Insect bites, 70
Insomnia, 29, 171
Intestine, large:
  alarm point to treat, 33
  nerve to, 28, 32
Intestine, small:
  alarm point to treat, 33

Intestine, small, *(cont.)*
  nerve to, 28, 32
Iron, what it does, 80, 81
Itching, 29, 71, 102
Ivy poisoning, treatment for, 68

J

Jaundice, 29, 129
Joint, stiffness:
  black cohosh therapy, 65
  "creaking," 89
  enlarged, 105
  vibration therapy, 187
Juices:
  body cleansing, 112
  contents of, 112
  dosage, 113
  handmade, 114
  types:
    alfalfa, 116
    asparagus, 117
    beets, 117
    cabbage, 118
    carrot, 119
    celery, 119
    cucumber, 119
    dandelion, 120
    endive, 120
    green peppers, 121
    lettuce, 120
    parsley, 120
    potato, 121
    spinach, 121
    tomato, 122
    turnip, 122
Juniper berries, dropsy treatment, 70

K

Kidneys:
  alarm point, 33
  buchu berry therapy, 67
  cell salt therapy, 91, 96
  nerve to, 28
  parsley juice for, 120
  stones, treatment for, 68, 117
  tension releases on feet, 42
Knee:
  nerve to, 28

Knee, (cont.)
  swelling, 94
  tension release points, 46
  treatment of, 43

L

Laryngitis, 29, 171
Leg:
  cramps, 68
  "give way," 102
  nerve to, 28
  tension release points, 45
  treatment for, 43
  twitching, 92
Lettuce juice therapy, 120
Lips, nerve to, 28
Liver:
  alarm points, 33
  beet juice therapy, 117
  carrot juice therapy, 119
  nerve to, 28
  treatment point on feet, 42
Lumbago, 29, 98, 171
Lungs:
  alarm points, 33
  in calcium deficiency, 96
Luyties Co., 85

M

Manipulation, soft tissue, 166
Mann, Felix, 34
Marshmallow, 71
McFadden, B., 191
Menstruation:
  cell salt therapy, 101, 106
  beet juice therapy, 117
  pain in, 89, 104
  parsley juice for, 121
  prolonged, 91, 104
Milk:
  cause of illness, 113
  not the "perfect" food, 79
Miscarriage, prevention for, 121

N

Nails, green pepper juice for, 71, 75
Nakatani, Yoshio, 26

Nausea:
  cell salt therapy for, 102
  peppermint therapy for, 71, 75
Neck:
  cell salt therapy for, 92
  glands, 28
  nerves, 28
  somatherapy for, 155, 157-158
  tension release points, 48, 49
Nerves:
  cervical, 32
  lumbar, 32
  optic, 28
  parasympathetic, 26
  sacral, 32
  sympathetic, 26, 32
Nervous system:
  aid to metabolism, 122
  aquatonic therapy for, 194-195, 205-207
  stability of, 25
  vibration stimulation of, 187
Nervousness, 29
  cell salt therapy for, 99
  rheumatism, cause, 65
Neuralgia, 29, 69, 70, 76, 91, 104, 121, 197, 198, 199, 207
Neurasthenia, 29
  aquatonic therapy for, 197, 203-205
  asparagus juice for, 117
  ice-water spray for, 207
  spinach juice for, 121
Noise, sensitivity to, 107
Nose bleed, 97, 184
  nerve to, 28

O

Onion, 71

P

Pain:
  abdomen, 98, 103, 104, 184
  arms, 29, 184
  back, 104
  cell salt therapy, 84, 93
  chest, 29
  cupping, for, 173
  extremities, 100, 108
  eyes, 103

Pain, (*cont.*)
feet, 184
forearm, 29, 184
friction rub for, 199
hands, 29
knees and legs, 29, 94, 102, 106
muscles, 70
sciatic, 29
teeth, 70, 93
vibration to relieve, 187
when sitting, 29, 96
Pancreas, 28
Parotid gland, 32
Parsley juice, 120
Pepper (green) juice, 121
Percussion, 183, 185-186
Pharynx, 28
Physical therapy, 166
Phytotherapy, 59
Piles (*see* Hemorrhoids)
Pituitary treatment point on feet, 42
Pleurisy, 29
cell salt therapy for, 87
fasting for, 129
herb therapy for, 69, 72
Pneumonia, 29
alarm point test, 35
cell salt therapy for, 98
Potato juice therapy, 121
Poultice, 71
Prince's pine, 73
Prostate:
nerve to, 28
treatment for, 117
Proud flesh, 73
Puberty, 95
Pulse test, abdomen, 18
Pyorrhea, cabbage juice therapy for, 118

R

Radcliff, 177
Rash, 102
Raspberry, 73
Rectum:
nerve to, 28
pain in, 184
Reducing, cabbage juice therapy, 118
Reflex, 26-27

Rheumatism:
asparagus juice for, 117
celery juice for, 119
cell salts for, 87, 96, 102-103
clay pack therapy for, 192
cucumber juice for, 119
herb therapy for, 65, 66, 69, 70, 71
signs and symptoms of, 65

S

Sacroiliac, 29
Sage, 74
Salt, craving for, 96
Scalds, 73-74
Scalp:
swollen, 105
tender, 95-104
Schussler, William, 79
Sciatica:
cell salt therapy for, 108
herb therapy for, 71, 100
how to relieve pain, 43
nerve, 28
pain in, 29
potato juice for, 121
somatherapy for, 172
vibration therapy for, 187
water therapy for, 200
Scotch douche, 200
Scurvy, 99
Sex:
drive lost, 102, 197
glands, 33, 42
Shingles, 29, 67, 207
Shoulder:
nerve to, 28
somatherapy for, 155, 159
spinal concussion for, 184
tension release points, 48, 49, 50
Sinus trouble, 28, 29, 116
Sitz bath, 202
Skin disease:
cabbage juice therapy, 118
cell salt therapy for, 93, 95
cucumber juice therapy, 119
herb therapy for, 70
itching, 95
reactions, 19, 25
rolling, 173-178

Skin disease, *(cont.)*
    sallow, 88, 92
Skunk cabbage, 74
Slippery elm, 74
Snake bite, 75
Solar plexus, 27, 162-163
    nerve to, 28
    tension release for, 54
Somatherapy, 141
Soreness, cell salt therapy for, 84
Sore throat, 29
Spasms (muscles), 85, 101
Spearmint, 75
Spinach juice, 121
Spinal column:
    curvature of, 29
    diagram of, 28, 29, 140
    technique for therapy, 20, 145, 155-156,
        196-197
    what it does, 26
    what it feeds, 28
Spleen:
    nerve to, 28
    tension release point, 42
Sprains/strains:
    aquatonic therapy for, 194
    cell salt therapy for, 97, 106
    somatherapy for, 172
Squaw root, 66
St. Anthony's fire, 80
St. Vitus' dance, 104
Sterility, 29, 121
Stings, clay pack therapy for, 192
Stomach:
    alarm points for, 33
    how to soothe, 75
    inactivity, 70
    nerve to, 28, 32
    problems of, 29
    sour, 102
    spinach juice for, 121
    treatment point on feet, 42
    ulcer, 99
Sweat:
    blue thistle tea for, 65
    how to induce, 71, 75
    neck and head, 95
    night, 96, 108
Swelling, 29, 71, 108
Sympathetic nerves, 26, 32, 196

T

Tape worm herb therapy, 73
Teeth, 28, 70, 95, 106
    dandelion juice for, 120
    grinding of, 102
Tension:
    how to test for, 52, 194
    treatment of, 39, 42, 177
Tests:
    abdominal pulse, 18
    alarm point, 18
    tension, 19
    umbilicus, 17
    vasomotor, 19
Thigh:
    tension release points, 46
    treatment of, 43
Thirst, 94, 97
Throat:
    constriction of, 104
    sore, 29, 96, 108
"Thrush" therapy, 71
Thyme, 75
Thyroid:
    nerve to, 28
    tension release point, 42
Tincture, how to make, 63, 73
Tiredness, 29, 37, 38, 74
Tomato juice, 122
Tongue:
    coated, 94
    nerve to, 28
Tonsillitis, 29, 74, 98, 129
Tonsils, nerve to, 32
Toxemia, 128
Trachea, nerve to, 28
Trigger points, 18, 19
    purpose of, 36
    where found, 37
Tuberculosis, alarm point test, 35
Tumors (external):
    leek therapy, 71
    witch hazel, 75
Turkish bath, 199
Turnip juice, 122
Twitching:
    eyelids, 95
    face, 104

U

Ulcers, 29
  carrot juice therapy for, 119
  leek therapy for, 70
  leg treatment, 64, 69, 73, 75, 90
  stomach, 69, 101
Ureters, nerve to, 28
Urinary problems, herb therapy, 73

V

Vagina:
  discharge, 94, 107
  "dropped," 89
  therapy, 70
Varicose veins, 29, 97, 105, 106, 119, 122, 189, 191
Vasomotor test, 18, 19, 22, 23, 24
  stimulation, 185
  what it reveals, 116-123
Vegetable juices, what they are good for, 116-123
Vertigo, 95
Vibration technique, 186
Virginia snake root, 75
Vision impaired, cause of, 88
Vitality, 80

Vitamin deficiency:
  buckbean therapy for, 68
  skin rolling for, 174
Vocal cords, nerve to, 28
Vomiting:
  blessed thistle for, 65
  capsicum for, 69
  cell salt therapy for, 91, 92, 97, 105, 107
  peppermint therapy, 71, 75
  Virginia snake root, 75

W

Water therapy (see "Aquatonics")
Weakness, in legs, 100
Weather, influence of, 101
Whiplash injury, ice-water spray for, 207
Wild cherry therapy, 75
Witch hazel therapy, 75
Worms, treatment of, 74
Wounds, treatment of, 74

Z

"Z" zones:
  key rules for using, 36
  tests for, 18, 19
  why they work, 26

WHEN IT HAPPENS

WHEN
IT
HAPPENS

BY

Susane Colasanti

VIKING

VIKING
Published by Penguin Group
Penguin Group (USA) Inc., 345 Hudson Street, New York, New York 10014, U.S.A.
Penguin Group (Canada), 90 Eglinton Avenue East, Suite 700, Toronto, Ontario,
Canada M4P 2Y3 (a division of Pearson Penguin Canada Inc.)
Penguin Books Ltd, 80 Strand, London WC2R 0RL, England
Penguin Ireland, 25 St Stephen's Green, Dublin 2, Ireland
(a division of Penguin Books Ltd)
Penguin Group (Australia), 250 Camberwell Road, Camberwell, Victoria 3124, Australia
(a division of Pearson Australia Group Pty Ltd)
Penguin Books India Pvt Ltd, 11 Community Centre, Panchsheel Park,
New Delhi – 110 017, India
Penguin Group (NZ), Cnr Airborne and Rosedale Roads, Albany, Auckland 1310,
New Zealand (a division of Pearson New Zealand Ltd)
Penguin Books (South Africa) (Pty) Ltd, 24 Sturdee Avenue, Rosebank,
Johannesburg 2196, South Africa

Penguin Books Ltd, Registered Offices: 80 Strand, London WC2R 0RL, England

First published in 2006 by Viking, a member of Penguin Group (USA) Inc.

3 5 7 9 10 8 6 4

Copyright © Susane Colasanti, 2006
All rights reserved

LIBRARY OF CONGRESS CATALOGING-IN-PUBLICATION DATA
Colasanti, Susane.
When it happens / by Susane Colasanti.
p.   cm.
Summary: High school seniors Sara and Tobey attempt to figure out what is important
in life as they try to balance their preparations for their futures with their
enjoyment of the present.
ISBN 0-670-06029-1 (hardcover)
[1. Interpersonal relations—Fiction. 2. High schools—Fiction. 3. Self-actualization—
Fiction. 4. Schools—Fiction.] I. Title.
PZ7.C6699Whe 2006 [Fic]—dc22
2005026405

Printed in U.S.A.
Set in Fairfield and Gill Sans

PUBLISHER'S NOTE

FOR DERRICK,
who proves that soul mates
really do exist.

The creative visualization used to manifest this book was inspired by . . .

The Visionaries

Anne Rivers Gunton, who saw my destination from way down the road; Regina Hayes, who knew the best path to travel; Jill Davis, who noticed there was a journey in the first place

The Yin

Laila Dadvand, for always knowing our fate; Allison Granberry, who will never ever settle; Sara Dhom, summer camp goddess extraordinaire; Nancy Bennett, the most awesome science teacher in this solar system; Michelle Shaw, my soul sister in the search for true love; Eileen Harvey, the sweetest Gram that ever was

The Yang

Jim Downs, for your unwavering support, all those walks, and believing in trust; Tim Stockert, a fabulous source of positive light; Joe Torello, who understands about five-dollar bills at Serendipity; George Pasles, the definition of eccentric creativity; Mike Ippoliti, kindred organization freak spirit; Shawn Lindaberry, for making Tobey the ideal boy that he is

The Saviors

Chad Parker, for saving those original pages when they morphed into rectangles; Andrew Hertzmark, boy-behavior analyst expert; Sharon Gannon and David Life, continuing to redefine New Year's Eve; David Ippolito, who helped me feel whole again, and for those magic changes on The Hill; Shakti Gawain, meditation guru; Universal Energy, for always showing me the way

The Sound

This would have been a different story without these musicians, who always took me where I needed to go: James Taylor, R.E.M., John Mayer, Eminem, Simon & Garfunkel, Sting, Coldplay, John Lennon, Led Zeppelin, Dave Matthews Band, Fleetwood Mac, and, of course, The Cure.

last days of summer
august 28, 7:23 p.m.

"So."

"Yeah?" I say. But I already know what she's going to say. She's asked me the same exact question every day this summer. And the answer is always no.

Maggie's like, "Did he call?"

"You need to get over yourself," I say, "because it's not happening."

The prospect of starting senior year next week without a real boyfriend is the worst. Not some math dork or physics geek I end up liking just because he's there. I mean a boyfriend who's everything I want. The whole package.

"Sara," Maggie says. "Do you realize what this means?"

I decide to ignore her. Maggie has this idealistic image of romance that I don't think exists in real life. I mean, I've been trying to believe it does all summer. But Dave never called.

"This can only mean that he's planning something huge," Maggie says.

"Colossal," Laila says.

"So huge it's gonna blow your mind," Maggie says.

Dave's this new guy who transferred to our school from Colorado at the end of last year. This gorgeous Greek-god type on the basketball team. Ever since he sat next to me at the junior meeting—out of all the prettier, more popular girls he could have sat next to—I've been waiting for him to make a move. We talked a few times after that, but nothing major happened. So when he asked for my number on the last day of school, of course I wrote it in his yearbook, thinking he was going to call me like the next day. But then . . . nothing. Maggie keeps insisting that he likes me, but if he's so interested, why didn't he call?

I hate that a boy is making me feel this way. And I hate that I'm letting it happen.

I go, "Next topic!"

Maggie turns to Laila. "How long do you think it'll take him to ask her out?"

"He'll do it the first day," Laila says. "Second, tops."

"Can we get back to the game?" I say. "Can't Fight This Feeling" plays through the Putt-Putt Mini Golf speaker system.

Laila goes, "Fine. Favorite scary-movie scene."

"Oooh!" Maggie says. "That's a good one!"

"I try," Laila says.

I smack my hot-pink golf ball way too hard.

"I know mine," Maggie says. "It's from that one

Freddy movie where he's under the girl's bed? And he slices through it and . . . like she falls underground or something. I forget how it went. But I woke up with scratches all down my neck."

"Hey!" Laila says. "I remember that! Wasn't that, like, in eighth grade?"

"I think so."

"Wild," I say.

My golf ball bounces off a plastic pink flamingo and, confused, rolls back to me.

Even though we're all best friends, we basically only know each other about eighty-five percent. That's why we made up the Game of Favorites. Once we got past our standard favorites, we moved on to asking the most random questions. Where you find out the meat-and-potatoes stuff you usually never get to know about another person.

I would go next, except the only scary-movie scene I can think of is the one where Dave dies of laughter over my even considering the remote possibility that he might like me. So I tap Laila's golf club with mine and say, "I pass. Your turn."

Laila has to think about this one. Her golf ball glides past the flamingo and stops right next to the hole. She plays mini golf perfectly. Just like she does everything else perfectly. She even had the perfect summer, interning at Overlook Hospital. She's going to be a pediatrician. Every single person in her family is a doctor. Except her brother. But that would be because he's eight.

"Okay," Laila says. "Remember how we rented *An American Werewolf in London* last Halloween?"

"Yeah?"

"And remember when they realize they're walking on the moors when they're not supposed to?"

"Um . . ." I glance at Maggie. She makes a face like, *I have no idea what this girl is talking about.*

"So scary," Laila says.

Maggie looks me over. "So how much weight did you lose?" she asks.

"Like five pounds."

"And what did you eat again?" Laila says.

"Just . . . you know. Less." All I wanted to do was fit into my jeans from tenth grade. And now I'm there.

"Don't do that again."

"Why not?"

"If you had any idea how much starving yourself damages your metabolism—"

"Hey, Laila?"

"Yeah?"

"But I look good, right?"

"Yeah."

"So there you go," I say. "And I didn't starve myself. I ate stuff."

"Like what?" Maggie says. "Two rice cakes and a carrot?"

"For your information I also had some lettuce." The truth is, I imposed a personal embargo against my daily Dunkin' Donuts fix. But Laila and Maggie don't know how bad my addiction to icing was, and I'm embarrassed to admit it. It's shocking what cutting out junk food can do for you.

We walk over to the next course that has this impossible windmill.

"Okay," Maggie says. "Goals for senior year."

"Simple," Laila says. "I'm going to be valedictorian."

"Oh, what, salutatorian isn't good enough?"

"No. It's not."

Laila's always had this problem with being second at anything. Her dad is this total control freak. Laila can't do anything after school and she's only allowed to go out on weekends and she can't even date anyone. I don't know how she survives.

"Actually?" I say. "You're supposed to state your affirmations in the present tense. As in, *I am valedictorian*." I've been reading this book called *Creative Visualization*. It's all about creating the life you want by imagining that it already exists. Since my second goal this year is to achieve inner peace, I'm focusing on what I want my life to be.

Laila's like, "Wait. Is that more of your Zen enlightenment hoo-ha?"

"Yeah," I tell her. "It is. And it works."

"Well, good luck overcoming the legacy of Michelle," Maggie tells Laila.

"Seriously, it's like she has this special-order brain that comes preprogrammed with every piece of useless information you need to ace high school." I rub my golf club on the plastic grass. "But if anyone can beat her, it's you. You go."

"Thank you, I think I will. Next?"

"I'll go," Maggie says. "I want to be smart."

"You're already smart!" I insist.

"No, I'm not. Not like you guys."

I concentrate on examining the waterfall at the end of the course. Because what she's saying is kind of true. Not that we would ever tell her. It doesn't even matter, though. I'd trade my brain for Maggie's body in a second. Not only is she a drop-dead gorgeous blonde, but she's had a string of drop-dead gorgeous boyfriends since seventh grade. Maggie also has more clothes than anyone I know, including the popular crowd. She was even friends with them until junior high. As long as you meet their two requirements of being beautiful and rich, you're considered privileged enough to hang out with the inner circle. But Maggie's also sweet and loyal and will fiercely defend me to anyone who looks at me the way they did. They even told her to stop being friends with me because it was damaging her reputation. Good thing Maggie iced them. And I'm embarrassed to admit it, but their rejection still hurts.

"I'll prove it," Maggie says. "Who'd you get for history?"

"Mr. Sumner," I say.

"See? I got Mr. Martin. They even have smart and stupid history!"

"You're not stupid!" we both yell together.

"Whatever."

"So," I say. "How—not that you aren't already smart because you are—but how are you going to do that?"

"You'll see," Maggie says. "Okay, Sara. What's your goal?"

Here's the thing: I want to reinvent myself this year. I've been a nerd since forever. My life for the past three years has been the same tired routine. Same honors classes with the same set of ten kids, same endless piles of homework, same waking up the next day to do it all over again. I'm tired of waiting for my life to begin. Something has to happen. Like an amazing boy. I know he's out there. I just have to find him. And it would be awesome if that boy was Dave.

"I'm going to find a real boyfriend," I say. "Someone who's the whole package."

They both look at me.

I'm like, "What?"

"Nothing," Laila says.

"What?"

"Nothing. It's just . . ."

"*What?*"

"I'm just wondering where you intend to find this perfect male specimen. Haven't you already gone out with all the halfway acceptable guys we know?"

"She's only had two boyfriends," Maggie says.

"Exactly. She's exhausted the supply."

"Yeah, well . . . that's why I'm thinking about getting to know guys in other classes," I say. "How random was it that Dave sat next to me at the meeting? It just proves that I could sit next to anyone I want. Like in assemblies and pep rallies and stuff."

"You don't go to pep rallies," Laila says.

"But I could! That's the point!"

"Those guys aren't smart enough for you," Laila says.

"Love isn't based on intelligence," Maggie huffs. "It can happen with anyone."

"Like who?" Laila demands.

"Hello!" Maggie yells. "Like Dave!"

I go, "Whose turn is it?" Because I don't want to jinx the Dave thing.

"It's yours," Maggie says.

For this one, you have to time your swing so your ball goes in between the windmill slats. If you don't, it's all over. Suddenly it feels really important for me to get this. Like it's a sign. If my ball gets past the windmill, it means that Dave likes me. If it doesn't . . .

I position my golf ball.

I examine the windmill.

I think to the universe, *Please make it real. Please make it happen.*

I move my golf ball to the right. And I swing.

It's a hole in one.

CHAPTER 2
first days of falling
september 1, 9:14 p.m.

Tomorrow is the first day of the rest of my life.

I finish the first set of curls with my thirty-pound free weights. I examine my biceps for signs of bulk. I decide they're huge. At least, compared to how they used to be. I started lifting on the last day of school in an attempt to improve the situation of my toothpick arms. I need to look good onstage when my band starts playing serious gigs this year. Everyone knows girls want a guy to be cut, with pumped arms and veins popping out, arms that will flex as he lifts himself on top of her. . . .

But I digress.

I do three more sets of fifteen reps and examine my arms again. Definite improvement. I do a hundred sit-ups and fifty pushups and saunter into the bathroom like I'm the biggest stud ever. But this facade shatters when I catch an accidental flash of my reflection in the mirror.

I usually avoid the mirror as much as possible. I some-how developed an insane hope that working out would also improve the condition of my face. I always get zits in the most conspicuous locations, and the fluorescent bulbs in here make me look burnt out like I smoke ten packs a day. Attractive.

Furious, I get into the shower. I should have called her over the summer. Yeah, right. To hear how loudly she would have laughed at the prospect of such a slacker asking her out? No, the way to go with this is to be friends with her first. Be charming and notice details and give her tons of attention. Girls love that. Then she won't be able to resist me when we take it to the next level.

I turn off the water and grab a towel. I'll finally see her tomorrow. Should I try talking to her right away? Or would that look desperate?

I need to mellow out.

Back in my room, I chuck the towel on the floor and pull on boxers. I wonder if she's into boxers or briefs. Or boxer briefs. Cynthia was a fan of the boxer briefs, but the other girls I've hooked up with didn't seem to have an opinion. Then again, Cynthia was the only one I had sex with. So maybe boxer briefs are a safe bet.

I peer into my dresser drawer at my ancient underwear. If I were seeing my underwear for the first time, what would I think? It all looks kind of damaged. Do I need to get new underwear? I hate having to ask my mom to buy it for me. Everyone wears underwear, but it's humiliating to admit this fact to your mother. Even if she does do my laundry.

Suddenly I have a profound idea. I can buy my own underwear! She doesn't have to know anything! Why haven't I thought of this before? I haven't had my car long enough to realize that I can go around and do this kind of stuff.

Are relationships always this complicated?

Technically, Cynthia wasn't my girlfriend. So I don't exactly consider what we had a relationship. It was all about sex. We didn't have much in common except for our mutual lust for each other. Which was fine with me, until I got sick of the emotional void. My friends don't get it. How I'm a complete anomaly when it comes to girls. I mean, I've hooked up with random airhead groupie types. But nothing ever lasted more than a couple months. They were too lacking.

I know what I'm looking for. Something that feels right. Something real.

I dig through the pile of Converse in my closet, old guitar equipment that I got at garage sales, and stacks of magazines until I reach the shoe box. The shoe box has all of my most personal stuff in it. I lean back against the wall and open the box. It's a total rush. I take out my first guitar pick, remembering how it felt to finally know how to use it. There's an E-string that broke during our first rehearsal in ninth grade. I keep all of my lyrics about girls and sex in here, in a smaller notebook separate from my main notebook. Because my mom has no problem with going through my backpack and looking through my stuff. Even though I've told her a million times that an admirable quality of parenthood is the ability to respect your kid's privacy.

I turn to a page with the song I wrote for Her. It's like she's renting all the real estate in the girl department of my brain. I don't even know her that well, even though we've always gone to school together. After they segregated us in seventh grade based on how smart they thought we all were, I didn't see her again until we had art together last year. I didn't have the balls to talk to her until the year was almost over. And then I heard she was going out with Scott, who is a total dweeb, but still. So I never asked her out.

There's something about her that's different from other girls. She's crazy smart. I dig that. And she's kind of shy. Not like the other girls I've dated who came right up to me and asked me to go home with them when I hardly even knew their name. Talking to those girls is cake. But talking to Sara is impossible. Not only is she smart, but she's hot. Girls with the beauty-and-brains thing going on are the most intimidating girls in the world.

What if I get this song ready for Battle of the Bands? I could dedicate it to her. She'll be so turned on. Then I'll smile and dazzle her with my eyes. Girls always tell me I have great eyes. But Battle of the Bands isn't until November. I can't wait that long.

I put the notebook back in the shoe box and stash it way back in my closet. I toss some magazines on top of it and cram random shoes against it.

I get this surge of adrenaline, like I could play for hours. I call this feeling my hot zone. When I'm in the hot zone, I know I can do phenomenal stuff.

I pick up my guitar and turn the amp down. My parents are probably already asleep. I guess that's what life is for most people. Marrying someone who seems decent enough, buying a house, having kids, and turning in at ten every night. They consider bridge games with the neighbors and the all-you-can-eat buffet at Sizzler entertaining ways to spend a Saturday night. Why does life have to be that way? I assume my parents were madly in love at some point, but now they just look tired all the time. I don't want to settle for that.

I jam on my guitar. The way I feel about Sara right now is the way I always want to feel.

I'm making it happen. Tomorrow.

CHAPTER 3
homeroom survivor
september 2, 7:49 a.m.

When Caitlin slams into my backpack running past me and screaming about Aruba, she doesn't even stop to say sorry. This is the way it's been between the princesses and the brains since forever.

I tell myself it'll all be over in nine months. Nine months, thirteen days, and approximately eight hours. Not that I'm counting.

Those of us who got here early are penned up in the cafeteria until homeroom. Trying to sit like I could *so* not be any less concerned that I'm sitting by myself on the first day of senior year is just not working. I lean forward with my elbows on the table. Then I shift back and try to sit straight on the uncomfortable bench. I don't know where to put my hands to make them appear unconcerned. Laila's not here yet, and Maggie went to the bathroom. At least I have my sketchbook with me to partially calm me down.

My sketchbook is actually a combination archive of

my artwork and designs, scrapbook of important events, and collection of journal entries. But its main purpose is for me to practice my architectural sketches, so I can make a portfolio of my work for college applications. I want to be an urban planner, which means double-majoring in architecture and environmental science next year. This will hopefully occur at New York University. Which is not exactly easy to get into. Which is why I've been working like a maniac for the past three years. My motivation for kicking academic butt is to escape this middle-of-nowhere New Jersey small town, this realm of nothingness. Living in New York City will be the ultimate existence.

Anyway, I take my sketchbook everywhere I go. I sketch whatever inspires me. You never know when it will happen.

I decide that it's important enough to document my first-day-back thoughts. I turn to the next blank page. I sneak glances at everyone around me. They're all running around frantically, acting like they care what everyone else did over the summer. I hate myself for caring that no one comes over to my table.

Not like I expect them to suddenly realize I'm alive. I'm used to being invisible. Why does it still bother me? Why does it even matter if Caitlin & Co. treat me like I don't exist? I have real friends—two of them—which is more than most people get to have. I've been telling myself to get over it for years. And I'll never achieve inner peace if I don't. So I need to move on.

But I can't.

Plus, how can I survive another year of the same expectations and stress? And if I see Joe Zedepski drop his calculator one more time I swear I will lose it. Just put your calculator in the middle of your desk instead of right at the edge where you know it'll fall off. How hard is that?

I try to visualize my future life. The place where everything feels right and good things always happen and I can be the person I want to be. I imagine my ideal, completely confident self in a pink bubble, floating into space, letting the universe make it happen.

But my visualization skills are working at less than maximum efficiency today. Because it's time for homeroom. And first impressions are everything.

I'm a nervous wreck.

I peek into the room, pretending to be waiting for someone. At least Dave's not in here. But a lot of his friends are, like Caitlin and Alex. If I manage to come off as cool, or at least as someone with a sense of style, it'll get back to him. Then maybe he'll ask me out. But if I act like a dork in any way, he'll know about it by third period. This is a small school, and word gets around fast. This school is way too small for anyone to even think they can keep anything to themselves.

I walk in with shaky legs. I find a seat. I pretend to look for something in my bag.

"Okay, people!" Ms. Picoult yells. "Your schedules are ready! Come on up!"

Ten seconds later, her desk is completely surrounded by kids complaining that their schedules are messed up and demanding to see a guidance counselor. Ms. Picoult yells that no one is to enter the guidance office until their lunch period. Chaos ensues. Snarly seniors rant that the people who program classes have no skills.

I move to the front of the room. My schedule is the only one left on her desk. I pick it up, expecting the worse. Miraculously, it looks okay.

Name: Sara Tyler	Grade: 12	Year: 2003-2004		
Period	Class	Instructor	Room	
0	Homeroom	Picoult	110	
1	PE	Spencer	Gym	MWF
1	AP Physics Lab	Blythe	300	TR
2	Calculus	Perry	308	
3	Drafting	Slater	Art Studio	
4	AP English	Carver	Auditorium	
5	AP English	Carver	114	
6	Lunch		Cafeteria	
7	U.S.History(Hon)	Sumner	225	
8	AP Physics	Blythe	302	
9	Music Theory	Hornby	Orchestra	

But of course there's a problem. It's the curse of first-period gym. I've had gym first period every year. I've tried to get out of it before, and there's no way. They just tell you that all the other classes are full and this is the way it is and there's nothing you can do about it. So now I get to experience the thrilling sensation of sitting around in my sweaty underwear all day for a whole other year. Fun times.

I sit down to fill out the seventy-three forms we have to do. Caitlin's sitting next to me, filling out her forms and talking to her posse. After a few minutes, she suddenly turns around and stares at my kneesocks. I only tried on a million outfits last night before I decided on these retro kneesocks and my new denim skirt and my favorite sky-blue T-shirt.

I go, "Hey."

Caitlin looks right through me like I'm not even there. Then she turns back to her friends. One of them laughs.

I raise my hand to go to the bathroom.

In the hall, some seniors are huddled together, clearly too cool for the mundane intricacies of homeroom. I'm about to walk right by them. But then I notice Dave is one of them.

I freeze.

Should I go up to him and say hi? Or just walk by and wave? If I don't do something now, I probably won't see him for the rest of the day. And I can't stand not knowing if he likes me. But look at what just happened with Caitlin. She obviously thinks I'm lacking. Now if I go up to Dave, it could be catastrophic.

I'm still debating what to do when Dave and his group walk down the hall, away from me. He never even saw me standing there.

My life is over, and it's not even first period yet.

CHAPTER 4
cafeteria survivor
september 2, 6th period

If the sign in the cafeteria that says WELCOME BACK! were being honest, it wouldn't say that. It would say SUCKS TO BE YOU!

Everyone in the cafeteria is so fake. Especially the girls. They're all kissing and hugging other girls they annihilated behind their backs last year. It's all so ridiculous. As if we couldn't wait to get away from each other last June. But it's not entirely their fault. They've been programmed by society to believe that if you're popular and pretty and perky you'll lead a fulfilling life. Don't they know it's always the geeks that turn out to be the most successful later on?

I'm still hesitating by the door. If Mike and Josh didn't have this lunch period, I'd definitely bail for Subway. Well, maybe it is entertaining to watch them play Cafeteria Survivor as if a million bucks were actually at stake.

Rules of Cafeteria Survivor

1. Always look like you know what you're doing. Everything you do is intentional. Even if your tray tips over and you spill your entire lunch all over yourself, remember: You meant to do that.

2. Always look like you're having the best time. If you're sitting with people you hate because there's no one else to sit with, act like you like them. Anything is better than sitting alone.

3. Always try to sit with other people, even if you're hovering at the end of a table. However, if you are forced to sit by yourself due to severe ostracism, read something and sigh a lot. This will create a mysterious aura about you, one that sends out the message: My life is so extremely hectic that I really need to break away from civilization right now. Please do not disturb. Thanks so much.

4. Always complain about the food. Do this even if you like it. Note: An exception can be made for pizza that actually looks and tastes like pizza. But only if the crust is not soggy.

5. Do not, under any circumstances, get voted off the island.

I think the last rule sums up the basic difference between them and me. I don't care if I get voted off the island.

Emerging from the line, I scan the tables to scope out the best location for people-watching. It's one of my hobbies. Seeing how people interact, imagining how they're feeling, sometimes overhearing bits of conversation . . . it always gives me ideas for lyrics.

I head toward the far windows. I put my tray down on an empty table. When Mike and Josh get here, the main thing we have to discuss is recording our demo. We've been working all summer to save up for studio time. Also, we need to decide what we're playing for Battle of the Bands.

I sit down and contemplate the fries.

"Hey, Tobey!" a girly voice screeches at me.

I look up to see an enormous pair of breasts bouncing my way. They're attached to Cynthia. I haven't talked to her since last April. That's when she gave me this ultimatum that she had to be my girlfriend or else. And I said I wasn't looking for a relationship. But the truth is, I didn't want to get serious with her.

"Hey, Cynthia," I say to be polite. But I want her to go away. I'm in such a different place now. It's crazy that I ever wanted her, even if it was just a physical thing.

She puts her hands on the table and leans over. You can totally see down her low-cut tank top.

I guess it isn't that crazy.

"What's up?" she says.

"Chillin'."

"Yeah, so . . . some of us are getting together at Zack's

tonight. His parents are still in Barbados." Cynthia inches across the table so her face is right in front of mine. "In the mood to party?"

"Not so much," I say. "Sorry."

Her smile instantaneously dissolves. I feel a twinge of guilt for making her feel bad. But I was pretty clear about things before.

"Oh," she says. "Whatever."

There's a second of regret when she walks away and I get a look at her ass in those jeans. I remember what her ass looks like out of those jeans. But then I remember Sara. And how Cynthia can make me feel great, but only for a few hours.

Josh comes racing up to the table. "Tobey! What up? Long time no see!"

He saw me three days ago.

Josh smacks his tray down and grabs my arm. "Whoa, dude! You're, like, huge! You been working out?"

Josh is a bit of a spaz. It's one of his best qualities.

"Ha," I say.

"Dude! You are so not going to believe what happened to me yesterday! I was down the shore at my brother's place and you know how . . ."

And his stories are endless.

I'm still letting him ramble on when Mike arrives.

"Hey, man," Mike says.

"Hey."

Mike is my best friend. He's into everything I am. Music, writing poetry and lyrics, playing backgammon and chess, brainy chicks. We also like the same old-school bands like

The Cure and R.E.M. We mostly have the same musical influences. Josh digs our style, so he kind of goes along with whatever we do.

Suddenly Josh yells, "Senior year, men! We rule the school! Par-tay!" Then he proceeds to bounce up and down on the bench.

All the drastic bouncing makes Mike spill Coke on his shirt. It's like there always has to be some kind of conflict between them. Josh is this total spontaneous, wild drummer type. His personality tends to contradict Mike's, who's constantly planning and analyzing everything. And I'm like the sensitive, introspective one. Together, we make one killer band.

"Dude." Mike puts his hand on Josh's shoulder. "Chill. What's the matter with you?"

"What's the matter with me, baby? What's the matter with you?" Josh jokes in his best Danny Zuko voice. The school play last year was *Grease*, and Josh played John Travolta's character. And he was actually really good. His goal is to be an actor. My goal is to be a musician. A lot of our conversations involve complaining about how the world keeps telling us to give up now while we still have a chance to make something of ourselves.

Mike ignores him. "Have you seen her yet?" he asks me.

"No," I say.

Subtle is not part of Josh's vocabulary. He's all, "Woo-hoo! Tobey's in love. He's in lust! Tobe's got—"

"Hey. Dude? Chill." Something in Mike's voice makes Josh actually shut up and eat his lunch.

Mike knows all about the Sara thing. Josh knows, too,

but it's different with him. Josh lives for relationship drama. He's notorious for public displays of mortification with ex-girlfriends in random hallways. But like me, Mike's also looking for something real. I just don't think he knows it yet. He loves the chase. He's never satisfied with what he gets.

"Let's see your schedule," Mike says to Josh.

We all get our schedules out and determine that the only things the three of us have in common are lunch and gym. The only other thing I have with Mike is history.

"Did you get that new bass?" Josh asks Mike.

They're talking, but I tune them out.

I finally see her.

She just walked in with Laila. She's hugging her notebook and looking different, but the same. Better, if that's even possible. I mean, she was hot before, but now she's . . . I almost have an apoplexy when she turns around and looks toward my table. Every fantasy I've had this summer comes back to me. Every scenario from all those sweaty nights in bed, listening to my iPod.

Mike feels the vibe and follows my stare. "Whoa. What did she do?"

Josh takes one look and says, "That's what's up."

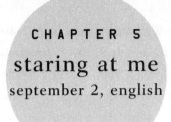

staring at me
september 2, english

When I see Scott in AP English, I completely forget what it was about him that made me be his girlfriend last year. Before I realized I wanted more and dumped him.

He looks at me. I quickly look away. I lucked out. Laila is saving a seat for me in the front. So I can avoid Scott, who's in the back wrestling with his bag, which I'm sure is already overpacked with books. I've had enough guy trauma for one day.

"Good morning, genius prototypes," Mr. Carver booms. "Welcome to the most demanding class of your entire high-school career."

Um, yeah. That seems a bit pretentious. I swear, the guy is on such an ego trip about English. I had him last year for honors. He thinks whatever he teaches is all that and a bag of Munchos. As if they even give us good stuff to read. It's like the reading list was established in 1927 and hasn't been updated. Ever.

Laila slips me a note. We started passing notes

about the Caitlin situation in calculus. Right before she had to restrain me from strangling Joe Zedepski. He already had his calculator out. His huge graphing calculator that we don't need yet because it's only the first day. The one he just had to put right at the edge of his desk, teetering precariously, just waiting to fall off. Anyway, it's most excellent that I have two classes with Laila. Plus we have lunch with Maggie next.

I unfold the note in my lap. It says:

> Sara,
>   Forget her. She's a scumbag.
>   Your number-one fan,
>   Laila

I write back:

> Laila,
>   Forget who?
>   Your fan club president,
>   Sara

Laila's right. Caitlin's not worth it. And if Dave doesn't even like me, then it doesn't matter, anyway.

On our way to lunch, the hall is beyond clogged. While we're inching toward the cafeteria, I practice a visualization exercise. I picture myself with my ideal boyfriend.

Then I put the image in a pink bubble and let it float out into the universe. True love is in my immediate future.

We get pushed through the doorway.

"There," Laila says. She points to a half-empty table.

We put our stuff down and get in line. I grab a tray and utensils and a bunch of napkins. I slide my tray toward a culinary destination of . . . what the frig is that? Fried turtle? I decide to pass and get a sandwich instead. And there's fries, so it's not a total disaster.

"Where's Maggie?" Laila says.

"I don't know."

We sit down. Laila is all hyper about filling me in on the details of her upcoming dissections in AP Bio. That nervous-stomach-first-day-of-school feeling is competing with my hunger.

Maggie throws her bag down on our table.

"Where were you?" I ask. "I was getting scared that you weren't in this lunch anymore."

"I was working on my goal," Maggie says.

Laila goes, "Huh?"

"You know. To be smarter."

"Yeah, I remember," Laila says. "I just don't get how you could instantaneously become smarter between fifth period and now."

"I tried to get into your history class," Maggie tells me.

I'm like, "Are you still on that? Don't worry about—"

"They wouldn't let me in. See? I told you. It's all planned according to brain size."

"Excuse me," Laila retorts. "But if you weren't smart, would we be hanging out with you?"

"Heck no," I add. "Then I'd have more time to spend with my boyfriend."

"And what boyfriend would that be?" Maggie asks me.

"You know. Jake."

"Okay." Laila says. "For the last and final time? Jake Gyllenhaal? Is not your boyfriend. He's a movie star. And sorry to tell you this, but last I heard he was dating someone who's not you."

"Yeah, well . . . my brain's bigger than hers."

"And I'm sure that's what he's interested in," Maggie says. "A girl with really big *brains*."

"Can we please just focus on real people?" Laila begs.

"Hi," Dave says.

Who is suddenly standing right next to me.

I gag on a fry and have this uncontrollable coughing fit that lasts for about a year.

"Oh, hi," I squeak. I gulp my iced tea. I try to wipe grease off my fingers, but I can't get the napkin to work right. I look at Maggie. She's just drinking her juice, unfazed. But if there were a thought bubble over her head, it would be screaming, *I told you so!*

"Is this seat taken?" Dave says. He's referring to the space next to me. Which is empty.

"Uh, no," I stammer.

Laila starts eating her meat loaf, enraptured with the nutritional information on her milk carton. I know that if she looks up at me, she will explode.

Dave puts his tray down. He sits next to me. Really close on the bench. Which is unnecessary, since no one is sitting on the whole rest of the bench.

I try to breathe normally.

Dave goes, "So, how was your summer?"

"Good," I say. "Um. This is Maggie."

"Hi."

"Hi."

"And, um . . . do you know Laila?"

"No, but I've heard of her." He looks over at Laila and smiles.

"Oh?" Laila is skeptical. "What did you hear?"

"Just that you're brilliant." Dave turns to me. "Both of you." He stares right at me. His eyes look like he's trying to show me how much he likes me without saying anything.

"Maggie's also brilliant," Laila says.

Maggie snorts.

Dave is just, like, *staring* at me.

I can't believe that the cutest boy ever is talking to me. To *me*. Maybe he really did want my number when he asked for it.

I feel myself turning red and stand up. "I'm, um— do you want anything? I need juice." I leave without waiting for an answer, because now my face is bright red and it's just too embarrassing.

I get back in line to buy juice that I don't want. I'm dying to know what Dave is saying to them. I can't believe I'm such a freak. I give myself instructions like

Do not turn red and *Just relax*. Remember, he came over to you. Chill. Be in the moment. Be Zen.

While I'm digging change out of my pocket, I drop a dime. I bend down to pick it up and bang my head against someone who went to pick it up at the same time.

I rub my head and stand up. I'm looking at Tobey Beller.

He holds my dime out.

"Oh—sorry! Sorry!" he stammers. "Are you okay?" He looks mortified.

"Sure," I tell him. "Thanks." I take my dime back.

"You have to watch these things every second," Tobey says. "They're always trying to get away."

I laugh. "Totally! These dimes just don't know how to act."

The thing about Tobey is he has these amazing blue eyes. You could stare at his eyes for days and still want more. I used to talk to him in art last year. It was the only class I've ever had with him since junior high. I kind of got the feeling he liked me, but he never did anything about it so I wasn't sure. It was probably just those eyes that got in the way of my typical logical thinking patterns. Anyway, slacker rock-star wannabes aren't my type.

I pay for my juice and get ready to go back to my possible future boyfriend. I'm so nervous that my heart feels like it's going to beat right out of my chest and run down the street the second I see Dave. Obviously, my path to inner peace is a long, complicated one.

I creep back to the table and sit down. Maggie is laughing at something Dave just said.

He turns to me. "Did you hear the one about the three guys driving through the desert?"

"No, I missed that one." I glance at Laila for signs of what Dave said while I was gone. But she just smiles at me. She's obviously loving every minute of this.

Dave goes, "These three guys are driving through the desert, and their car breaks down. So they decide to get out and walk. The first guy says, 'I'm taking these Doritos in case we get hungry.' And the second guy says, 'I'll carry our water bottles.' But the third guy starts taking off one of the car doors. So the first guy goes, 'What are you doing?' And the third guy says, 'I'm taking the door with us.' The second guy's like, 'Why?' And the third guy says, 'In case it gets really hot. So I can roll down the window.'"

The joke is so corny that it's hilarious. I laugh until my face hurts.

Suddenly Maggie's like, "I have to go to the bathroom," and she gets up. "And so do you." She grabs Laila's arm and pulls her away. I know that Laila just went before lunch.

"So, what do you like to do on weekends?" Dave says.

"Um . . . I like to read," I tell him.

"Really?" he says like it's the most interesting thing he's heard in his life. "Me, too! What are you reading right now?"

"Besides the five books for AP that are due tomorrow?" I say. "I'm reading *It*."

"What?"

"*It*."

"What?"

"Oh, no, that's the name of the book. *It*. By Stephen King."

"He rules. Did you read *The Shining*?"

"Oh my god! I love that book. I've read it a million times."

"Really?" Dave smiles at me.

"No. Just three. And the movie rocked."

"Yeah, it was cool. So, you like movies?"

Who doesn't like movies? "Of course."

"Do you want to see one this weekend?" Dave asks.

He did it.

He actually asked me out.

I start to turn red.

I tell myself: *Do not turn red! Stop it!*

But it's too late.

Dave notices. "I'm sorry, I didn't mean to . . . "

"No, it's okay." I try to hide my face behind my juice bottle. "It's just really hot in here." *It's just really hot in here?* Please tell me I didn't just say that.

"So," he says. "What do you think?"

He can't possibly still want to go out with me. "About what?"

"About going out with me Saturday."

It takes every bit of my willpower to remain sitting

on the bench instead of jumping up and dancing on the table. This unbelievably gorgeous guy likes me! Apparently, spending the summer visualizing that a Greek god is into you really does work.

"Sure," I say.

"That sounds convincing!" Dave says. But I can tell he's teasing me.

"No! I really want to."

This makes him smile. "So do I." He's looking at me again with that look.

It is at this precise moment that Laila arrives back at the table.

"Hellooo!" she trumpets. "Lunch is over. That's why everyone's leaving, in case you haven't noticed."

looking at juice
september 2, 12:50 p.m.

"You should go," Mike tells me.

"Where?"

"What do you mean where? Go get in line!"

"But she's—"

Mike shoves me over. "Go!"

I'm stuck to the bench. This is not the way I imagined it would happen.

"What's good, yo?" Josh says. "Move!"

I get up. I walk toward the line. I've just spent the last five minutes watching that jock clone Dave and his over-inflated ego sit next to Sara. Talking to her. Talking to her friends.

Where the hell did *he* come from?

I get in line. She's ahead of me. Looking at juice.

I have no idea what to say to her.

The next thing I know, she's bending down to pick something up. Here's my chance. I run to her, almost knocking over the girl in front of me. I see a dime on the floor.

I bend down to get it. Our heads smack together. Well, to be more accurate, I smack my head against Sara's like a socially inept moron. Smooth move.

I hold out her dime. She's rubbing her head.

"Sorry!" I say. "Are you okay?"

"Sure," she says. "Thanks."

I can't even remember what I say three seconds after I say it, but apparently it's funny. She laughs.

I said something funny and made Sara laugh.

I rule.

"See ya," she says.

"Okay," is all I can think to say. No wonder she practically runs back to Dave.

I go back to my table. Josh is gone.

"Well?" Mike says.

I just sit there.

"Dude! What happened?"

"Nothing."

"How can that be possible? This was your chance to make a move."

"I know."

"So?"

"I don't know."

"Man," Mike says. "That's messed up."

Now Dave's making everyone laugh. Dave just moved here. He shouldn't be allowed to go over there and make everyone laugh. I've known Sara and Laila and Maggie since third grade. I've watched them grow up. I know their histories. Dave doesn't know anything about them.

"We need strategy is all," Mike says. "No problemo."

When Laila and Maggie leave, I panic. What's he saying to her? What's she thinking? Is there a worse form of agony than this?

She smiled at me. But then she was gone. How did life move ahead without me?

CHAPTER 7
the idea of him
september 4, drafting

"This sketch is so not happening," I say.

Mr. Slater watches how I'm struggling with the T-square. I can tell he's trying not to laugh. He goes, "What's up?"

"My brain is on strike. I've had to start over, like, ten times already." We're starting the year with mechanical drawings, and each one is a fresh slice of torture. Today we're doing these Escher-type sketches of shapes that have no beginning or end.

"Take it easy," Mr. Slater says. "You'll get there." Which is of course what he would say. He's like this mid-life non-crisis hippie dude who never gets upset about anything. He has long black hair with gray streaks that he wears pulled back in a ponytail. This is a drastic fashion statement, considering we live in upscale rural-slash-suburbia where you're not allowed to wear your hair like that. Unless you're a girl. There's actually a magazine called *Weird New Jersey* that did an article on Mr. Slater a while ago. Apparently, he was supposed to be like the next Frank Lloyd Wright or something. But then his college roommate stole his big design plan and became this totally famous architect in New York. And Mr. Slater got stuck with us. Somehow, I don't think his life plan worked out.

"I'm nervous," I tell him. I almost rip up my paper in a fit of frantic erasing.

"About what?"

"A guy." I tell Mr. Slater everything. All of us love him. He's totally supportive and gives great advice. Which is the antithesis of my mom.

"Oh?"

"This guy Dave."

"Who's Dave?" Mr. Slater says. "The new kid?"

"Yeah," I say quietly.

Mr. Slater sits down on the stool next to me. "Why's he making you nervous? Did something happen?"

"No . . . it's just . . . it's not really him, it's more like . . . the idea of him."

He waits.

"Like, I want him to be who I imagine he is." I reposition my T-square. "But what if he's not really like that? What if he's just some guy?"

"Is that a bad thing?"

"It's not what I'm looking for."

Mr. Slater scratches his chin. "Tell me again what happened with your dad?"

I'm used to Mr. Slater's non sequiturs by now. I've had art classes with him every year. He has this special talent for remembering the most mundane details of our lives and then showing them to us when we least expect it in this way that makes us understand our lives better.

"I don't really know," I say. "I think they were too young. My mom was only sixteen when she had me. Remember?" He nods. "My dad was a senior, but his parents took him out of school, and they moved away before I was born. I don't remember ever seeing him."

"Do you want to find him?"

"No."

"Well, the only way to know who Dave is for sure is to get to know him."

"True."

"Mr. Slater!" erupts a screech from across the room. "My T-square broke!"

Mr. Slater smiles. "Good luck," he tells me.

"Thanks." It's not that he said anything astounding. But his chill approach to life always helps me minimize stress.

But two corroded sketches later, I'm back to feeling nervous. When it was all just a fantasy with Dave, I was so impatient and excited. Now that he asked me out for real, it's like I still want it to happen but at the same time I don't. And I have lunch soon. With Dave.

And I have an actual date this weekend.

With Dave.

☯

By the time Laila and I are walking to lunch, I'm a nervous wreck.

"So," I say. "Do you think Dave's sitting with us again?"

"That boy is completely infatuated with you," Laila says. "Wild horses couldn't keep him away."

"What?"

"I have no idea what I just said. I think Mr. Carver permanently damaged my medulla oblongata."

"What?"

"Hey," Dave says. He's waiting for me by the door.

"Hey," I go. But I can't really make eye contact with him. Even though we've talked on the phone the past two nights for a really long time, talking in person is way different. There's something about him that's like looking at the sun. He just looks *so* good. It's a miracle I don't spontaneously combust whenever I get within thirty feet of him.

Dave leans toward me and whispers, "Can I talk to you?"

"Uh . . . sure." I look over at Laila. "I'll be right in."

"Take your time," she says.

Laila goes in and sits down at our usual table. Maggie's there, saving us seats. I love how we already have a usual table.

Dave says, "I was wondering if you want to sit with my friends today."

"Um . . ." I look in at Maggie and Laila.

"'Cause last night? We were all hanging out at the mall, and Caitlin was saying how you seem cool but, like . . . she doesn't really know you and stuff."

"Oh." I'm trying to look like it's no big deal. But everyone knows when the boy you like wants you to meet his friends, it's a big freaking deal. Particularly if it's Caitlin, who is normally oblivious to the fact that you exist. So of course I want to sit with him! But then I remind myself of the first rule of sisterhood: best friends before boyfriends. I can't just bail on Laila and Maggie like that. I decide to compromise. "What about next week? I promised Maggie and Laila—"

"No problem," Dave says. "Are you buying?"

I wave my lunch bag in his face.

"That would be your lunch." He smiles. His dirty-blond hair falls over his eyes. He flips it back in this sexy way.

"That would be, yeah." My mouth is all dry.

"I'll be right back." He goes to get in line.

I sit down across from Maggie.

"Watch out, guys," Maggie says. "It looks like octopus today."

"What *is* that stuff?" Laila examines her tray.

"I told you," Maggie says. "Octopus."

"Is it noodles?" I ask.

"You guys aren't listening! *Oc-to-pus!*" Maggie screams. "It's octopus!"

"Appetizing," I say.

Laila goes, "Could Mr. Perry be a bigger asshole?"

"I know!" He actually gave us a pop quiz today in calc, and it's only the third day of school. Who does that? "And then he acts all shocked when no one's ready? Please."

"We really have to watch out for that guy," Laila says. "I have a feeling he may be even more sadistic than Mr. Carver."

"Like that's even possible," I say. "Wait. Let me tell you how—"

"Sara?"

I look up to see that Caitlin has graced me with her presence. And that would be the royal plural, since the two most popular guys are with her. Even though Dave told me what she said, it's still hard to believe she's not here on some twisted mission to humiliate me.

I glance over at Maggie. She's looking at them like she's my bodyguard and they've just threatened to kill me.

"Yeah?" I cautiously say to Caitlin.

She goes, "You're talking to Dave, right?"

The way she smiles at me seems so legit you would think she's being nice. I want to believe what Dave said, but any second now she'll probably tell me to lay off him because he's already reserved for a gorgeous girl who actually deserves him. Instead of a nobody nerd like me.

"Yeah?" I say. Alex, who's captain of the basketball team, and Caitlin's boyfriend, Matt, smile down at me.

Alex goes, "Sweet. I always thought you were cool."

"Totally," Matt adds. "Just, you know, shy."

Did the most popular guys in school just call me cool?

Caitlin is still smiling at me like she's seeing me for the first time. Maybe she doesn't even realize how she usually ignores me. "You should come sit with us," she says.

Is the most popular girl in school really asking me to hang with her? This can't be real. But I say, "Yeah," anyway. It appears to be the only word I know.

Dave comes back with his lunch. He puts his hand on my shoulder and sits down next to me. While he's talking to Alex and Matt, I look over at Laila. She gives me this disapproving glare. I don't even look at Maggie. I'm sure I already know what she's thinking.

"So I was about to tell Sara that we should all hang out sometime," Caitlin says to Dave.

"Sure," he says.

"Cool." Caitlin smiles. "We'll talk."

"Later, dude," Matt says to Dave.

"Later."

Caitlin grabs Matt's hand. "Let's go, Pooky."

I'm like, *Pooky?*

They drift off with an air of importance.

Laila looks over at Dave. "Well, Pooky," she says, "you better start eating. Your octopus is getting cold."

Dave gives Laila a strange look. Like he's annoyed or something. It's only for a second, but it's like he's mad at her for making fun of his friends.

He takes a huge bite of whatever it is and gags. "Uh! What is this stuff?"

"I thought octopus was your favorite," I say.

"Yeah, but this is something else. Ostrich strips, maybe."

"No, no," Laila says. She samples another bite. "Eel skins. Definitely eel skins."

"You guys are weird," Maggie announces. "I'm getting a sandwich."

"Chicken," Laila says.

"I don't think there's chicken," Maggie says.

"I'll go," I say. "I need a new sandwich. The jelly totally leaked through on mine."

"Get me one? Here." Dave takes out a twenty and hands it to me. "My treat."

As I'm walking to the line, I have to pass a table of jocks. I hold my breath, speed up, and watch the floor. But then I glance over at them anyway. One of the girls grabs another girl's arm and points to me. Then she whispers something, and they smile at me. One of them even says, "Hey, Sara," as I walk by.

I know Laila and Maggie aren't feeling me right now. Snobs who ignore you forever and then suddenly start acting like they've been your friends all along don't interest them. And somewhere deep down, I know they shouldn't interest me, either.

But after being a nobody for so long, it feels awesome to be a somebody. A girl could get addicted to being treated like she matters.

CHAPTER 8
not that i'm desperate
september 4, 7:23 p.m.

"I don't fucking believe this."

The Cure's *Disintegration* plays on repeat mode.

Mike examines the chess board.

"I just don't fucking believe this happened," I say. "How did this happen again? What exactly did I do wrong?"

"Well, since you asked," Mike says, "it's like this: One, you were too much of a wimp to say anything to her. Two, you went back to school with no plan. Dave had a plan. He got Sara. You got *nada*." Mike leans back, balancing on the back legs of the chair. "Zilch. Zero. You didn't have the balls to go up to her. Dude. I warned you this would happen."

"Thanks. I feel so much better now." I move a pawn up two spaces.

"I don't even get it. You had no problem with Cynthia, and any guy would kill to nail her. What's so hard about talking to Sara?"

"She's different. It's complicated."

"Okay," Mike says. "You fucked up. But there's hope."

"There is?"

"Totally, man. Look, I'll tell you what to do, but if I tell you, you have to swear that you're gonna do it."

Mike's practically the only person I trust for advice on getting the girl. His whole philosophy of dating has been about quantity, not quality. So he's had a wide variety of experiences. You can most definitely trust a person with experiences.

"And just what am I supposed to do?" I say.

"Promise you'll do it first."

"Whatever. She's already going out with Dave."

"Man, what's with you? Why are you being such a pussy?"

"What if she doesn't like me?"

"You don't get it. He just asked her out, what, *Tuesday*? It's not like he's suddenly her boyfriend in two days. You have just as much chance as he does."

"Right. Only he's the one who's with her." I move my rook. "Fucking asshole."

"You have to play it like you're the most incredible guy out there." He moves his rook. "It's all about strategy."

Mike is so kicking my ass right now. He's like this chess mastermind. We're both smart types in general, but no one else really knows this. He tries to reject academic restraints like me. At least, until his mom threatens that we can't practice at his place anymore. Then he's forced to do his homework.

It's this big mystery to everyone why I choose to be

such a massive slacker. The guidance counselor is always like, "Your grades are not reflective of the work you could do," and "Don't you want to make something of yourself?" As if we're actually going to encounter any of this in real life. Maybe if classes weren't so useless I might work up an interest. They don't get that the reason so many of us aren't into school is simply because it's boring. Why can't they make it relevant to our lives? Anyway, I make decent grades by acing all the tests and quizzes. They're always cake. Not doing homework kind of balances the whole thing out, and I end up with a B-minus or C average every year. Which is fine with me.

So now I'm trying to convince the ultimate class brain that I'm smart. Or at least smart enough for her to want to be with me.

I sigh in defeat. "Dave's got her. I should just accept it and move on." But the thought of moving on from something I never had in the first place is depressing. "I can't move on."

"Shit, man. Force her to notice you."

"How?"

"You can strategize it so you just happen to run into her."

"Uh-huh."

"Like . . . you can see when she goes to her locker to switch books. Then you just figure out which way she walks after. And you can try to find out her schedule."

"So that's what I'm supposed to do? Pretend to run into her?"

"Just . . . talk to her! The same way you talked to all the others, man!"

But that's the thing. All the other girls I've been involved with approached me first. I didn't really have to convince them to like me.

"See what she does," Mike explains. "If she likes you, talk some more the next day. But if she's totally repulsed, then you know she doesn't like you."

"This is your major plan?"

"No, dude. This is my typical chick-catching method. For single girls. In your case, we need something more extreme."

"Like what?"

But Mike is hesitating. "I bet if I tell you, you won't even do it."

"I'll try anything at this point." I don't have to look at the chess board to know I'm losing this game. "Not that I'm desperate."

"No, of course not. You?" Mike snorts.

"Yeah, okay. Let's go already."

"If you don't do it, you have to wash my car."

"I don't even know what it is yet!"

"Too bad. That's the deal."

I'm so obviously desperate. "Okay, fine. Just tell me what to do."

"And wax."

"Fuck you!"

"And wax."

I pick up my king. "Fine," I tell him. "But it can't be, like, some crazy shit you know I would never do anyway."

Mike pretends to look hurt. "Am I not your best friend?"

"Let me try to remember."

"Look, people pay for this kind of advice. Self-help books are written about this stuff, and I'm telling you for free."

"That's why I let you hang out with me," I say.

"So. Is it a deal?"

"Wait. What do I get if I do it?"

"Same thing."

"Deal."

"Okay," Mike begins. "Here's what you do."

CHAPTER 9
this remote island
september 5, 5:32 p.m.

"Okay." I turn over this huge shopping bag in the middle of Maggie's king-size bed. I swear, her bed is bigger than my room. "I brought my flares, my low-rise, my skinny jeans . . . oh, my size-eight low-rise—"

"I thought you were a size six."

"Yeah, but size eight makes my butt look smaller."

"And this is a good thing because . . ."

"Because my butt looks bigger than California in all the others?"

We're deciding what I should wear for my big date with Dave tomorrow. Or Maggie's giving me things to try on and then deciding for me.

"Oh, please." Maggie picks up the flares. "You look fabulous in these."

"Are you sure?"

"Would I give you bad wardrobe advice? Here." Maggie holds them out. "Put these on with, um . . .

hang on." She dives into her enormous walk-in closet. "I am now locating the shirt that will drive Dave crazy."

I laugh. But it's not funny. This reminds me of reason number seventy-three why I'm nervous about tomorrow. I know it's only the first date, but what if Dave's expecting a lot more than I'm used to? I wonder if he can tell I'm a virgin.

I lie down on Maggie's bed. I pile all the pillows on top of me. I'm freaking out. This is nothing like what I had with Scott. That was definitely *not* a case of zsa-zsa-zou. Whenever Scott tried going further than I wanted, the decision was easy. I just smacked his hand away and he didn't push it. But with Dave . . .

"Okay." Maggie emerges with a stack of shirts. She holds out a red backless thing. "Try this first," she says.

"What," I go. "Seriously?"

"What's wrong with it?"

"It's not exactly . . . me." I don't want to hurt her feelings, but sometimes we have really different ideas about what's sexy. When it comes to clothes, Maggie subscribes to the Less Is More school of seduction. Whereas I'm more into the Jeans and a T-Shirt Always Look Cute way of thinking. Then again, this is new territory. I've never dated a Calvin Klein ad before.

I grab the shirt. I'm trying to figure out how it goes on when a door slams down the hall. Then there's yelling. Maggie's parents are fighting. It's been happening a lot lately.

"There they go again," Maggie says. "My dad just

got home from a business trip. This is gonna be a long one."

Her dad is always traveling. He's, like, this systems-analyst guy who gets hired by all these different companies as a consultant. He makes a ridiculous amount of money, which is why Maggie has her own credit cards and her mom doesn't even work. I love Maggie like a sister, but I'm so jealous of her it's wrong. But maybe her life isn't all that.

"You can totally work that," she tells me.

I look at myself in the mirror. I'm wearing a belt that's masquerading as a shirt. "There's no way," I tell her. I yank it off.

Maggie hands over a pink silk top with sequins. "Girl, you don't realize how sexy you are. That shirt and anything else can be you if you let it." That's the thing about Maggie. She dates all these gorgeous guys on her terms and has never been dumped in her life. She's had sex with two guys already and doesn't regret any of it. It's like love is this fun adventure for her, while for me it's all about wanting something you don't have.

Until now.

"Any tips?" I say.

"Sure." Maggie plops herself down on a gigantic floor pillow. "What do you want to know?"

"Well . . ." Of course Maggie's told me all about the guys she's slept with. But before, sex seemed like this remote island. Now that it's a definite possibility, I need details. "What's it like? The first time?"

"I'm sorry. Since when do we sleep with guys on the first date?"

"I don't mean for tomorrow! It's . . . for future reference."

"Do you think you're gonna sleep with Dave?"

"I don't know." I smile at the floor. "Maybe."

"Look at you!"

"So what's it like?"

"Well, at first it hurts."

"A lot?"

"It depends." Maggie shifts on the pillow.

"Were you nervous?"

"Not really. I wanted to and . . . it was the right time for me."

"How did you know?"

Maggie shakes her head. "I was . . . I don't know. I just wanted to."

It's not like I don't want to. But I've never reached the point where I've wanted to more than I didn't want to.

"Does it hurt the whole time?" I say.

"No. Just at first. But then it gets better."

"So . . . what if like four months from now he's getting impatient, and I'm still not ready?"

"Then you don't do it."

"But what if I think I'm ready and we're almost doing it and then I realize I'm not and I freak out right when he's about to—"

"Chillax! You're thinking about this way too much." Maggie throws a lacy turquoise top at me. "That's the problem with you genius types. You overanalyze every-thing."

"I don't think I'm overanalyzing. I just—"

"Look, stop worrying so much. Just go with the flow." Maggie scrutinizes my outfit. "I like the pink on you. But try this one—it's much tighter."

I take the tiny shirt and try to squeeze myself into it.

"It only matters what *you* want," Maggie says. "Don't let him force you into anything."

"Right."

"Don't forget mints tomorrow. And—oh yeah! This is the shirt!"

"No way."

"Why not?"

"It's too tight." I peel it off.

"That's the point. You're wearing it."

"No, I'm not. I like the pink one."

"But the turquoise is so you."

"Um, no."

"Oh—you should get some condoms so you have them when you're ready. You have no idea what's out there. And you can't always expect him to have them." Maggie has condoms, plus she's on the pill. She believes in doubling up on birth control.

"What if he wants me to put it on?"

"Yeah?"

"How do you do it?"

"Oh, it's easy," Maggie says, like it's nothing. "First, you have to make sure you're putting it on the right way or else it won't unroll. Then you squeeze the tip to let the air out so when—"

"I get it."

"Then you just unroll it. But make sure you unroll it all the way down. You don't want it to come off, believe me."

All this seems like too much. Figuring out which way to unroll a condom in the dark and how much it's going to hurt and how I'm going to feel after. Is it worth all the drama?

I steer the conversation back to the date. "Okay, so mints. What else?"

"Don't act all shy when you see The Look. You know you're dying to make out with him."

"Finally," I say. "Familiar territory."

"Oh, yeah, like Scott ever gave you The Look," Maggie scoffs. She's convinced that a person can't be smart and passionate and president of the chess club. Two out of three, maybe.

"It wasn't his fault I wasn't more attracted to him," I sniff.

"It also wasn't his fault he wasn't attractive. Big whoop."

"Oh! He's cute!"

Maggie raises an eyebrow at me.

"Sort of," I mumble. I glance at the clock. "It's getting late." I shove my jeans back in the bag. "I better go."

"Hey," Maggie says when I'm in her doorway.

I turn around just in time to catch the pink shirt that's flying toward me.

On my way down the hall, I pass her parents' room. Their voices are lower, but they're still fighting. I consider listening at the door, but that's tacky. Anyway, I don't want to know. I'm not ready to find out that the only parental role models I've ever had aren't happy after all.

CHAPTER 10
living proof of the impossible
september 5, 9:43 a.m.

I never thought talking to a girl would ever be this hard.

At least we have Music Theory together. The problem is that we were put into pairs the first day, and so I never get to talk to Sara. She sits all the way across the room with Laila. I could always go up to her after class or something. But it's not that simple. How exactly do you get a girl who likes someone else to like you instead?

Mike's philosophy is if a girl likes someone and you want her to like you, you should watch what the guy who she likes does. Then whatever you see him doing around her, do that. The logic is that since the girl likes this guy so much, she's automatically into the kinds of things he does. Mike's big plan for me is to do the same exact thing that Dave did. So all I have to do is go up to Sara, talk to her for a few minutes, and then ask her out. Since it's only been three days since Dave dropped the bomb, I'm not technically scamming on some other guy's girl. And Dave is an asshole who doesn't deserve to be with Sara. And Sara isn't some random girl.

But I still haven't come up with a feasible enough excuse to talk to her. So I've decided to accidentally-on-purpose cross her path in the hall. Josh found out from Fred that Sara has drafting third period. There's only one way Sara can walk to drafting. So I've scoped out the staircase where some serious serendipity is about to go down. Today's the day.

When second period is almost over, I start packing my bag on the sly. The instant the bell rings, I sprint out of class. The halls are clear. I station myself at the bottom of the small staircase that leads down to the art studio.

I wait.

People moving by bump into me.

I wait some more.

And then I see her.

I start to walk up the stairs.

She starts to walk down.

She looks at me.

I smile at her.

My lip sticks to my front tooth.

I say, "Hey."

And that's when I trip. My books go flying all over.

I never thought it was possible to fall up stairs. But here I am. Living proof of the impossible.

I put my hands out to break my fall. My fingers slip on a stair. Some kids behind me run up, pushing me over. I bang my head against the wall. Random pages from my binder, which popped open when it smacked against the floor, are scattered for what appear to be miles in every direction.

Sara bends down to help me up. "Are you okay?" she says.

I get up quickly like it's no big deal. "Yeah, I'm fine."

"Every time I see you, you're bumping your head!"

And every time I see you, I wish my headboard was bumping against the wall. With you in my bed.

The bell rings.

"Are you sure you're okay?" Sara says.

"Yeah."

"Do you want help picking up your stuff?"

"Oh. Did something fall?"

Sara laughs. This is a good sign. Most girls don't get my sense of humor.

"That's okay," I tell her. "Thanks, though."

"Okay, well . . . see you."

"Later."

I watch her walk away. Here was my chance and I blew it. And I looked like a spaz for nothing.

Could I *be* a bigger loser?

By the time all of my papers are shoved into my binder, I realize I should be in pre-calc. I'm mad late. Well, what do they expect? We do have lives here. Whoever established that there should be only five minutes between periods was obviously designing this rule for a school with like ten students. Sometime around 1908. Not that I'm ever in a rush to get to class on time. But still.

The teachers couldn't be more clueless about our lives. The more I think about this as I walk to class, the more annoyed I get. Like, now I'm late, and Mr. Perry is going to ask me for a pass, and I don't have one, and he's going to be all, "Why are you late?" And what am I supposed to say? "Oh, sorry, Mr. Perry. I was just acting like this deranged stalker, and then I had to humiliate myself in front of the one girl I'm dying to get. The humiliation part took longer than I thought." Yeah. That'll work.

I walk into class like I'm not guilty of anything.

Everyone stares at me.

I sit down.

Mr. Perry quits speaking in the middle of a sentence. He glares at me.

It's very quiet.

I open my notebook to a new page. I write the date like nothing's wrong.

"Tobey?" says Mr. Perry.

"Yeah?"

"Do you have a pass?"

It's like they all read from the same script.

"No," I say. But what I really want to do is jump out of my chair and yell, "Don't you think that if I had a fucking pass I would have fucking given it to you when I walked through the fucking door?!" Then slam my notebook shut and stomp out the door in a triumphant huff. But he'll harass me more if I do that.

Then he goes, "Why are you late?"

"Sorry," I say.

Everyone is still staring at me.

"I appreciate your apology, but that doesn't answer my question."

"I was in the bathroom."

"Without a bathroom pass?"

"That's right. It was an emergency." I shake my head dramatically. "Trust me. You don't want to know."

Everyone giggles. Mr. Perry looks embarrassed.

"Next time you're late, make sure you have a pass." He goes back to talking about something that is, I assume, of vital importance to our lives.

After a few minutes of everyone writing down what he writes and no one raising their hand to answer his questions, Mr. Perry says, "Take out your homework. Let's go over number nine."

Everyone rustles in their notebooks and produces pages that may be homework or are just posing as homework until Mr. Perry discovers that they are, in fact, not homework. I don't even bother to pretend to look for something that I would never have.

Mr. Perry looks at me. "Where's your homework?" he demands.

"I don't have it." I never have it and he knows it. How long is it going to take him to get it?

"Why not?" he barks.

"I wouldn't want to shock you with unprecedented behavior."

It's so quiet I can actually hear the water running in the fountain outside.

Mr. Perry slowly walks over to me as if twenty other kids weren't in the room.

He is pink.

He is fuming.

He leans on my desk and says, "I don't like your tone."

"I wasn't aware that I had a particular tone," I say.

"Don't get smart with me!" he threatens.

I'm vaguely aware that this is escalating into a situation. Mr. Perry should come with a Parental Advisory sticker. If he thinks being late and not doing homework is such a life-or-death situation, this dude seriously needs to brush up on his current events.

Mr. Perry picks up his hall pass, which is a huge protractor with his name on it, and whips it at me. "Go to the guidance office," he says. "I'll be there after class."

I take the pass. I close my notebook. What would be the point of protesting?

When I get to the guidance office, Ms. Everman notices me right away. She's practically the only adult here who cares about what happens to us.

"Hi, Tobey." She smiles. "Want a Jolly Rancher?"

"No, thanks."

"Are you here to see me?"

"Well, yeah, but not by choice," I tell her.

"Hmm, sounds interesting. Why don't you have a seat?"

I sit in the big stuffed chair. Her office has lots of posters and plants and stuffed animals. The radio plays classical music.

"So," she says. "What's up?"

"I was late to pre-calc, and Mr. Perry told me to come here and wait for him."

Ms. Everman scrunches her eyes up like she's confused.

"Why would he want you to come all the way here just because you were late?"

"I didn't have a pass."

"Okay..."

"You always have to have a pass with Mr. Perry or he has a conniption."

"Why didn't you have a pass?"

"Because I was just late."

"Why were you late?"

There's no way to explain this without telling Ms. Everman the whole story about Sara. I mean, that's what guidance counselors are for, but it's too embarrassing to go into it with her. So I say, "I lost track of time."

"But you're wearing a watch."

"I just . . . wasn't paying attention."

"Yes, that seems to be the story again this year." Ms. Everman picks up one of those squishy stress balls from her desk. "I've already gotten complaints from a few of your teachers that you're not doing homework. Are you planning to keep up the same trend this year?"

"You know me. Homework is against my religion."

"And what religion is that?"

"Dadaism."

"Dadaism isn't a religion," she says. "It's a cult."

"You mean they didn't tell me this whole time?"

"Tobey, if we could be serious for a few minutes here, I'd really like to know what you intend to do about graduating with a decent transcript."

"Other than doing it?"

"What makes you think you'll get into a good college without doing all your work?"

"I always have at least a C average. You know that."

"Yes, but why are you satisfied with that? Especially when we both know you could be doing so much better?"

"I'm fine with it," I tell her.

Ms. Everman sighs and shakes her head. "There's a lot more to life than just getting by, Tobey."

"It works for me," I say.

"A person with an SAT score of 1450 should have a much higher GPA." She smiles. "But I'm sure we can find some colleges that would be thrilled to have you."

"But—"

"Stop," Ms. Everman interrupts. We've had this conversation before. She's been on my case about college since I met her freshman year. I told her I wasn't interested in going to college. She told me that I'd realize the error of my ways. Which so far hasn't happened. "I'm serious. Just think about it. Hard."

"Okay." I give her a wide-eyed, optimistic look.

The look works. "You know where to find me," she says.

In Music Theory, I'm all frustrated from the conference with Mr. Perry and the dean and then writing an essay entitled "Why What I Did Was Wrong and Will Never Happen Again." And now my pen is getting all blotchy. Cheap pens suck. I write a reminder on my hand to get decent pens after school. Then I glance over at Sara. She's laughing at something Laila said.

And that's when it suddenly hits me. A plan that will actually work. I won't have to pose as a deranged stalker with zero potential anymore. Sara can see me for who I really am.

It does involve some initial risk, though. In order for it to work, I have to talk to Laila.

when you connect
september 6, 3:34 p.m.

I decide that the only way I can possibly calm my nerves before Dave is supposed to pick me up in three hours, twenty-five minutes, and seventeen seconds is to work on my sketchbook. So I fill a glass with water, grab my colored pencils and watercolors, and go sit on the front porch. Everything else I need is already sitting on the wicker couch—glitter, glue, scissors, *Jane* magazines, CD player, and *Creative Visualization*. I'm at the part where I have to make a treasure map of my ideal relationship. The concept is that if I physically create a description of the boy I want, if I can see him that clearly in my heart and in my mind, then I'll be more open to him coming into my life. Of course, I already think this guy is Dave, so I'm imagining how I want him to be from the little I already know about him. When he's my boyfriend, I can show him this later, and we'll laugh about how I knew him even before I knew him.

With my favorite James Taylor CD playing, I use

yellow to paint a border around the page, which makes the whole page look like it's lit up. So far my treasure map is a collage of words I cut out of magazines and glued at all different angles around the page. Words like "romantic" and "smart" and "cute" and "introspective." I shade around some of the words with a pink colored pencil. I smudge the pink into light blue.

I spread glitter over the border. Then I write about the way I want to feel when I'm with this awesome boy. Like I'm the most beautiful girl he's ever seen. Like I'm the most important thing in his life.

I flip through this month's *Jane*, looking for more words and images to describe him. I cut out a couple sitting on a hill, watching a sunset. I cut out "irresistible" and "funny." I cut out a yin-yang symbol. James sings how the secret of love is all about opening up your heart. And then I imagine an absolutely perfect date happening tonight, with romance and excitement and the euphoria that happens when you connect with the person you're meant to be with. Not that I've ever experienced that feeling. But I can imagine how intense it is.

At the diner, I'm feeling really confident. Dave told me I looked great when he picked me up, and he held my hand for half the movie. He even said how he'd been looking forward to tonight all week. So I ask the thing I've been dying to know all summer.

"Why didn't you call me this summer?"

"I was staying with my uncle in Boulder. I had a summer job set up there before I moved, so it was just easier for me to go back than try to find something here."

Knowing that there was an actual reason he didn't call me is the best part of the night. "If I'd been here," Dave says, leaning toward me and reaching for my hand across the table, "I would have definitely called you."

I am insanely happy.

But I'm still nervous about the inevitable kiss later. I wish that I wasn't nervous so I could be hungry. When I'm telling the waitress what I want, I'm all weirded out about Dave watching me. For some reason, I always feel self-conscious about ordering food.

"So," I say.

Dave smiles at me.

I smile at him.

And I can't think of one single thing to say.

"I'm so glad we had that storm yesterday," Dave says. "The heat was killing me."

"Isn't it hot in Colorado?"

"Not really. Or when it gets hot, it's not that humid kind of hot. It's a dry heat, so you don't really feel it."

"Oh, yeah! I remember that from earth science. It's like . . . when air is dry, it has less water vapor, so there's room for your sweat to evaporate."

"So why don't you feel as hot?"

"Because when your sweat evaporates, that's how you cool off."

"I knew that." He smiles at me. "I was just seeing if you did."

Then Dave talks about basketball, explaining the rules and special techniques and stuff. I'm so not into sports, but I let him go on because he's gorgeous. Then our food arrives. And the worst thing happens. When I reach for the mustard, I knock over his soda. Dave jumps out of the booth before it pours all over his lap. But his sleeve is soaked.

"Oh!" I yell. "I'm sorry!"

"It's okay," Dave says.

I pull a bunch of napkins out of the napkin holder. "Here, let me—"

"No, it's okay. I got it."

When he comes back from the bathroom, I still can't think of anything interesting to say.

Then Dave's like, "What are you thinking about?"

"I like that photo," I tell him. It's of an old cobblestone street somewhere that feels like Europe. With lots of plants hanging out of the windows.

"Oh." He points behind me. "I like that one."

When I turn around to see it, I'm like, *He has to be joking*. It's a loud, annoying painting of a boring landscape. Totally impersonal and with stupid colors. It reminds me of the guy on PBS who does these really gross paintings and you're supposed to paint along with him. As if you would want to.

"Yeah, right," I laugh.

"No," Dave says. "I'm serious."

"Oh!" I look at it again. "Well, yeah. It's nice." It is

not nice. It is horrendous. But everyone knows that people in a relationship should have different interests. You can't expect someone to like all the same things you do.

"You know," he says, chewing, "I didn't think you would go out with me."

"Why not?"

"Like, you went out with Scott, and he's . . . really . . . smart."

"So then why'd you ask for my number?"

"I always thought you were cute. Remember when I sat next to you at the junior meeting?"

I nod. If he only knew how many details I remember.

"I was hoping you liked me. But I didn't know if I was smart enough for you."

"But you're smart!"

"Yeah." He squeezes my hand. "But you are absolutely brilliant." He lets my hand go and touches my cheek. "And really cute, too."

I am insanely happy.

When the check comes, I remember what Maggie said to do. She said that since Dave asked me out, he should be the one to pay. And that I shouldn't offer to pay for my half the way I usually do.

I bite my lip. My lips are dry and crackly. And of course I didn't bring any Chap Stick. So I have to think of a way to lick them without Dave noticing before we kiss later.

Dave pays. I exhale.

I kind of blank out during the ride to my house.

Neither one of us is talking much. I'm way too nervous about the kiss. He must be, too.

We hold hands walking to the porch. Then we're standing on the porch. The light is on. I look over at my neighbors' yard to see if anyone's watching.

"Thanks for dinner. And the movie. I had a good time."

"You're welcome," Dave says. "I had a good time, too."

I look up at him. His brown eyes look black in the night. I can't tell what he's thinking.

I wait for the rest to happen.

Dave leans toward me. I lean toward him.

And then he kisses me.

On the *cheek*.

Dave says, "So . . . see you Monday."

"Yeah," I say. "See you."

Even after he's gone, I'm still standing there. Still waiting for my real kiss.

CHAPTER 12
more determined than ever
september 6, 7:58 p.m.

"That's a fucking awesome plan," Mike announces. He twangs the strings of his bass, tuning up again.

"Why do you have to have a plan?" Josh asks. "Why can't you just ask her out?"

This makes Mike defensive. The man likes his plans. "What's wrong with having a plan?" Mike says. "Three years ago when everyone thought The Cure was going to break up, *Bloodflowers* came out. Why? Because they had a plan. And they acted on it. And now look."

"Fine," Josh says. "But when Tobey freaks her out acting like a psycho and she hates him, can I say I told you so?"

"You *are* sort of obsessed," Mike tells me.

"I don't know what my problem is," I say. I've been trying not to think about the fact that Sara and Dave are out together right now. I keep messing up my chords. I keep forgetting how the lyrics go. And I'm the one who wrote them.

"Dude," Mike says. "Stop stressing. Remember what

you're capable of. Cynthia's wet panties were on the floor before you could say ribbed or glow-in-the-dark."

"You my hero, dog," Josh says.

I only think about having sex with Sara once every three seconds. But talking about her that way with the guys seems like I'm disrespecting her. I've told them everything about the other girls I've been with. But it's different now.

Josh clashes the cymbals. "Are we doing this or what?"

We're working on our set for Battle of the Bands. Actually, we only get to play one song. Two if we make it to the final round. But we're still narrowing it down.

We go through this Led Zeppelin number Mike's convinced will rule. Then Mike says, "This is the one." I kind of disagree, though. His vocals aren't sounding all that.

"I think one with a drum solo would be better," Josh says from behind the drums.

"Oh, really?" Mike says. "And why's that?"

"It's heavy drum sessions that shake up the scene. Everyone knows this." Josh taps his sticks together.

"Then how come—"

"Michael!"

The sound of Mike's mom indicates that practice is over. Since it's Saturday, we can practice until she gets home from doing errands. We also get the garage from after school until she gets home from work. Then it's time for dinner and homework. At least, it is for Mike. His mom hovers over him like a dark cloud with a perpetual absence of silver lining. If he doesn't do all his homework, we can't use the garage. She even checks it over and everything. So his grades are pretty good. But he's a slacker at heart, like me and Josh.

The door swings open. Light from the kitchen filters in.

"Hi, boys."

"Hi, Mrs. Panalba," Josh and I say together.

Her heels click across the cement floor as she walks toward us. "How's the world-famous MindFlame this evening?"

I get a little thrill whenever I hear anyone say the name of our band. I thought of it myself. It's a whole lot better than What Jesus Would Do, which is what Josh wanted. Or Mike's idea, the Jeans Creamers. I guess our band is sort of weird. We've been described as "out there." But I really feel like we're on the verge of a breakthrough. Plus, we have a reputation for kicking ass with our classic rock covers. So the gigs we play are mainly class reunions and pre-midlife-crisis birthday parties and even some pool party and barbeque-type events in the summer. Which don't suck since we always get paid really well. Josh has been lining up more gigs for this year. And of course Mike is organizing plans to record our demo.

"Making progress," I say.

Mrs. Panalba rubs Mike's face. "What's this on your face?" she says.

"Ma!" Mike yells. He jerks away. "Get off!"

"What is that?" She touches his face again.

"Nothing!" Mike slaps her hand away. "God!"

"Aren't you using the Clearasil I got you?"

"*Ma!* Jeez!"

"Okay, okay." She heads back toward the kitchen. "Take care, boys."

"We'll try," Josh says.

Mrs. Panalba gives Josh a funny look. She closes the door.

"I swear, it's like her sole purpose in life is to humiliate me," Mike says.

Josh shrugs. "Yeah, but that's parents."

We start packing up.

"You guys wanna chill at the mall?" Mike says. He gets off easy on non-school nights. And my curfew isn't until one.

"Sure," I say.

"I can't," Josh says. "I'm still on lockdown."

Josh is grounded, like, every other week. He's always doing something stupid. This time it was chucking his dad's bowling ball through the window while demonstrating his stance to this chick he was trying to impress. Real impressive.

Mike and I decide to take my car. As I drive, Mike yammers on about all his elaborate plans for the band's inevitable success.

When we're sitting at the food court with enough fried food to feed a small country, Mike says, "We've gotta get your mind off things." He's looking at something over my shoulder. "And I think I know how."

I turn around. And that's when I see them.

Cynthia and Marnie are slumming it in line at Cinnabon. If this were last year, it would have been perfect. I was nailing Cynthia, and Mike's been trying to get with Marnie for a long time.

I'm tempted for a second. How easy it would be. How good she looks. But hooking up with Cynthia again would be such a pain. She'd start nagging about how she wants to be my girlfriend. Then she'd start demanding to spend more time with me. It's a road I don't want to go down again.

"I'm out," I say. I stand up and get my garbage together.

"What? Are you serious?"

"Yeah."

Mike looks at me like I'm insane.

"Can you get home okay?" I say.

He glances over at Marnie. "Definitely."

"See you."

"Later."

Walking across the parking lot, I'm more determined than ever. There's no way I'm giving up. It has to happen.

CHAPTER 13
yin and yang
september 8, 12:33 p.m.

"How many calories does a banana have?" Caitlin says.

"Eighty," Heather says. She picks some fuzz off Alex's shirt.

I can't believe I'm sitting at Dave's table and his friends are actually treating me like I'm good people. And Dave made me feel included right away. I felt sort of bad ditching Maggie and Laila, but they said it was okay as long as I still eat with them sometimes.

Dave puts his arm around me. "Are you gonna eat your Ho Ho?"

I was so looking forward to this Ho Ho. But peeking at the other girls' trays, I detect a substantial lack of desserts. I don't want to be all eating my Ho Ho with everyone staring at me.

"No," I say. "You can have it."

Glancing around the cafeteria, I can tell that a lot of other kids are noticing me sitting over here. It's nice to finally feel accepted.

By Music Theory, I'm drifting happily along in a pink bubble.

"What's up with Tobey?" Laila says.

"What do you mean?"

"He's been staring at you since he walked in the door. Don't you notice anything?"

I look over at Tobey. He quickly looks away.

"Drool much?" Laila says.

"I was only seeing if he was looking at me!"

"Protest much?"

"Okay, people!" Mr. Hornby says, clapping his hands together. "Let's move on to scales!" He sits down at the piano and begins to play. We're supposed to hum along. While we hum, I look at Tobey. He's really tall, like maybe six-one, which you can tell from the way he's folded up in his chair. His hair is dark and his skin is pale. Like yin and yang. I'm drawn to those eyes again. They're big and deep blue. Almost a violet color. And he has these really long eyelashes.

Tobey catches me looking at him. When he sees me, his eyes get even bigger. He looks serious and contemplative. If I didn't already know about him, I'd think he was extremely intelligent. Which is usually the main thing that turns me on about a guy. But Tobey's a total slacker. His confidence is amazing, though. His expression says, *I'm looking at you because I want to and I don't care if you know it.*

It's really weird, but for a few seconds we're both

just staring at each other. Why is it that when I look at him now, it's like I'm seeing him for the first time?

I look away.

I forget what we're supposed to be doing. Laila jams her elbow into my side, and I start humming along like I didn't miss anything. For the rest of the class, I refuse to look over at Tobey. But I can feel him staring at me.

After class, I take a long time getting my stuff together. I'm seeing if Tobey will try to talk to me again. My stuff only consists of a notebook and a book and a pencil, so I pretend to look for something in my notebook. I'm in a state of panic until I see Tobey leave.

Why am I so disappointed that he didn't say anything to me?

As Laila and I are walking out, she goes, "What was *that* about?"

"What?"

"Oh, please. Like you don't know."

"I don't."

"Like you weren't staring at him for the whole class," Laila says. "What? Did he reprogram your brain so now you can't think straight?" Laila says this in a nasty tone. That's because she hates anyone like Tobey. People who don't do anything and still pass classes severely annoy her. She can't understand why anyone would want to slack off like that. I mean, Laila's so dedicated to being first in our class that she doesn't even mind not being allowed to date. Plus, she apparently has no interest in romance. Which could be because she's convinced her parents stopped having sex in 1987. But Laila would definitely not understand why I already feel like there's something between me and Tobey. Not that I even understand.

"Hmm? I really don't know what you're talking about." It feels like I'm floating out of the room instead of walking.

"Fine. Be that way," Laila says. "You know you'll tell me eventually." She whisks off to her locker without saying bye.

I lift my bag out of my locker and try to figure out what I need to take home. But I can't even remember what I did today. I think it's Monday. So Laila, as usual, is right. But here's the question: Why is the boy who is taking over my brain Tobey instead of Dave?

"Hey," Dave says. "Need a ride home?"

"Oh," I say, startled. I wasn't expecting to see him again today. "Yeah." I rearrange my sketchbook so I can also fit my enormous calc book in my bag.

"Here," Dave says, gently pushing me up against a locker. "Let me get that for you." He takes my bag and puts it on the floor.

He leans into me. He runs his hands down my waist. He presses up against me.

He puts his lips on mine.

This is it. He's finally kissing me. For real.

I'm not sure if the kiss is life-altering, the way I was hoping it would be. But at least it's finally happening.

something real
september 8, 3:41 p.m.

"Laila?" I say.

She's working her lock combination.

"Laila?"

Laila has that jumpy reaction you get when someone scares you.

"You scared me," she says.

"Sorry. It's just that you didn't hear me."

"So that's a reason to scare someone?"

I really hope that Laila gets easier to deal with in the very immediate future.

"Can I talk to you?" I say.

"You already are."

"Not here. Can we go somewhere?"

"Uh ..." She eyes me suspiciously. "Like the courtyard?"

"Okay."

"Just give me a minute."

I stand there watching Laila cram her bag with more

books and notebooks than I've probably had in my entire life.

"That's amazing," I say.

"What?"

"How much you have to take home. Isn't your bag mad heavy?"

"Yup." Laila slams her locker and spins the number wheel on her lock. "Let's go."

We walk to the courtyard, which is in the opposite direction of the main doors. This is a good thing because it means we don't have to risk running into Sara and the asshole.

Outside, we sit on a bench.

"So," Laila says.

"So," I say. I clear my throat. "I'm not really sure where to begin."

"The beginning's always a good place."

I try to remember what I'm supposed to say. I had this great speech all planned. But after the way Sara was looking at me in class just now, I'm all distracted.

"I know Sara's going out with Dave, but . . . do you think I'd have a chance with her?"

"Um. I don't think you're exactly her type. No offense."

"It's just . . . she's been sort of looking at me in class so . . ."

"She was probably just trying to figure out why you were looking at her."

So I guess I wasn't all that inconspicuous. "But do you think there's a chance she might like me?"

"I couldn't tell you."

"You don't know?"

"Look," Laila says. "Sara's my best friend. Even if she told me she liked you? I couldn't tell you."

"She said she likes me?"

"No, I said *if* she said she did, I couldn't tell you." Laila sighs. "Why do you want to know, anyway?"

"Wouldn't you want to know if someone liked you?"

"No."

"Why not?"

"It would be useless information. I'm not allowed to date."

"Oh."

Anyone else would be completely mortified to admit what she just said. But Laila sits there, scuffing her sneakers against the ground like it's nothing.

"Is that it?" she says. "You want to know if she likes you just to know?"

"No." I squint at the sun.

"Then why?"

I turn to look at her. This is Sara's best friend. Maybe if she sees that I'm for real, she'll help me. But Josh is right. I don't want to come off like some demented lunatic, all liking a girl so much who I don't even know.

"The thing is . . . I think I might . . . like her."

"Yeah," Laila says. "I think I got that part."

"I know it sounds crazy and she obviously likes Dave, but I like her."

Probably for the first time in her life, Laila says nothing.

"That's why I want to know if you think I have a chance with her."

"That's interesting, because last time I checked you weren't even friends."

"We're not. I mean, we talked last year. Sort of." I sound like an idiot. But I don't care. "And she's too good for Dave. The guy's a dickhead. He's—" I could go on. But now's not the time.

"I don't really know Dave, but Sara didn't even sit with us in lunch today. I get the feeling he needs a lot of attention."

"I'd definitely be more flexible about that."

"But you don't even know her," Laila says. "How can you like someone you don't even know?"

"But see, that's the thing. I feel like I already know her. Haven't you ever felt so connected with someone that you just click right away?"

"No."

"Oh. Well, you should try it sometime." I give her my most charming smile. "It'll change your life."

Laila gives me a weird look. "Why are you telling me all this?"

"Because I'm hoping you'll help me. And I trust you."

"You do?"

"Yeah. Shouldn't I?"

"No, you can. I won't tell anyone."

"Thanks." Now for the hard part. "There's this other thing I want to ask you. . . ."

"Yeah."

"Would you switch partners with me in Music Theory?"

"What? No! And be with Robert? Are you completely insane?"

"Not completely. Just enough to ask you for a huge favor that would change my life."

"No, that is way beyond a favor. I'd say this request would require you to be my personal slave for the rest of the year."

"Hey, if this works out, I'll be your personal slave for life."

"Why should I help you?" she says.

I try to find the right words to make her see that this has to happen. "It would give us a chance to find out if this is what I think it is."

"And what's *that?*"

I take a deep breath. "Something real," I say.

Laila doesn't say anything.

"So?" I slide off the bench. I kneel on the ground. I reach out for her hand. She laughs. "Will you do it?"

"I'm not saying I like this," Laila says.

"Of course not." I shake my head violently.

"You don't even know her. And you're weird. And you're not her type."

"All true." I nod vigorously.

"I'm only doing this because Sara's my best friend." Laila stands up and hucks her bag over her shoulder.

"Deal?" I say.

"Deal," she says.

We shake on it.

I race to the music room. Mr. Hornby's still there, all hunched over his desk. I've never really talked to him. He's notorious for throwing a tantrum at the most minor thing. I heard he even takes off points for yawning. So I have to be extra careful how I play this. Of particular difficulty will be constantly reminding myself not to call him Mr. Horny. Which is naturally what everyone calls him. And it's probably true because he has, like, ten kids.

I knock on the open door.

"Yes?" He looks up from a stack of papers.

"Sorry to bother you. I was—"

"Did you just get here?"

No. I've been under the piano this whole time.

"Yeah. I'm . . . I have a quick question for you."

Mr. Horny grumbles. He motions me over.

I go over to his desk and sit on the chair across from him.

"What can I do for you?" he asks.

"It's about class. I was wondering? If I could switch partners."

"Is there a problem with Robert?"

"No. Well actually yeah. Not that he's a problem."

Mr. Horny waits.

"It's kind of complicated," I say. In my rush to get here, I forgot to figure out what to say.

"I think I know what's going on."

"You do?" How can he possibly know? Is it that obvious?

"I'm not as out of it as you think," he says. "I am rather observant, you know."

"Oh—yeah, absolutely." So the guy's been watching me lust over Sara this whole time?

"It's not easy being in your position." He sighs. "I've been there myself."

Mr. Horny is, like, the last teacher I want to hear this from. Not that I want to hear about any of my teachers' sex lives.

"I should have seen this coming," he says.

The guy is good. He must have hormonal fluctuation radar. My readings fly right off the chart every time I look at Sara.

"Robert's not, how shall I put this delicately, the sharpest crayon in the box."

"Huh?"

"You have an outstanding talent, Tobey. I realize that Robert's not up to snuff."

"Oh." This would be my current partner, Robert Garten. From that horrible incident in the locker room last year. I still feel bad for him. And how Dave was a part of it all.

"Can you hang in there until the end of the marking period? He'll be transferring out of the class at that time. I think he's realized he's not too musically inclined."

"Uh . . . I was sort of hoping for tomorrow."

"Well, I'll be making changes at the end of the marking period, but I can't do anything until then. In the meantime, maybe some of your talent will rub off on him."

The end of the marking period isn't until next month. I have no idea how I'm going to last that long. But I have to play it cool.

"Maybe," I say.

Mr. Horny opens a notebook. "Let's see. There are some other changes I want to make, so let's get all of this down. Who should I pair you up with? If I switch Paula with Graham—"

"Actually, I had an idea."

"Oh?" Mr. Horny looks up from his page. "What's that?"

"Well . . . I was thinking that Laila and Sara are both really smart and they're together. And that's kind of hogging all the brainpower, you know?"

He laughs. "I get the picture."

"And I'm trying to do a lot better this semester, for college apps and all. So if—"

"Aha!" he announces like he just solved the Bermuda Triangle mystery. "I can put you with Laila." He starts to write that down.

"No!" I yell.

Mr. Horny raises an eyebrow at me.

"I mean, I was thinking that it would be . . . better if you put me with Sara."

"Any particular reason for that?"

"Yeah." The lie comes to me quickly. "She told me—she—we were talking about my music and she's really into what I'm doing and we're both into Vivaldi's quartets and—"

"Ah! I like those myself. Fine." He writes that down.

"Okay, well . . ." I get up.

"Thanks for being honest with me, Tobey."

I only feel a little guilty.

☯

I drive to Mike's house. I barge into his room without knocking.

"Don't mind me," Mike says. "I just live here."

"Dude," I say. "It's done."

"What?"

"The plan! Sara's my partner!"

"Shit!"

"I know. But not until next month."

"No worries," Mike says. "Until then, you always have girlongirl.com."

CHAPTER 15
my everything
september 8, 5:17 p.m.

The phone rings while I'm resisting the impulse to
blowtorch my calculus book.

"Hello?" I say.

"You are so not going to believe this."

"What?"

"Tobey likes you."

"What?"

"Tobey? You know, the guy who's been staring at
you? The same guy you've been staring at? Does any of
this sound familiar?"

"How do you know?"

"He told me."

"What!"

"Yeah. It's crazy. But not entirely surprising."

"Laila. *What happened?*"

"He came up to me after school and said he wanted
to talk. So we went out to the courtyard, and he told me

he liked you. And he wanted me to switch partners with him in class so he could be with you."

"Oh my god."

"I'm just saying."

"Doesn't he know I'm going out with Dave?"

"Yeah, but he doesn't really care."

"Dave kissed me."

"When?"

"After school. In the hall."

"So you were probably kissing Dave at the exact moment Tobey was telling me he likes you. Fascinating."

"Oh my god."

"How was it?"

"What?"

"The kiss."

When I told Laila and Maggie about Dave kissing me on the cheek, I explained that I was sure the real kiss would be life-altering. "It was . . . nice," I say.

"Nice? Just nice?"

"Yeah. . . ."

"What happened to earth-shattering?"

"Life-altering."

"Whatever."

"I don't know."

"Wow. So it looks like Mr. Looking for Something Real Guy has a chance after all."

"What?"

"Tobey said you're his *something real*."

"What!"

"Then he—damn. I have to go. My mom is kvetching because I haven't spent the last five minutes doing homework."

"Wait!" I yell.

"What?"

"What did you tell Tobey about switching?"

"I told him it was fine with me. I doubt Mr. Hornby will go for it, though."

"Why?"

"Please. You know how he is about—"

"No, I mean why did you say okay to Tobey?"

"Oh," Laila says. "Why not?"

"Spill."

"What are you telling me? You don't want to be with Tobey?"

"No. Yes. I mean, no! I'm not saying that."

"So what's the problem then?"

"Why would you even agree to talk to him?" I say. "Since when do you sit around talking to guys like Tobey?"

"Everything is not as it seems," Laila says cryptically.

"What's that supposed to mean?"

"I'd love to fill you in on all the details, but my mom is literally pulling the phone away from my ear as we speak. I'll talk to you tomorrow."

"Laila!"

"Have fun with all the calc."

After she hangs up, I call Maggie and tell her everything Laila said.

Maggie's like, "Tobey who?"

"Tobey Beller! You know . . . from art last year?"

"Oh, yeah! He has gorgeous eyes."

"I am aware of this."

"But so does Dave."

"I am aware of this also."

"So, what . . . are you interested in Tobey now?"

"No! I like Dave. Obviously. How long did I wait for him to ask me out?"

"Dave is totally gorgeous."

"I know."

"And he adores you."

"I know. And he kissed me after school!"

"Yay! How was it?"

"Nice."

Maggie is quiet.

"Hello?" I say.

"Not life-altering?"

"I just wanted it to be . . . I don't know. It's like I have these really high expectations and then . . ."

"I used to do the same thing," Maggie says. "Not that there's anything wrong with that."

"So what happened?"

"After a while you find out that no guy can live up to your fantasies. I haven't found one guy yet who meets all my criteria. But Dave's awesome. I'm sure it'll get better."

"You're probably right. I shouldn't expect one guy to be my everything."

But the truth is, I still do.

CHAPTER 16
the problem with dave
september 23, 3:02 p.m.

"I think I get the syncopation thing in measure thirteen now. Can I try and explain it?"

I nod. I keep my eyes on the floor. Robert keeps talking, but I'm not listening. I'm trying really hard not to look across the room. But I can't help it. Sara's right over there. In a few weeks she'll be over here.

It would be easy to tell her how Dave really is. I almost told Laila when we had the talk, but I want Sara to like me for who I am. Not for who Dave isn't. Not because Dave beat up Robert and got away with it. Not even because I know what Dave really thinks about her.

The thing about Robert is that he's totally on the fringe. He has zero status. I'm getting to know him for the first time now. And he's actually a decent guy. Which makes what happened even sadder.

It happened one day last April when I decided to stay after to use the weight room. I was changing in the locker room when Dave and some other guys from the basketball team came in from practice. Robert was also in the locker room for some reason. He was changing near the door, but I was all the way back by the showers. So Robert was the first thing the guys saw when they came in.

"Hey, dickhead," I heard. "How's it going?"

When I heard this, I knew there was going to be trouble. Not like I could have done anything about it. Matt was the one who said it. I didn't have to see those guys' faces to know who was saying what.

Apparently, Robert was trying to ignore them, because then Matt sounded tight.

"I *said*, how's it going?"

"Fine," Robert said.

Then the whole team started imitating Robert's voice in this whiny falsetto. "Fine! Fine! Fine!" I knew Robert must have been nervous and scared. I hated myself for being too tired to go over and defend him. I stayed hidden in my corner of lockers.

I guess Robert was done changing and tried to leave, because then Alex said, "Hey, dickhead, going somewhere?"

"He's got a hot date," Matt said.

"Probably with another fag." Dave was the one who said this.

"Just let me go," Robert said.

"Oooh!" Alex said. "The fag's getting restless."

"He needs to relax," Matt said.

"We can help him relax," Dave said. "Right, guys?"

"Sure," Matt said.

And then I heard a smack. Robert cried out.

"I think he likes it," Dave said.

"Leave me alone," Robert said.

"Why?" said Matt. "You're not having fun yet?"

"Just let me go," Robert said. "Please."

"No problem, man," Dave said.

And then I heard something slam against the lockers. Hard.

I knew it was Robert.

For the next few minutes, I sat on the floor and hated myself. How could I let them do those things to him and just sit there? Why didn't I try to do something? But I knew that there was nothing I could do to defend Robert. And if I went over there, Robert would know that I know. And I know how that kind of embarrassment feels. The absolute worst is when someone else was there to feel your pain.

Then I guess Robert ran out, because the guys started talking about other things. I felt trapped in the locker room. I decided to wait until they left, and then I would go.

So I sat there on the floor and heard everything. They were talking about dates for the weekend and how Dave wanted to ask Sara out. Dave said how he had noticed her for the first time during our junior assembly. His friends were telling him everything they knew about her.

"So why don't you, man?" Matt said.

"I don't know," Dave said. "Maggie's a lot hotter."

"Yeah, but dude," Alex said. "She's friends with Sara."

Dave yelled, "Bonus!"

Everyone laughed. I could hear hands slapping high fives.

Dave said, "You guys don't think she's too . . . you know."

"What?" Matt said.

"She must be a virgin," Dave said.

"Dude," Matt said. "It's the nerdy ones that are the best."

"Yeah," Alex said. "All that built-up sexual frustration. She's like a volcano ready to explode!"

"Plus, she could do your homework and shit," Matt said.

"Yeah, but Maggie looked so fucking hot in that mini-skirt today," Dave said.

"She was totally smokin'!" Alex said. "There was definitely no underwear involved."

"Here, it's like this," Matt said. "Do you wanna waste time trying to convince Sara that her virginity is a sin, or do you wanna go with the used goods?"

"I could always pop another cherry," Dave said.

"Everything comes easy for the D-man." As Alex said this, his voice got louder. I knew he was about to walk past me, so I pretended to be going through my stuff.

Alex jumped a little when he saw me. "Hey! What the hell are you doing in here?"

"Changing. But I'm done, so . . ." I tried to walk out like it was no big deal.

"Who's back there?" Matt said. He walked back to where we were. "Shit. He's been in here the whole time!"

"No, genius," Alex said. "He just walked in."

Matt and Alex looked at each other like they knew I could tell on them about Robert and were figuring out what to do with me. But all that happened was Alex saying, "You tell, you die."

"Whatever," I said, and got out of there. It's one of the

biggest regrets of my life that I didn't stick up for Robert.

As I passed Dave, he glared at me. I remember thinking he was the most fucked up out of all of them.

"Does that sound right?" Robert says to me now.

Since I didn't hear a word he said, I just nod. Even if he repeated everything it would probably be wrong. I don't feel like going over the whole thing again.

Suddenly, I feel her eyes on me.

I glance over at Sara. She looks away.

She was definitely staring at me. Again. I've caught her doing it every day since I talked with Laila. And girls tell each other everything. That was part of the plan.

I think she likes me. And I think Dave is turning out to be less than all that. So why should I wait until we're partners to do something when I could be finding out how she feels right now?

CHAPTER 17
the problem with popularity
october 4, 7:11 p.m.

I have nothing to wear.

I've already tried on everything in my closet at least twice. Nothing looks good. Tonight we're doing a double date with Caitlin and Matt. Nothing I have even remotely resembles the insanely stylized world that is Caitlin's wardrobe. I'm sure that shirt she was wearing yesterday was more expensive than all of my clothes put together.

I'm huffing and stomping around my room in a frenzy. And then I remember. Mom just got this fierce halter top. She was trying to show it to me when she was in a rare good mood the other day. At the time, I was too fixated on the eventual return of her typical nasty mood to care that she was treating me like an actual human being for two seconds. But now I want that shirt.

I turn the doorknob and pull my door open slowly

so it doesn't make that sticking noise. Sounds of a low grumbly voice and ridiculously outdated music and Mom's fake laugh all mean one thing.

Howard is here.

Howard is Mom's current man. She calls him her boyfriend, but I think calling him her boyfriend somehow negates the reality of his wife.

I hate Howard. And I hate the way Mom acts when he's around.

As I'm sneaking down the hall to her room, the floor creaks. There's this one creak that's impossible to avoid. It shouts me out every time.

"Sara!" Mom screeches. "Come say hi to Howard!" So now with only like fifteen minutes left to get ready, I have to go deal with this.

He's sitting on the couch drinking wine. She's sitting on the rocking chair drinking wine. By the time Dave picks me up, the wine will be finished and they'll both be in her room. Which means I really need to get that shirt now. She won't even notice me leave with it on. Then I can put it back tomorrow with no problem.

I peer around the corner into the living room. "Hi," I say.

"Hi there," Howard says. "How's it going?"

I look at the floor.

Mom clears her throat.

I mumble something that may or may not pass for "fine."

"What's new at school?" Howard says.

The sad part is, he really is this clueless.

"Nothing," I tell the floor.

"Why don't you talk to Howard?" Mom says. I can hear the fake smile she has plastered on her face. They both make me want to scream. I get so furious that I'm forced to be nice to this guy or the guy before him or the guy after him. What's the point of getting to know someone who's going to disappear from your life when you least expect it?

"I'm done talking," I say. I head back to my room. I'll try for the shirt again in a few minutes.

As I'm about to close my door, Mom smacks it open. She follows me into my room and slams the door.

"What's the matter with you?" she hisses.

"What?"

"Why can't you ever be nice to Howard?"

"Um . . . let me think about that."

"What's your problem?"

"*My* problem?" I say. "Are you serious?"

Mom crosses her arms. She glares at me. It's obvious that she doesn't really like me. She just keeps me around because she has to.

"Maybe it's that I want some privacy," I say.

"Privacy is a privilege," Mom says. "You don't earn it by being rude to guests."

"Guests? Is that what you're calling them now?"

Mom's eyes narrow at me. She's giving me that look she gets right before she starts yelling. But she'd never yell at me while he's here. It's like she needs him to think she's a good mother. Which is a game I don't feel like playing.

"I have to get ready," I say. "You can't just barge in here and start ramming into me."

Mothers aren't supposed to act like this. All uncaring about their kid. Only concerned with the way things look to everyone else. And I'm not sympathetic just because she's had a hard time.

Mom had me when she was sixteen. After my dad moved away, she dropped out of school and got her GED. Now she sells real estate and complains about how fucked-up her life is. She yells at me how I'm the reason she's so miserable. Like it's my fault she didn't use birth control. So now Mom is angry at the world and angry at me for stealing her childhood, and she's angry every single day. I don't think she's ever going to stop blaming me for something I didn't even do.

I'm tired of this. I need to feel like someone wants to be with me.

By the time Dave and I are walking from the parking lot to the mall, I'm over it. The nervous excitement in my stomach goes into overdrive mode. Even though I've hung out a few times with Dave's friends, this is the first official double date we've been on. And part of me still worries that I'll do something dorky.

We're meeting Caitlin and Matt out front. It's really nice out. It makes me feel like I can hold on to summer for a little longer. Which somehow exacerbates my nerves instead of helping me relax.

"Cool pants," Caitlin says when she sees me. "Where'd you get them?"

"They're just these random painter's pants," I say. "I don't even remember."

"That's hot," Caitlin says.

This astounds me. Now that I'm sort of popular by default, the cool kids suddenly like my style. The same style they've totally ignored for the past three years. I feel like that guy in *Can't Buy Me Love* who pays the most popular girl in school a thousand dollars to make him popular. All he has to do is hang out with her, and suddenly everyone thinks he's the hottest thing since TiVo. Watch my discount pants turn out to be the latest trend.

"So," Matt says. "What are we doing?"

"I don't know," Dave says. "Did you guys eat?"

"I'm starving," Caitlin says.

"Let's eat," Matt says.

We go inside and walk around the first floor for a while. I feel like I'm all that. Hanging out with the most popular kids in school. The same as every other Saturday night.

Caitlin pulls a pack of Orbit out of her bag. "Gum?" she says.

"No, thanks," I say. I don't get the point of gum. You just chew it? I mean, I can see if you're having a breath issue. But recreational chewing? And then there are those girls who cram a whole pack of grape Bubble Yum into their mouth and chomp it all loud with their mouth smacking open like a cow. Like Caitlin's doing. It's beyond repulsive. But she's Caitlin, so she can get away with it.

When we get to the escalator, I miss the first step and stumble.

Matt goes, "That walking thing's still a challenge for you, huh?"

Everyone laughs. I laugh with them. But I don't mean it.

Standing in line at the food court, I try to be myself. But I forget how I usually stand when I'm myself.

Caitlin gets a salad. This is apparently what size-zero stick-figure cheerleaders eat when they're starving. I really want a cheeseburger and onion rings. But so I don't look like a whale I get a salad, too. As if I can eat anything being this nervous.

"Oooh!" Caitlin squeaks. "And I love your shoes! Where'd you get them?"

She's talking about these bootleg discount striped shoes I found in a clearance bin. It occurs to me that maybe she's been making fun of me ever since we got here.

"Uh," I say. "Some random clearance bin."

This wipes the smile off her face instantaneously. I wait to see how she'll handle this tacky bit of information.

"Oh! Funny!" She laughs. She has this annoying squeaky laugh to match her annoying squeaky voice. "I thought you were serious!"

I crunch on my salad.

Dave and Matt totally ignore us. They're talking about basketball and video games and how they're going to make loads of money after college being stock-market wizards. Then Caitlin joins in, and they're all talking about something that happened last year that was apparently so funny root beer is coming out of Caitlin's nose.

I glance at the next table. It looks like a bunch of good friends, all comfortable in jeans and T-shirts. I'm sure none of them had to try on fifty different outfits before they felt even remotely acceptable to go out. The way I have to every time I go out with Dave. Everyone over there looks like they're having the best time. Over here it's like no one can risk busting a brain cell by talking about anything important. Now they're all making fun of people. It's like the Evil IQ-Under-100 Club.

I go, "Why did he do that, though?"

Dave's like, "You had to be there."

They continue to screech about the incident I wasn't there for like I'm not even here now.

I crunch on my salad some more.

Before this happened, I would have given anything to be here. But now that I am, I so don't want to be.

Then I see Robert Garten and Joe Zedepski sit down a couple tables over. I've seen Caitlin and Matt pick on them enough times to know that I shouldn't say hi. But I practically live with Joe at school, and Robert and I are acquaintances. So I say, "Hey, guys."

Joe waves. Robert looks scared.

Everyone at my table stops talking.

"What are you doing?" Caitlin says.

"Just saying hi." I look over at Dave for support. He knows I'm friendly with those guys. But Dave doesn't even turn to say hi to them.

"Ohhh-*kay*," Caitlin says. She rolls her eyes at Matt.

Matt scrunches his straw wrapper into a ball and throws it at their table. Then he says, "Losers."

And Dave *laughs*.

I can't believe he's such a follower.

When we're walking to the movie theater, Caitlin has a cow in front of this way-too-expensive store. "Ehmagod!" she squeals. "We have to go in!" She yanks my arm and pulls me toward the door.

"Yeah," Matt calls after us. "We'll be down here."

"Oooh!" Caitlin yells. "Come look at this!"

I reluctantly walk over.

She goes, "Can these pants be any cooler?"

"Not really," I say.

"Feel how soft they are!"

But I already know how soft they are. I felt them a few weeks ago when I came in here to pretend that I could afford to buy whatever I wanted. What's it like to be able to go into any store and get whatever you want and not even care about the price tag? Of course the price tag is the first thing I look at and I already looked at this one and that's how I know these pants are a hundred and ten dollars and there's no way.

I feel them. "They're so soft," I say.

"I'm getting them," Caitlin says. She flips through the rack and extracts a size that would be too small for Barbie. "Aren't you trying them on?"

"Nah," I say. "I already tried them on last week. They make my butt look big."

"Are you sure?"

"Yeah."

"Okay, well, come on!"

When we get to the dressing rooms, I look around for a chair so I can wait. But Caitlin grabs my hand when the door opener isn't looking and pulls me into the dressing room with her. She throws the pants on the bench and rummages through her bag. Then she pulls out a mint tin.

"Want one?" she goes.

"Sure."

But when she opens the tin, the mints look kind of weird.

"What kind of mints are those?" I say.

"Oh!" she laughs. "These aren't mints."

I look more closely at the pills. They have weird symbols on them. It reminds me of the scene where everyone gets high in *Garden State*.

"Uh . . . I'm all set," I say. "Thanks."

Then Caitlin knocks her bag over and everything

spills all over the floor. I bend down to help her pick stuff up. Including Heather's credit card.

"That's just . . . she lets me borrow it sometimes," Caitlin says.

"Don't you have your own credit card?"

"I'm . . . yeah . . . just not on me."

It's obvious she's totally lying by the way she can't even look at me.

"Actually," she says, "I don't really need these. Let's go."

By the time we find the guys snorting over porn magazines, I'm wondering what exactly I'm doing here. And what I saw in Dave that made me think he could be my ideal boyfriend.

CHAPTER 18
better for her
october 7, 12:40 p.m.

"Man," Mike says, "I have never seen you this hooked on a girl."

We're having lunch at the diner. Josh decided to stay in the caf to scam on some sophomore.

Mike is trying to get the ketchup to come out of the bottle. He shakes the bottle over his cheeseburger like he's trying to strangle it.

"Tell me about it," I say. "We finally talked yesterday, but it's not enough. She's still going out with that asshole."

Mike sticks a knife into the ketchup bottle. "Dude," he says. He shakes the bottle over his plate. The ketchup spurts out everywhere. But Mike doesn't see this because he's looking at me and saying, "Maybe you're making it—"

"Watch it!" I point at his plate, most of which is now covered with ketchup.

"Shit!" He starts scraping ketchup off his cheeseburger. "Do I want some fries with my ketchup or what?"

"The knife technique apparently works."

"Right."

"Maybe I'm making it what?"

"Huh? Oh. Well . . . maybe if you're making it too easy for her, she won't feel forced to do anything."

"Yeah. . . ." This is way too complicated. I can't figure out how to get her to see that I'm better for her than he is.

"I have this vague recollection of you in your prime," Mike says. "Back when you had balls."

I throw an onion ring at Mike's face. It hits his left ear. Then I take another onion ring and dip it in mustard.

"Never attack your master planner," he says. He takes a huge bite of his cheeseburger.

"Yeah, but your first plan sucked," I tell him.

"You're just pissed because you fucked it up. You must have looked really good falling up those stairs." Mike laughs. "Man, I wish I'd been there!"

"Hey! She talked to me, didn't she?"

"I hate to be the one to tell you, but that was out of pity."

"I don't know. . . . Talking's not enough. I have to do something drastic." I dip another onion ring in mustard. "Suggestions?"

"You need me to wipe your ass for you, too?"

"How much am I paying you for this advice again?"

"What about gym?"

"You know gym doesn't count. All we do is run together."

"You just need strategy." Mike thinks for a minute. "Does Sara ever see you with other girls?"

"Like who?"

"Like anyone. It doesn't matter. If she sees you with

another girl, she'll think there's competition. Girls always like guys more when they're less available."

Suddenly, I have my own plan. "You're a genius," I say.

"What?" Mike says. "You just realized this now?"

Our plans have been known to suck. But this one is pure brilliance.

☯

That night, I don't speak during dinner. I'm still in planning mode.

After dinner, Dad and I do the dishes. It's my turn to dry. Mom's upstairs. She has a headache. So at least we don't have to listen to Simon & Garfunkel or Cat Stevens or any of her other hippie jams. James Taylor's cool, though.

Dad washes the last dish. "Have you given college any more thought?" he says.

All anyone's been talking about at school is college applications. Mike is so frantic he's scaring me. Even Josh is buying into the hype. We have to work on application essays, like, every day in English, which is seriously cutting into my lyric-writing time. And Ms. Everman cornered me in the hall the other day. She apparently thought it was possible to convince me to apply between third and fourth periods. Even Mr. Hornby wants me to apply to Manhattan Music Academy, where he went. And Sara's in the top ten of our class. If I ever convince her to be with me, why would she want to get serious about someone who's not even applying to college?

"Your future depends on your education, Tobey."

"Dad. I know."

I bang a glass down in the drainer too hard. But it doesn't break.

"No," Dad says. "You don't know. If you knew, you wouldn't be sitting around."

"I'm not sitting around."

"I don't know what to do with you anymore."

"Well, it's your lucky day, because in only eight short months I'll be in New York. And then you won't have to be embarrassed about your loser son anymore."

"Tobey. It's not like that." Dad sits down at the table. "I've been trying to get you to understand for . . . You weren't like this when you were younger."

"That was before I got a life." I wipe my hands and throw the towel on the counter.

"Yeah, it's important for you to be your own person. But part of achieving balance in life also involves being a responsible person. You're responsible for your future."

"I know that. Don't you think I know that?"

"You don't—"

"Okay. Dad? This has nothing to do with you."

"It has everything to do with me!" he yells. He rubs his hands over his face. I can't remember the last time I heard him yell. When he looks up at me, it's like he's going to cry or something.

I sit down across from him. "Why do you keep trying to change me?" I say.

"This isn't about change. It's about who you are. Who your mother and I raised you to be." Dad leans forward in his chair. "You're brilliant, Tobey. But that intelligence doesn't mean squat unless you use it to create the best possible life for yourself. Being smart and not using that gift is a waste of your life."

"Wait. Are you saying that I'm wasting my life because I'm more interested in my music than conforming to a corrupt system's rules? I've been working on my music, Dad!"

"I know you have. But why can't you do both?"

"Not everyone is Ivy League material like you guys."

Dad sighs. "Have you thought about going to college and doing something with music?"

"I don't need college to do what I want to do."

He gets up. "I'm not telling you to give up on your dreams. Just think about college. It can help you achieve them." He shuffles toward the stairs.

I sit there for a long time. Thinking.

In my room, I pick up my acoustic guitar. I start to play this Bach concerto that always clears my head when I feel conflicted. It's one of the first things I learned to play. It kind of transports me back to this time in my life when everything seemed simple. When there weren't all these problems. And when I did have a problem, the solution was always simple: Follow your heart.

I go over to my desk and take out some paper and a pen. I make coffee. I sit back down. Then I do something I never thought I would do in a million years. I write *Life Plan* at the top of the page.

And then I begin.

CHAPTER 19
already over it
october 14, 9:25 a.m.

"That did not just happen," I whisper.

Joe Zedepski dropped his calculator. For the third time today. In the last ten minutes. It's a miracle the thing still works after all these years.

I write on the side of my page:

If I spontaneously combust, it's Joe's fault.

I point to what I wrote with my pencil. I glance at Laila. She's read it already.

She writes on the side of her page:

Can someone get this guy a pocket protector?

Maybe it's sleep deprivation from being up until two in the morning every night this week doing what should be an illegal amount of homework. Or maybe it's that I'm starting to feel like I'm with the wrong boy. But for some reason, I'm having a laughing fit.

At first I don't make any noise. I cover my face and

try to think sad thoughts. But it doesn't help. I'm cracking up uncontrollably. And Laila's going to start, and it's going to be bad. I can already see her trying to resist. We're always laughing at the worst times when it's mad wrong to be laughing. I'm sure it's stress related.

"Would you girls like to share the joke with us?" Mr. Perry booms.

This guy has no sense of humor. Like, if there was an actual medical condition for lack of sense of humor, Mr. Perry would have the most severe case.

We don't say anything. I pretend to take notes.

"Simmer down, please!" he says.

Which is of course even funnier than the pocket protector thing. So now it's even harder to calm down. I push my hair behind my ears. I nod a little to appear competent. I bounce my foot up and down. I try to get it together.

After class we meet Maggie in the hall. They both stand there, looking at me. Then Laila's like, "Are you sitting with us at lunch or what?" Maggie looks at me expectantly.

I've been dividing my time between their table and Dave's, over where life is all shiny and sparkly. The thing is, Dave said there isn't room for Maggie and Laila at his table. I guess it is pretty crowded at Dave's table, but it still feels like he's dissing my friends. And they feel it, too.

"Um . . ." I know deserting them is wrong. But I've wanted to taste the high life for so long. I'm not ready to give it up yet.

"You think about that," Laila says. She motors down the hall.

"Laila—"

Laila turns around. "And FYI? You'll never find something real at *that* table." And then she's gone.

"Mags—"

"Look," Maggie says. "I know how much you like him. I've been there. Just don't turn into one of those girls who ditches their bf's for some boy."

"Of course not! I just . . ." How can I explain what sitting at Dave's table means to me without hurting her feelings? "Maybe I . . . like, I could sit with you guys more and . . ." Even I can hear how lame I sound.

"Yeah," Maggie says, "maybe . . ."

And then she's gone, too.

After the first two hours of calc homework, I can't decide between ripping out every single page of the book to burn them individually or just burning the pages all together in one huge bonfire.

"I hate this!" I yell. I fling the book across the room. Since my room is about the size of a postage stamp, it hits the wall right away and thumps onto the carpet. My room is so small it makes me feel constricted and edgy, like there's no escape.

Like Dave makes me feel sometimes.

The past two weeks have been disappointing. Dave and I just aren't connecting the way I thought we would by now. We don't have that much in common and his sense of humor is lacking. Not like Tobey, who always makes me laugh. And Dave totally goes along with what Matt and Alex do. It's not like I suddenly hate Dave or anything. . . . I still feel like I want to be his girlfriend. But I can't help thinking about Tobey, too. . . .

Dave's lying on his stomach on my bed, reading his history book. History is his favorite subject. Stuff that happened a million years ago to dead white men. Thrilling. How can he actually like that stuff? How can I like someone who actually likes that stuff?

"Sara, take it easy." Dave gets up and kneels next to my chair. "You're brilliant. What could you possibly not get?" He rubs my arm.

I try to focus on the problem. But sitting at my rickety pseudo-desk makes it impossible. "I'm . . ." Mom's idea of a desk was to put a board over some cinder blocks. The cinder blocks are covered with burlap. I am not kidding. So here I sit, just like every night, churning out an endless deluge of homework. It's only October, but I'm already over it.

Dave is still kneeling next to me. He keeps rubbing my arm. "I think you need a break." He takes his hand away from my arm and gently runs it down my leg. "When's your mom coming home?"

Mom works late on Tuesdays and Thursdays, and it's Tuesday. We have at least another two hours alone. Not that it matters anyway. Every time Dave comes over, we end up making out, even with my mom in the next room. And my door doesn't even lock. And I know she knows what we're doing. But it happens anyway because she doesn't care.

"Later," I say. "Why?"

"I thought we could . . . you know."

I'm like, "What?" Even though I know what. It's the same thing he brings up every time we make out.

"Nothing," he says. "Just this." He starts kissing me.

It's weird how one minute I'm all tense and the next minute all my stress disappears. Dave is gorgeous. Dave is kissing me. Dave can make me feel better. I kind of get why some relationships are only based on physical attraction.

He pulls me over to my bed and we sit down. He kisses me harder. I'm having a hard time remembering why I was upset before.

But then he reaches down to the floor and unzips his bag. And takes out a condom. And puts the condom on the bed.

How tacky is that?

Dave says, "You know you want to." Then he smiles at me like he's the most irresistible thing ever.

How condescending is that?

"Um . . . actually?" I say. "I'm not ready for that."

His smile dissolves. "Why not?"

"I'm just not."

"Maybe you need some convincing," he says. He starts kissing me again. The bedsprings creak.

Nothing about this feels right anymore.

I push him away.

"What is it with you?" he says.

"What?"

"You always do this."

"Always? Like it's been that many times?"

"What are you so afraid of?"

"I'm not afraid," I say. "It's only been five weeks."

"Exactly. It's been five weeks."

"No, it's *only* been five weeks. That's nothing."

"How long do you need?"

"I don't know. Longer than this."

Dave stares at me. "You're never gonna have sex with me, are you?"

"Huh?"

"What's the problem?"

"Nothing."

"Why do you always say 'nothing'?"

"Because nothing's wrong."

"Look," Dave says. "I know something's wrong. So what is it?"

I miss being able to put on my pajamas and chill in front of the TV and actually get all of my homework done before midnight. I mean, making out with my boyfriend would be preferable if it felt right. I might even want to sleep with him. But something's still missing. "It's just . . . I need to get my homework done."

"But we always do homework."

"That is so not true," I tell him. "We always make out, and then I don't have enough time to do anything." I look at the condom. "And now . . ."

Dave looks at the condom. Then he leans toward me. "I really think we should," he whispers.

"Why? Why is this so important to you?" I know guys are obsessed with sex, but this is ridiculous. Dave's pushing it so much you'd think he's desperate.

"Because you're beautiful." He kisses my neck. "And sexy." He kisses my collarbone. "And I was hoping our first time could be together." He kisses my shoulder.

"What?" What did he just say? *Our* first time? There's no way he's a virgin!

Dave stops kissing me. He's like, "Oh, no, I meant . . . for you . . . it would mean a lot for . . ." But we both know what he meant.

Dave's actually a virgin!

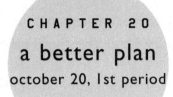

CHAPTER 20

a better plan

october 20, 1st period

Now that it's getting colder and it's so early in the morning, all the girls are wearing so many layers that you can hardly tell who's who. But I still see Sara right away.

Coach bustles out ahead of us. He yells a lot through his bullhorn. We never really know who he's talking to or what he's saying. He noticed that I was lifting weights over the summer because the first thing he said in September was, "Tobey! Bulking up?"

As I pass through the gates to the track now, he says, "Tobey! Still lifting?"

"Yeah," I tell him.

"Maybe you'll change your mind about spring track." Ever since freshman year when Coach got me to join track for a nanosecond, he hasn't given up on the idea that I'm coming back. I'm tall and thin, and these are supposed to be good qualities for running.

"I don't think so," I tell him. "But thanks."

"Well, think about it."

"Sure," I say, so he'll leave me alone.

As we start running, Mike says, "Are you gonna do it?"

"Yeah," I tell him.

Even though I thought of this plan a while ago, it needed some serious refining. I might even have to make more attempts before I get the results I want. We'll see how it goes today.

We run. I look around for Sara. We have to do three laps but the girls only do one, so I usually only have one chance to pass her.

I see Sara running ahead of us with Maggie. I speed up to get to her.

"You the man!" Josh yells after me.

I'm running really fast, psyched by my plan. When I'm right behind Sara and Maggie, I slow down. I try to hear what they're saying. These annoying loud girls are next to me. I turn to see who they are.

I couldn't have planned it any better.

Normally, I try to avoid Cynthia. I never run with her or even let her get close to me. But now I need her.

"Oh, *hi*, Tobey!" Cynthia says loudly. Even though we're over, she still acts all flirty whenever she sees me. She's all, "Wow, you're wearing shorts! Aren't you cold?"

"No," I say. I watch Sara's back. I can't tell if she's listening.

"Have you been working out?" Cynthia says. She grabs my arm. "Your arms are *definitely* bigger than before!" Cynthia digs her nails into my bicep. She keeps running right next to me, smiling up at me, clenching my arm.

That's when Sara turns around to look.

"Yeah," I tell Cynthia. "You can tell?"

"Oh, *definitely*! Do you work out every day?"

"Yeah," I say.

"You can totally tell," she says.

We get to the gate. The girls walk off the track, heading back inside.

"Bye, Tobey!" Cynthia calls over her shoulder.

I wave back and keep running.

Sara doesn't look back at all. She just keeps walking.

I let Mike and Josh catch up to me.

"Dude!" Josh says. "So what happened?"

"I don't know."

"Did it work or not?" Mike says.

"I think so," I say. But instead of feeling all excited about it, I feel kind of guilty. "But it didn't work out like I thought it would."

"Did she see you?" Mike says.

"I saw you!" Josh says. "Could Cynthia be any more in your pants?"

"She saw," I say. "She wasn't happy about it."

"Victorious!" Mike says. "You're in!"

I know what happened had some effect on Sara. I could just feel it when she looked at me, how she walked away. So I should be stoked. . . .

Music is the only thing that can take me away from the pain. It's my drug of choice. So that afternoon I ram on my guitar. We've decided to do a classic rock number for

Battle of the Bands next month and one of our own as an encore. Mike thinks we have a better chance of making it to the final round that way.

The last two times we practiced, Mike and Josh had to leave early to do homework. I hope that doesn't happen tonight. I need this.

But then Mike is talking about that Spanish project, and he's like, "Yo. I gotta bounce."

"Seriously, man," Josh says. "I haven't even started the outline."

Somehow I thought being in a band would be more exciting than this.

"Isn't it due tomorrow?" Mike says.

"Yeah," Josh says.

They start packing up their stuff.

It wasn't supposed to go like this.

"You guys can't leave yet," I say. "We didn't even get through 'Ahab's Fish.'"

"Dude," Mike says. "If I don't go right now? My mom's gonna freak. Plus, I have math and . . . I don't want to fall behind too much."

"Why not?" I say. "What's the difference?"

Mike walks up to me. He stands real close. "Why do you always do this to yourself?"

"What?"

"What are you up to on your project?"

"What makes you think I started it?"

"You're a trip, Tobey."

"I'm beginning to think you guys don't care about the band anymore," I say.

"Okay. Dude? I don't know about you, but I want to go to a decent college next year. I don't always have time to fuck around like you do." Mike bends down to tie his sneaker.

"I'm not fucking around. This is what I want to do with my life. You know that." What is it with everyone ganging up on me?

I take my guitar strap off.

"Look," Mike says. "You should reconsider about the whole anti-college stance. Even Josh is going."

"Hey!" Josh yells. "Thanks a lot!"

"You know what I mean," Mike says.

"Yeah," I say. "I get it."

What I get is that even my friends think I'm wasting my life. It's like everyone has this attitude that if you don't go to college, you're nothing. Screw that. If that's what it takes to show everyone who I am, then fine. Maybe I will apply. Just to show them.

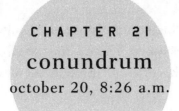

conundrum
october 20, 8:26 a.m.

Can I just say that gym is the absolute worst?

I have a new rant page in my sketchbook. I'm ranting about the lack of connection with Dave and how we hardly have anything in common and how conceited his friends are and, now, the torture that is gym.

Here's Why Gym Sucks
1. I can't catch.
2. I can't throw.
3. I'm totally uncoordinated.
4. I always get picked last for teams.
5. I hate sports.
6. I keep forgetting the rules.
7. I always have gym 1st period. Sweaty underwear is bad times.

And I hate changing for gym. Naturally, Maggie doesn't have to worry about simple everyday things like changing. This is because she's physically perfect. But I'm a different story. There's this whole complicated production I have to go through every single day to change for gym. I try to keep this entire changing procedure under three-point-two seconds.

First I sniff the shirt that's in my locker to make sure it doesn't smell too bad. Even if it does, I still have to wear it. But then I know not to stand too close to anyone.

Next I look around to see if anyone's watching. If no one is, I face the corner and quickly switch shirts. If someone's looking, then I have to wait.

Putting on sweatpants is the most complicated part because this is when my whole gross butt is hanging out for everyone to see. And I hate my thighs. I've tried wrapping a towel around myself, changing in the bathroom, or not changing at all. But then everyone makes fun of me more for being so weird. Even though Maggie insists I look totally thin, I don't really believe her.

Today we're playing pickle ball. Pickle ball is this game where you get in a pair with these big paddles and a whiffle ball. Then you take turns smacking the ball against the wall. I like this game because it's fun without being sweaty. And I can actually hit the ball sometimes.

"It's Agassi's serve, and Roddick waits eagerly to smash the ball to pieces." I hunker down in front of the wall, shifting my weight back and forth and swinging my paddle.

"But, wait!" Maggie screams. She slams the ball. I

jump up with my paddle over my head, but the ball is about ten miles away. "Roddick is experiencing technical difficulty. Please stand by for Agassi's win."

"Silence on the court!" I order.

After twenty more minutes of Agassi stomping Roddick, Ms. Spencer blows her whistle. "Okay, ladies!" she yells. "Let's hit it!"

We walk out to the track to run a lap. This is so we can benefit from the added humiliation of the boys checking us out in our scuzzy gym clothes. It's already freezing, and it's only October. Hasn't New Jersey ever heard of fall? Running in these arctic conditions makes my lungs ache and my throat burn. I refuse to believe it's good for you. At least there's the possibility of seeing Tobey to distract me.

We filter out onto the track. I reluctantly start running. Maggie's talking about her parents. How they're always fighting when her dad's home. How miserable her mom is when he's not.

"Did you find out what's wrong yet?" I say.

"No one tells me anything. But I heard my mom saying how if my dad's not attracted to her anymore, he should admit it and stop running away."

"What did he say?"

"I couldn't hear. I think . . ."

"Have you been working out?" a voice screeches behind me. "Your arms are *definitely* bigger than before!"

I turn around to see what's happening. I immediately wish I could take it back. Just turn back around and pretend that Tobey still likes me and only me.

Did Cynthia say "before"? Did he used to go out with her? She's such a skanky ho-bag! I thought Tobey told Laila he likes me. Which was the whole reason for switching partners in Music Theory next week. So what is this?

I turn back around. I speed up.

"What's wrong?" Maggie says.

"I'll tell you later," I mumble. I hate how jealous I feel.

I think about Tobey a lot. Way more than I think about Dave. Which is so weird since I don't even know him. But Tobey just seems so sweet. And those eyes. Sometimes I can't even sleep.

This conundrum calls for an emergency Burger King lunch conference.

It's tradition for Laila and Maggie and me to go to Burger King whenever we have something major to discuss. But it's not tradition for one of us to have a boyfriend waiting. We're deciding what to tell him on the way to the cafeteria.

"Just tell him we're going," Maggie says.

"I can't."

"What?" Laila says. "Like he has you on a leash? You're allowed to do what you want."

"What's the emergency anyway?" Maggie says.

"It's too complicated to get into right now," I say.

"Oh," Laila says. "I thought you might finally be ready to tell us about you and the object of your desire."

"Something happened with Dave?" Maggie asks.

I bite my lip. "Not exactly."

Dave's already waiting for me at his table. When I first started sitting with him, seeing him saving me a seat next to Caitlin and Matt was so exciting. Now it feels constricting. Like I don't have a choice about what I do. And the way I practically ignored Maggie and Laila just to have the opportunity to sit with him was bogus.

We go over to Dave. He's like, "I have no clue what this is supposed to be." He points to his tray.

"Emu," Laila says.

"Huh?"

"It's emu," Laila says. "A massive, flightless bird, indigenous to Australia. They must have had it imported."

"Is there anything you don't know?" Dave asks.

"Yes."

Everybody is quiet.

"Well, we're going to Burger King," I tell Dave.

"Oh, but . . . I kind of wanted to stay here today."

"You can. I mean . . . *we're* going."

Dave looks pissed. "Oh. Whatever."

Matt and Caitlin arrive like celebrities.

Caitlin says, "Hey, Sara!" Totally ignoring my friends.

I look at Dave. "So . . . bye."

He gets up. He kisses me on the mouth. Hard.

As we're leaving, I see Tobey across the cafeteria. He's pressing his hands over his face. I know he saw everything. I have this sudden compulsion to run over and tell him that the kiss didn't do it for me. That the whole reason we're leaving is to talk about him. I want him to know everything. But of course, that's stupid. Everyone knows once you tell a guy how much you like him, he loses all interest.

The walk to Burger King takes five minutes. Lunch hour isn't even an hour. It's forty-five minutes. We don't have a lot of time, so I start talking.

"Okay. Can I tell you guys something?"

"Anything," Maggie says.

"I didn't look at Tobey first."

"I knew it!" Laila shouts. She points at me. "I knew this was about him!"

"Could you say that a little louder? I think there might be someone in Africa who didn't hear you."

"So you're finally admitting it."

Maggie's like, "Can someone please tell me what's going on?"

We get to Burger King, and I run to the door. I'm letting Laila fill Maggie in on her side of it first. That way there'll be less interruptions when I tell my side.

After we get our orders and sit down in a booth, Maggie says, "I had no idea you liked him that much! You didn't tell me that before!"

I'm very absorbed in opening mustard packets for my onion rings.

"Must I remind you that we're pressed for time

here?" Laila chomps down on her Whopper.

I forget where I wanted to start. How do you explain something to your friends you can't even explain to yourself?

"Okay, I'll help," Laila says. "When we left off, Sara did not look at Tobey first. Which implies that Tobey looked at Sara first. Which then implies that he likes her, but we already knew this because he told me. So my guess is that we're here to talk about how you like Tobey. Since you stare at each other every single day. And since, as a bonus, as if getting to be partners with Robert in a few days isn't enough of a reason to celebrate, I get to watch you stare at Tobey every single day *and* wipe the drool. Did I miss anything?"

"No, I think that about covers it."

"So tell me this," Laila says. "What do you see in him? He has, like, a point-three GPA. Where's he going next year? Morris County Community College?"

I put extra tartar sauce on my fish sandwich.

"Just because someone isn't making straight A's doesn't mean they're stupid," Maggie says. She looks at me. "But why exactly do you like him? Other than he's cute, because Dave is cuter."

"The way I feel about Tobey is totally different."

"And what way is that?" Laila demands.

"There's just . . . this intensity that I don't have with Dave. It's like . . . like the few times I've seen him, he makes me laugh. . . . And he's so confident. . . . There's something in the way he *is* that keeps pulling me in." This is so hard to explain. How do you translate your heart? "And Dave was so mean at the mall. With Robert and Joe?"

"That was atrocious." Maggie chews an ice cube.

"Well, I don't know what his problem is with the lunch-table thing," Laila says. "He obviously doesn't want us sitting over there."

"Excuse me," Maggie says. "Not that we'd want to."

"I mean, I like other stuff about him, but . . . it always feels like something's missing."

Maggie nods. "There's, like . . . this void, right?"

"Yeah. It doesn't feel the way I wanted it to. It's like I'm forcing myself to be happy with him while I wait for it to turn into what I want."

"And what's that?" Laila says.

"Something real." I smile across the table at Laila. She's never even gone out on a date, so I can't expect her to understand everything I'm saying. But I know she gets this part of it.

Laila smiles back. "Well, it would be nice to have you back at our table full-time."

"I don't know *what* you see in those people," Maggie huffs. "Popularity is *so* overrated."

"Seriously," I say. "They come off like they're all that, and meanwhile Dave's a virgin."

"I still can't get over that," Maggie says. "The boy is truly gorgeous."

"Is he still being an ass about the sex thing?" Laila says.

He pulled that repulsive condom trick, like, a week ago, and since then he's been over twice. At least now he's decent enough to make out for a while before he starts begging. "I think he's embarrassed. He's still pushy, though."

"He's such a child," Maggie says.

"Tobey wouldn't be that pathetic," Laila adds.

"How do you know?"

Laila rolls her eyes. "Isn't it obvious?"

"What?" I go. "Now you like him?"

"I wasn't going to be the one to encourage you and Tobey getting together," Laila says. "But now . . ." Laila shakes her head. "When he was talking about you he had this look in his eyes, like . . . honesty and clarity and confidence. I haven't seen . . . I've never seen any guy here look that way."

Maggie and I stare at Laila.

"Oh my god," Maggie says. "Do you hear that?"

"What?"

"I think it's the sound of hell freezing over." Maggie laughs. "Is it just me, or did Laila admit she thinks a guy is cute?"

"I didn't say I like the whole guy," Laila insists. "Just the eyes part."

Maggie and I go, "Woooo!" Hearing Laila say anything remotely positive about any guy is huge.

"Too bad guys aren't like Mr. Potato Head," Maggie says. "Where you can pick and choose which parts you want. Then we might come up with a guy who meets your standards."

"Never gonna happen." Laila looks at me. "So what are you going to do?"

"I don't know."

"Don't you think you should break up with Dave?" Laila asks.

"Wait," Maggie interrupts. "Aren't you switching partners next week?"

"Don't remind me," Laila moans.

"You need to give it time," Maggie says. "Get to know Tobey and find out for sure if he's the right guy for you. And in the meantime you can vacillate between them."

"Vacillate?" Laila says. "What's with the SAT vocab?"

"It's part of achieving my goal."

We stare at her blankly.

"You know. To be smarter."

We stare.

Maggie puts her hands up in front of her like, *Wait till you hear this one*. "I'm reading the dictionary."

"What, like, cover to cover?" I say.

"No. I'm doing ten new words every day. Then I'm picking one to use at least three times that day, so I can memorize it."

"What about the other nine?" Laila says.

"Oh, yeah . . . I'm memorizing those, too."

Laila turns back to me. "I think you should dump Dave. If you already feel this way about another guy, what does that say about your relationship with Dave?"

Maggie nods. "And Tobey totally seems like someone who'd sit at our table."

Walking back, Laila and Maggie continue to discuss my situation. But I'm only half listening. Because what they said before is right. What I have with Dave isn't enough for me. I visualize slow-dancing with Tobey, a Dave Matthews Band song playing, being completely happy with him. I put the image into a pink bubble and let the universe decide.

But it's obvious that I've already made up my mind.

When Sara walks into the room, I'm nervous. I wipe a piece of lint off her chair.

I glance over at Laila. It looks like she's already having a fight with Robert. And class hasn't even started yet. Robert decided to stay in the class, but Mr. Hornby said he would still make the switch. I totally lucked out.

Now Sara is sitting next to me.

"Hey," I say.

"Hey," she says.

And just like that, I'm not nervous anymore. It's wild. She feels really familiar.

Everyone is doing the warm-up, which involves a lot of clapping and going "ta-tata-ta rest ta." You can tell that everyone in here really wants to be here. There's a comfort in being around fellow dorks with a similar purpose.

I pretend to listen to Mr. Hornby, but I'm too aware of Sara staring at the ripped knee of my jeans. I knew I should have worn less grungy ones.

Sara takes out *Vivaldi's Four Seasons*. Which is weird because Mr. Hornby just told us to take out *Remembering the Beatles*.

"Sara?"

"Yeah?"

"I think we're working on—"

"I know. I was just seeing something."

I'm such an idiot. She's not stupid. She knows what we're doing. Why did I have to say that?

"Sorry," I say.

"That's okay."

When we start working, I lean in close to Sara. She smells like flowers. But not in a perfumey kind of way. More like in an it's-just-the-way-she-is kind of way.

I can't get over how comfortable I am with her. We just click.

Then Sara looks right at me, catching me off guard. I am instantaneously transformed into this sweating, heart-pounding freak. I am no longer Tobey Beller. It's bizarre that I'm still able to speak in this condition.

"So," I say, "do you play an instrument?"

"I played the violin up until last year."

"You don't play anymore?"

"Not really. I haven't had as much free time this year."

It almost doesn't bother me that her lack of free time has to do with the asshole.

"Me neither," I say. "The world tour, recording my new album . . . gotta keep the fans happy."

She laughs.

Yes.

While we're doing the assignment, Sara seems impressed with my analysis of syncopation. And I caught that the sixteenth notes she was describing were actually thirty-second notes. So I'm feeling good that she sees I have a brain in working condition.

We finish before all the other pairs. I panic for a second, trying to think of something else funny to say. But Sara speaks first. "So, where are you applying?"

"Applying to what?"

"Ha-ha. Very funny."

"Do . . . you mean college?"

"Uh, yeah?"

"Oh." Now comes the part where I sabotage everything by telling her I'm still figuring out what to do about college. After which she politely excuses herself to run up to Mr. Hornby and demand that we switch partners back.

"Um . . . I'm still narrowing down my list. What about you?"

"Well, my first choice is NYU."

"You already know where you want to go?"

"Only since eighth grade."

"That's amazing." And intimidating.

"Not really. It's just a goal I've had for so long. . . ."

"Do you know what you want to major in?"

"I'm going to be an urban planner . . . mainly focusing on architecture and interior design. I'm into aesthetics."

I can't believe I've wasted all this time with brain-dead chickenheads.

"What about you?" she says.

"Oh. I'm ... not completely sure yet. No, I mean, I know my career will be music-related. I've played guitar since I was five and I'm in this band with—"

"I know."

"Oh. Yeah, so, I feel like we're on the verge of a break-through or something, something huge, and that's probably taking off. . . . And I might do recording sessions for sound-tracks . . . that kind of thing. . . . So I'm thinking of applying to music school. . . . Actually, Mr. Hornby wants me to apply where he went."

"Huh."

"Yeah."

What exactly did she mean by "huh"? Huh like, *That's really cool you are so beyond my realm of righteousness?* Or huh like, *Could you be any more of a slacker, how could you not have even applied yet?*

Sara looks over at Laila. Laila looks like she's about to attack Robert with the music stand.

"So," I say.

"So," she says.

"You know how to play Dots?"

"What's that?"

"You've never played Dots before?"

"I don't think so."

"Dude." I open my spiral to a new page. "Allow me. This is an essential skill to have. Your life won't be complete without the constant possibility of a burning Dots session on the horizon."

I expected that to get a laugh. But when I look at Sara, she's looking at me kind of weird.

"What?"

"Nothing," she says.

I start filling up the page with dots. "Okay, so when you do this, it's really important that both the rows and columns are even. So, like, you use the lines for the rows and make the dots this far apart—"

The bell rings.

Unfair. The one day in my life I want class to never end, and it's over.

"Don't panic," I say. "We'll pick this up next time."

"Don't lose that page!"

"I won't. See ya."

"Yeah. See ya."

After, I run into Mike in the hall.

"So?" he says.

"Yeah, you know. I worked my usual charm. I'm sure she'll be breaking up with Dave any minute now."

"And then she'll be dumping your ass after she finds out what a loser you are. Looks like you're in for some fun times."

CHAPTER 23
i enjoy a good pen
october 27, 2:54 p.m.

Normally I like to experiment with how long I can possibly stay in bed after the alarm goes off and still catch the bus. But today, half an hour before I had to get up, I bolted out of bed like it was on fire.

The highlight of the day was when I put this really complicated problem on the board in calculus that took forever and then it wasn't even the right problem.

All I've been able to think about since I woke up is this. And now it's here.

When I walk into Music Theory, Tobey's already there. Robert is sitting next to Laila.

Mr. Hornby comes up to me and says, "Sara, may I see you a minute?"

He pulls me over to the side of the room and gets this tone like we go way back. "I told Tobey that he would have a new partner starting today." Mr. Hornby jingles some change in his pocket. "He suggested switching partners with you. He knows how bright you are and says you have similar tastes in music. I think you'd be much better for Tobey—he could use the motivation. Laila and Robert are both fine with switching." He clears his throat. "Would you have a problem working with Tobey from now on?"

I remind myself how to speak.

"No," I say too loudly. Then I'm paranoid that Tobey heard and thought I meant no, I don't want to switch. "I don't mind."

"Great." Mr. Hornby smiles at me like he's relieved I didn't try to get out of it. "Thanks for being flexible, Sara."

"Sure."

While Mr. Hornby starts explaining what we're doing today, I go over and sit next to Tobey like it's nothing.

"Hey," Tobey says.

"Hey," I say.

And then my speck of confidence disintegrates like a meteoroid burning through the atmosphere.

Tobey's chair is facing mine because that's how we're working with our partners from now on. So there's nowhere to hide. He sits with his legs spread apart and his arms crossed. I look at his light yellow T-shirt that has ATARI in green, his faded jeans with the ripped knee, his black Converse high-tops . . . anywhere but his eyes. The muscles on his arms. Right at his crotch . . . look away!

I blush furiously like I have a sudden lethal fever. I know Tobey just saw me look at his crotch. Now he probably thinks I want him. Which of course I do, but I don't want him to know it yet.

Mr. Hornby finishes whatever it was he was saying. Everyone's taking out their sheet music. I pretend like I've been listening to him the whole time and get out the first sheet in my folder.

"Sara?" Tobey says.

"Yeah?" I put the sheet on my music stand.

"I think we're working on—"

"I know," I interrupt in a panic. I am mortified. Now he probably thinks I want him *and* I'm inept. "I was just seeing something." I pretend to analyze some notes in the third measure. Out of the corner of my eye, I see Tobey take out *Remembering the Beatles*. I wait a few more seconds before I take out my copy.

"So," he says. "I guess we're partners now."

"Yeah. I guess so."

I smile so he knows it's okay with me. He smiles back, and my heart does this entire gymnastics routine.

"Do you mind?" he says.

"No. It's fine."

I can't put my sheet music on the stand because he'll see my hand shaking, so I hold it in my lap.

We actually manage to get work done during class. Tobey's really into it because we're writing our own music soon. I love music and worship anyone who loves it even more than I do. So when Tobey tells me he already writes his own songs, I'm delirious.

I like how we work together. We help each other

without being annoying. We laugh at all the same things. And it's so weird, because we have this instant connection like we've known each other for a long time. I feel it really strongly at one point. I try to see if he feels it, too, but I can't tell.

Mr. Hornby comes over and sees that we've finished the assignment before everyone else. He looks it over and decides that it's wonderful. "It appears that the two of you work well together," he says.

"I think so." Tobey looks at me with a glint in his eyes. Totally hypnotic.

"So," I say. "Where are you applying?"

Tobey goes, "Applying to what?"

He has the best sense of humor. And he does it so seriously you would never know he's joking. But then it sounds like he doesn't even know what he wants to do. And he doesn't exactly answer my question. I knew he was in a band and I can already tell he's an awesome musician, but how can he seriously think this rock-star fantasy will actually come true?

Laila is yelling at Robert. Something about how he messed up two whole lines of notes. I feel bad that she has to put up with him. But not bad enough to switch back or anything. I owe her big-time.

"So," Tobey says.

"So," I say.

"You know how to play Dots?"

I get this immediate tingle of excitement. I'm a game fanatic. But everyone else pretty much stopped wanting to play them after junior high.

"What's that?" I say.

"You've never played Dots before?"

"I don't think so."

"Dude." Tobey opens his notebook. He writes *Dots— Sara and Tobey—Volume One* on top of the page.

I look at his T-shirt again. I bet it feels really soft.

I don't know what it is about him. Or what it is with all this. It's like nothing's happening, but at the same time everything is.

"What?" he says.

I think I might have been staring at him with my mouth hanging open.

"Nothing," I say.

Tobey draws a few dots on the page. Then he's like, "Oh, man. This pen sucks." He digs another one out of his bag. "I hate blotchy pens."

"I know!"

"I enjoy a good pen."

"Totally."

No one's ever gotten me about my obsession with quality pens. Scott couldn't even see the difference between a 99-cents store pen and a Gelly Roll. It used to drive me crazy.

Class ends way too soon. I wish I could stay here for the rest of the day, playing Dots with Tobey.

As soon as he leaves, I dash over to Laila.

"Thank you *so* much," I say. "I majorly owe you." I feel exhilarated but exhausted.

"You're telling me?" Laila is clearly only feeling the exhausted part.

"How was it with Robert?"

"Infuriating. He can't tell the difference between a quarter and an eighth note. I'm like, *It's practically November. What have you been doing all year?*"

"You said that?"

"No, but I should have."

"Are you sure you want to do this?" I ask her. "Because I can come back with you."

"No, can't. Something real is happening. Resistance would be futile." Laila sounds resigned to fate.

"You're always so sure about everything. Don't you ever have doubts?"

"Sure," she says. "But don't tell anyone I'm human. My dad would kill you."

CHAPTER 24
mr. applied guy
october 28, 12:39 p.m.

"My dad's gonna kill me," Josh says. "I'm majorly failing Spanish."

"That's nothing compared to how my mom's grounding me," Mike says. "I have like a D in history."

"That's outrageous," I say.

"Just because you don't care about college. . . ." Mike rips open his pack of butter-crunch cookies. It's the only decent thing available for lunch today.

Mike would be right if he were talking about the old me. Mr. Slacker Guy. But the new me is making some changes so she'll realize that I'm smart enough for her. I am now Mr. Applied Guy.

The other day in class, it felt like I could get Sara. Like it was actually possible to win her over. I could feel it. This one time when she looked at me, it was like . . . I wanted to throw her down on the floor and do it right there. And I know I wouldn't have that usual panic I always had after sex with Cynthia. Where I felt this urgency to leave as soon as possible without making her mad. With Sara, I would actually want to hang out after.

"For your information," I say, "I talked to Mr. Hornby about it yesterday."

Mike puts his cookie down. "About what?"

"About college."

"Why?" Josh says.

"Well . . . I'm thinking about applying now."

Mike is looking at me like I just announced that, in reality, I hate guitar and would rather spend all my time playing Yu-Gi-Oh! I understand his shock. I feel like I'm a different person. Completely driven by testosterone and desire to impress this phenomenal girl.

For as long as Mike's known me, I've always said that college is wrong for me. That living life passionately is the only way to learn anything worth knowing. But then Sara gave me that look when I said I didn't know what my plans were. It was just for a second, but I caught it. It was what disapproval would look like if it could look at you. Which normally wouldn't bother me. But coming from her . . .

Mike picks his chin up off the table. "You're serious."

"Yeah. Mr. Hornby says Manhattan Music Academy is awesome. It's where he went, and he said he'd write me a recommendation. He thinks I can get in if I just get my grades up this semester."

Josh looks at Mike. "I think he's serious."

I lean back and cross my arms over my chest. "Mr. Hornby thinks I'm good enough to go for it. He says I'd definitely have a shot with my audition and demo tape."

"No doubt," Josh says.

"I want to check out the app requirements after school, so can we practice like half an hour later?"

Mike and Josh stare.

"Okay," Mike says. "What happened?"

"What?"

"How did this happen all of a sudden?"

"Can't a guy change his mind?"

"Uh, a guy can. But you? About college? Not so much."

"You know all your plans for getting Sara?" I say.

"All brilliant and rock solid," Mike says.

"All fucked up and creepy?" Josh clarifies.

"They're fundamentally flawed, I can't—"

" 'Flawed' being the key word," Josh points out.

Mike ignores Josh. "How?"

"I can't force her to like me. Or pretend to be some other way. If I keep throwing myself at her, it's like I'm giving off a vibe of desperation. Girls are always repelled by that."

"Have you been watching Oprah again?" Josh says.

"Screw you! I'm serious. Running after something like that doesn't work."

"My plans were excellent," Mike insists. "But here's the thing: Do you really think Sara would go out with you if she wasn't with Dave?"

"Why wouldn't she?"

"I don't know. She never noticed you before. Face it— you're not exactly her type."

Of course I've thought about this. It would be going against every high-school social code of ethics for Sara to go out with me. National Honor Society brains don't develop sudden interests in fringe slackers. And I know she cares about what other people think. But we have a connection. There's no denying it.

"Anyway, she's still getting to know you," Mike says. "Chicks are like that. They base how much they like you on an emotional level. They have to be into your *personality* first, and then they decide they want you. But if a guy thinks a girl is hot, he'll learn to like her personality later. It's two different worlds, man."

"Jesus!" Josh groans. "You've both been watching Oprah!"

I'm still thinking about what Mike said after school when I'm in the guidance office. I wonder if it really is that different for guys and girls. I mean, yeah, guys are after sex more. But don't we basically all want the same thing? To find someone who makes us feel satisfied?

I find the course catalog for Manhattan Music Academy. I take it over to the table and sit down. The best part about this college, other than it being a kick-ass music school, is that Sara's first choice is NYU. They're like down the street from each other.

I flip to the admission requirements page. The minimum GPA requirement is 3.0. Shit. I have a 2.9.

"Hi, Tobey."

I look up. Ms. Everman is looking down at me.

"Hi."

"Is that a course catalog?"

"Yeah, well . . . Mr. Hornby was just telling me about Manhattan Music Academy. . . ."

"What instrument do you play?"

"Guitar."

"Acoustic or electric?"

"Both, actually."

Ms. Everman nods. "When's the application deadline?"

I scan the page. "December fifteenth."

"So you've finally seen the light."

"Something like that."

"Too bad you didn't see it earlier. But we might be able to do something. And doesn't MMA have auditions in February?"

"Yeah."

She sits down next to me. "What's your GPA?"

"I think it's like two-point-nine."

"You'll need to pull straight As this semester, which may be possible if you get your act together. The question is . . . are you ready to do this?"

"Yeah."

"Yeah kinda? Or yeah you really want to?"

"I'm ready."

Ms. Everman smiles. "Great. How about starting right now?"

☯

When I pull into Mike's driveway, my brain is swimming with the application I have to fill out and the recommendation letters I have to get and the demo tape I have to put together and the essays I have to write and the audition I have to get ready for and . . . it all seems like way too much. I'm finally getting why everyone is freaking out to the point of having nervous breakdowns. Plus, Ms. Everman helped me find some backup schools I have to apply to. I have no idea how I'm going to get all of this done and get my grades up and be ready for Battle of the Bands by next month.

I walk into the garage in a daze.

"Whudup," Josh says. "How'd it go?"

"Does the word 'frazzled' mean anything to you?" I put down my guitar case.

"I feel you, man." Mike shakes his head. "My mom is on my case something severe."

"She seriously needs to chill," Josh says. "The damage is done. It's not like colleges are looking at our grades anymore. They just care about what we did up until this year."

"Not really," I say. "Supposedly they really do look at our grades this semester. That's why I actually have a chance of getting into this place."

"But your grades suck," Josh smacks a drum.

"They're called average."

"What are you saying?" Mike asks.

"I have to get my grades up. Like, starting now. Then I'll have a chance."

"But what about last marking period? Didn't you bomb?"

"It was fairly heinous. But Ms. Everman said she's going to talk to my teachers to see if I can make up the work I missed. I had to promise to do it all, though. And then they might change my grades."

"No way!" Josh yells. "Why do you get to do that?"

"Apparently if you pull a one-eighty, they make exceptions for you."

"Let me get this straight," Mike says. "You're going to make up all the work you missed? And do all the work from now on? And do all the application stuff? *And* practice?"

"Well . . . yeah."

"Congratulations." Mike comes over and shakes my hand. "Welcome to the real world."

you just know
november 3, 10:13 a.m.

I'm all jittery in drafting. I had this intense dream last night about Tobey. The kind of dream where it feels so real it's like you're still in it for the rest of the day. I'm high on butterflies and sleep deprivation.

My hand, apparently with a mind of its own, smacks against my water bottle. Water spills all over the workbench. My calc notes are immediately saturated.

I run over to the paper towels and pull out half the roll. I frantically blot my notebook. Then I raise my hand. I'm dying to talk about this with someone who can give me advice. Mr. Slater's, like, the only adult I can talk to.

Mr. Slater comes over. "What's happening?" he says, all chill as usual.

"See," I whisper, "I'm having this problem."

I glance across the table at Scott. Why does he even have to be in this class with me? It's like I'm being stalked by relationship karma.

Scott stops sketching. He slowly looks up.

We look back at him.

Scott picks up his sketchbook and charcoal and moves the whole operation to another table.

I quietly go on. "You know how I'm with Dave?"

Mr. Slater nods.

"Well . . . there's this other guy I feel really connected to."

"How do you feel about Dave?"

"I don't know. Not the same as before. He's not who I thought he was."

"What do you mean?"

"All summer I wanted to go out with him. And I thought about him all the time. I had this idea of him that . . . But he's like . . . It turns out that he goes along with whatever his friends want, and we don't have that much in common, and . . . we're on different wavelengths when it comes to sense of humor. He's just . . ."

"How do you feel about this other guy?"

I get this huge smile on my face. "He's . . ." I'm trying to take all of these feelings I have about Tobey and translate them into words. It's like trying to describe how different colors feel.

I look right at Mr. Slater and say, "He's something real."

"That's deep." Mr. Slater nods thoughtfully. "Then what's the purpose of staying with Dave?"

"I don't want to hurt him. And everyone knows you have to work at relationships."

"Good relationships aren't so much work that you're

unhappy more often than you're happy, though."

I pick at my charcoal stick.

"Sara, when do you think your relationship with Dave will end?"

"What?"

"Are you guys going to the same college next year?"

"No," I say. That's another thing. Dave isn't that smart. And even though I was fighting it because Dave is so gorgeous, the truth is I need to have a boyfriend who's at least as smart as me.

"So your relationship would have to end then, wouldn't it?"

I don't say anything.

Mr. Slater goes, "Even if you had a long-distance relationship, which, by the way, in my experience, never works out, one day your relationship will probably end."

"Why?"

"Do you want to be with Dave for the rest of your life?" Then he rips off a piece of paper and picks up the smallest charcoal stick from my set. He writes something. He passes it over to me.

It says:

Time will tell.

"And while you're waiting," he says, "don't settle for anything less than what you really want."

He's so right. It's like I forgot about what I'm looking for. I remember the boy I described on my treasure-map page before my first date with Dave. And how I've been waiting so long for him to come into my life.

I take my sketchbook out of my bag and turn to that page. All of the words there describe one person.

And that's when I realize that it's finally happening. Because when it happens, for real, you just know.

"It's so cool that they only have booths here," I say.

I asked Dave to come with me to the diner for lunch. I wanted to have some privacy so I could try to talk to him about this. But I don't know if I can do it yet. . . .

"Why?"

"Because! Then you don't have to sit at a table if they're all full." I play with the retro sugar shaker.

"No, I mean, what's the difference where you sit?" Dave says. "You're still sitting down to eat. Why does it matter if you're sitting at a table or a booth?"

He's so completely clueless it's unbelievable. This is just one of many examples that proves Dave and I aren't soul mates. In the past three weeks, Dave hasn't understood the following: why I have to work on my sketchbook every day, why I like lamps instead of overhead lighting, why games are so much fun, why I get so upset if I get a B in anything, and why I'm still not ready to have sex. And now he doesn't get it about how anyone who's even remotely into diners would want to sit at a booth instead of a table. And yeah, I realize that these are little things. But they all add up to the big picture of my life. And if you don't get them, then you don't get me.

And if he was ever going to get me, wouldn't I have been gotten by now?

"It's about aesthetics," I tell him.

"What do you mean?"

This isn't something you should have to explain. If you have to explain about how something's supposed to feel, it takes away all the magic. So I go, "Never mind." My sad voice depresses me even more.

And something else has been bothering me for a while. Dave usually drives me home every day and then stays at my place for a few hours. Lately, I'm feeling that confined feeling even more. I miss my alone time.

"By the way," I tell him, "you don't have to drive me home every day. Sometimes I just need to be alone for a while."

We don't talk for about seventeen thousand years.

Then he goes, "Okay, let's start over."

As if it were that easy.

I keep eating. I don't look at him. But then I feel bad, so I go, "Let's play the Game of Favorites."

"Fine," he says. "You start."

"Um . . . favorite movie scene of all time?"

"Let's see. . . ." Dave's thinking, but I already regret suggesting this. This game is only good to play with people you want to get to know better.

After he tells me this way-too-long-and-boring description of a movie I have no interest in seeing, he goes, "What's yours?"

"Lloyd holding the boom box over his head."

"Who?"

There's no way he doesn't know this. "Dave. You know that huge poster I have in my room? Of John Cusack holding the boom box up?"

"Oh . . . yeah?"

"Remember—I told you about this already." But did Dave ever ask about that huge poster in my room? Wouldn't that be, like, the first thing you ask someone about if you're seeing their room for the first time? But Dave hardly looks at my stuff. And he doesn't really ask that much about me. It's like he only cares about what his friends think of me.

And now he only has one thing on his mind when he's in my room. He doesn't even bother with the pretense of doing homework anymore. He starts kissing me the second I put my bag down. And when we hook up, he's so impatient.

"What movie's that from again?" he asks.

"*Say Anything . . .*"

"Oh, yeah. Now I remember." He talks and chews at the same time. "I hated that movie."

"You *hated* that movie?" It's only my favorite movie in the whole entire universe.

"Yeah. I mean, okay, so two people like each other. But then there's all that stuff about her dad keeping them apart? I don't buy it. If they really loved each other so much, why didn't they just get together?"

"It's not that simple."

"And I don't get the whole thing about that scene. Like, what's so big about a boom box?"

Obviously, this is the last straw.

When I get home later, I put *The Eminem Show* in my CD player, put on the same headphones Marshall wears, and crank the volume. Then I get out my sketchbook and my favorite pen. My favorite pen is pastel blue and writes really smoothly. It feels like liquid silk slicking over the pages.

I want to write down what I'm looking for. And why it feels like I'm not finding it with Dave. I write and write until my hand hurts. When I look at the clock, it's one in the morning. But I'm not even tired.

I change into my fuzzy pajamas with the satin trim I always wear when I'm upset. I turn out the light and get into bed with my iPod.

And I think about Tobey.

soul mates
november 7, 3:23 p.m.

There's a high probability that I'm bringing this up too soon. I never meant to push it like this. But I can't help myself.

So I say it.

"Do you believe in soul mates?" It's such an atypical guy question. But there's no other way to explain what's happening with us. And Sara knows I'm not your typical guy.

Sara is examining the Dots board. It's the paper I started to fill in a couple weeks ago. Now the paper is covered with dots in neat rows and columns. The goal of Dots is to draw more squares than the person you're playing against. When it's your turn, you get to draw one line, connecting two consecutive dots. You can't do diagonal lines. If you complete the fourth side of a square when you draw your line, then you get that square and you put your initials inside. Every time you finish a square, you get to draw another line. The fun part is when you're on a roll and you make a whole bunch of squares in one turn. We've been continuing the same Dots game whenever we finish early in class.

"Yeah," Sara says. "Absolutely." She connects two dots. "Don't you?"

"Yeah. I do." My face is like an open book. She must totally know how I feel.

Sara blinks. She looks down at the Dots board. Her cheeks are sort of pink.

"It's your turn," she says.

"Oh. Right."

I pretend to examine the board. But I'm really trying to figure out what possible words I could put together to equal the magical thing she needs to hear to know that we belong together.

"I think it's important not to settle," Sara says.

"You should never settle." But what I really want to say is, *So then why are you with an asshole like Dave?* "Settling is a guaranteed approach to unhappiness."

"Exactly. Like people who go out with anyone just to be with someone. It's like they'd rather be unhappy than be alone."

"Or even just staying with someone when they know there's someone else out there who's better for them."

Sara smiles this little half smile. She nods slowly. "There's that, too."

"There is that."

"Sure is."

Then we're just sitting there, staring at each other. Which has been happening a lot lately. It's like whatever wall there was between us, however she was holding herself back from me . . . all of that pretense is gone.

"And when you find a soul mate," Sara says, "it's unde-niable. You have to be together."

"That's my philosophy." I look back at her. "You have to go with the flow."

"Exactly. I think the universe guides you to make the right choices."

"Do you believe in fate?"

"I guess, but . . . it's more about creating the life you want so you can make that fate a reality. You know?"

"Yeah." I love how she's so Zen. "Can I have your number?"

Sara doesn't say anything for a long time. I can see her breathing. My heart pounds with dread. I try to convince myself that I shouldn't be surprised when she says no.

She flips to a new page in my notebook. She rips the bottom corner off.

She's doing it.

Sara writes her number down. She folds the paper. Then she turns my hand over, presses the paper into my palm, and bends my fingers around the paper.

"Okay," she says.

Yes.

"It's my home number," she says. "I don't have a cell."

"Me neither. I think they're heinous."

"Same here!"

"Who needs to talk to other people that much?"

"I know!"

The bell rings.

"Are you staying after?" I ask.

"It's possible."

"If you were possibly staying after, where would you be?"

"I'd be in the physics room. Possibly."

That's where I find her half an hour later.

"Hey," I say.

"Hey."

I walk over and stand next to her. It's hard to resist touching her. We look out the window.

"Remember when you could see the Twin Towers over there?" she says.

"That was the only reason I'd come in here. It was such a rush."

"Yeah."

It's very quiet. No one else is around.

We stand there for a long time without talking. Like, three whole minutes.

I look at her.

She looks at me.

I say, "Favorite tree?" Sara told me about the Game of Favorites. It rocks. In class, we alternate between Dots and Favorites. So far we've had the same favorite things almost every time. It's bizarre how much we have in common.

"Weeping willow."

"Why?"

"They always look so sad."

"True."

"Favorite ice-cream flavor?"

"Mint chocolate chip."

"Mine, too!"

"No way."

"Way."

"How are you getting home?"

"Oh, um . . . I'll wait for the late bus."

Here's what I really want to say:

Let's go under the stairs so I can rip your clothes off.

Here's what I actually say:

"Can I drive you?"

"Okay. Thanks."

All of my organs slam against the front of my stomach.

We walk down the hall so closely I can feel her body heat. We're the only ones still here except for a few teachers with no lives.

Mr. Hornby passes us. "Aha! Discussing that piece from class today, are we?"

"Exactly," I say.

"Terrific." Mr. Hornby scoots down the hall.

At the front doors, I button my coat. Sara's trying to zip her hoodie, only it won't zip.

"Here." I put my hands over her hands on the zipper. I slowly pull the zipper up. "Watch your hair."

"Yeah." She lifts her hair out of the way.

All I can think about is kissing her.

We walk to my car. All of these ideas about what could happen on the ride home spin around in my brain.

"What kind of car is this?" Sara says.

"It's a Chevy Malibu. Are you into cars?"

"Not especially."

"Me, neither. That's why I have this one." I open the door for her.

"Thanks."

"You're welcome." I make sure her scarf is in before I close the door.

When I start the car, music blasts from the speakers. I quickly reach over and turn it down.

"Who is this?" Sara says.

"You don't know R.E.M.?"

"No, but I've heard of them."

"I'll let you borrow it. They're phenomenal."

"Thanks. Hey, so, what are you doing over break?"

I pull out onto Pine Street. "Oh, you know, the usual. Survive too many family visits. Do the expected holiday crap." I glance over at her. "As if Thanksgiving won't be enough torture."

"Totally!" she yells. "Sitting through another fake happy family scene is the worst form of torture that exists. Well, except maybe for gym."

"I can think of worse forms." Like how I have to watch Dave put his hands all over you every single day. That asshole.

Sara's quiet for a while. Then she says, "Yeah. I can't stand my mom."

"Why?"

"She ignores me. It's like I'm not even there. Or if she remembers that I exist, all I hear about is how I ruined her life."

"That's messed up."

"Tell me about it. It's so hard to deal with a single parent. They take out all their anxiety on you. It's like, she's so angry all the time. And I didn't even do anything!"

"That's so wrong."

"Yeah."

"Where's your dad?"

"I don't know. My mom had me when she was still in high school, so . . ."

"You don't see him at all?"

"No, and I don't want to. I have no interest in maintaining a relationship with someone who didn't love me enough to stick around."

"That's rough. My dad's been on my case about college, but he's decent people." I pop the R.E.M. CD out and put in The Cure.

"Please," Sara says. "I wish my mom noticed how hard I work. I could be Laila and she still wouldn't say anything."

Trees whizz by in the silence. But it's not like the kind of uncomfortable silence I always had with Cynthia where it felt like we were both struggling to think of something to say. It's a peaceful silence. Like we don't have to constantly be talking to prove that everything's okay. It just is.

I pull into Sara's driveway. I panic that she might not ask me to come in. Then I panic that she might.

"Well . . ." I want to say so much all at once. Everything's all scrambled together.

"Thanks for the ride," Sara says.

"Of course."

"So . . ." She looks over at me.

All rational thought processes disintegrate. I start to lean toward her.

"Thanks again," she says.

"Anytime," I say.

I lean over some more. . . .

CHAPTER 27
real love
november 7, 4:46 p.m.

I recognize The Look. And this overwhelming feeling that goes with it. I already know I'm not going to be able to focus on my homework tonight. Or probably for the rest of the year. I'm just sitting here with Tobey in his car, but just this much is already too exciting.

I try to remember how to breathe.

I try to remember that I already have a boyfriend.

I have to get out of this car.

My eyes scan his. I want to memorize every detail of his face. I never want to forget how this feels.

Tobey is still leaning toward me. The force of the energy between us is so strong. It would be so easy to kiss him right now. Every part of me wants to.

But it wouldn't be right. Not yet.

"I guess I better go," I say.

He stops leaning.

It takes all of my strength to push open the door.

I go around to Tobey's side and stand there. The

world spins around me. For the first time I can remember, I'm not freezing outside in November. It actually feels warm.

I stare at Tobey. He looks back at me with such an intensity I expect the glass to shatter.

I press my hand against his window. He presses his hand on the other side of mine.

For a while, we stay like that. With our hands pressed together, separated by glass.

It's good that the next day is Saturday, because I would be a total zombie if there was school. I think I fell asleep around four thirty. All I could think about was Tobey. And what to tell Dave. Not that Dave would be trying to hear it right now. I've been kind of pulling away and avoiding him. Then I told him I needed to take a break this weekend for some alone time.

The bad part about today being Saturday is that I'm still waiting for Tobey to call. I've been waiting all morning. I glance at the clock. It says 12:32. Why hasn't he called? Maybe he sleeps really late. And we don't have call-waiting, so I'm not calling anyone until I hear from Tobey. I called Laila and Maggie last night, so they know everything. Maggie totally thinks I should go for it. Laila said I shouldn't have even gotten a ride home from Tobey until I broke up with Dave. Which completely goes against what she was saying before, but whatever. It's obvious that I have to dump Dave.

I decide to do a new page in my sketchbook about yesterday and another one about how to tell Dave it's over. That should kill a couple of hours. Then it'll be afternoon, and Tobey will probably call by then. But what if he feels shot down because I didn't kiss him yesterday? Doesn't he know how much I like him? I'm sure he knows that I wanted to kiss him, but I can't kiss him and still be Dave's girlfriend. Even if it is just a technicality at this point.

After an hour of staring at my blank sketchbook page, it's obvious that capturing the feelings of yesterday on a page is impossible. I decide that working on my dream-home design would probably be more effective. I pick out a thin charcoal stick and outline the master bedroom.

I glance at the clock. It's 1:46. *Is he thinking about me at all?*

I sketch the walk-in closet and bathroom. The bathroom is huge with separate areas for the sink and bathtub. And post-modern faucets with water flowing over a chrome plate into the tub, like a mini waterfall.

It's 2:17. Why doesn't the boy call?

I throw my pencil down on my desk. I stomp into the living room, fling myself on the couch, and pick up the remote. Seventy-three channels and nothing's on! Not even a repeat of *Dawson's Creek* makes me feel better.

3:05.

I try to eat an apple. But I'm too nervous to eat it all. I throw the other half out.

3:11.

Maybe I should take a nap. Why don't boys come with a user's manual?

I lie down on my bed and toss my blanket on top of me. I close my eyes. Tobey is all my eyes can see. Even when they're closed. Which just reminds me that he still hasn't called.

By the time I get up, the clock says 5:48. I'm going to be insane if the phone doesn't ring right now.

Right now right now right now.

No response from the phone.

Does he even remember who I am?

Trying to do my homework would be pointless. I camp out in front of the TV for the next few hours.

Then the phone finally rings.

I try to adjust my voice so it won't sound like I think it might be him. "Hello?"

"Hey," Tobey says.

This tidal wave of relief crashes over me. "Hey, you."

"Sorry for calling so late. My dad was going over college stuff with me all day."

"Oh . . . that's okay. It's not that late." I glance at the clock. It says 9:25.

This was officially the longest day of my life.

"I wanted to tell you that I had a great time yesterday," Tobey says.

I swear, he's, like, the perfect boy.

"Me, too."

"Really?"

"Yeah."

"Cool," he says. "So, what'd you do today?"

"Not much. Just . . . work and . . . stuff."

"That's cool."

"Yeah."

"So, I was wondering. If . . . you were thinking about . . . like, do you think you should tell Dave about . . . um . . . ?"

"Yeah," I say.

"Yeah?"

"Yeah."

"Cool."

I think I just agreed to break up with Dave.

So the next day at the arcade, I go, "We need to talk."

Maggie taps the eight ball. It falls into the corner pocket.

"Let me guess," Laila says. "No, wait. I don't have to. I'm sure it's about Tobey."

"Yeah."

"I thought you decided—"

"Can I just tell you what happened?"

"Something happened?" Maggie says. "Like, *happened* happened?"

I bite my lip to stop the smile, but the smile wins. "Yeah," I tell the orange ball.

They race to my side of the pool table and crowd around me.

"Tobey called me last night. And I agreed to break up with Dave."

Maggie's eyes are huge.

Laila goes, "So when are you dumping him?"

"I'm seeing if he can drive me to the mall after school tomorrow. I'm going to do it there."

"Good," Laila says. "I like the public-place approach. That way if he gets in your face, he'll look like a psycho."

"Anyway, it's not like he'll be surprised," I say. "Things haven't been right between us for a while."

Maggie nods. "It's a case of fake love. It's classic. I used to do this all the time."

I go, "Huh?"

"You know, fake love. As opposed to real love."

"Define." Laila puts down her pool stick.

"It's like fake love is what you had with Dave," Maggie explains. "You wanted to be in love with him so badly that you convinced yourself it was possible. And he's not really who you wished he was, but you wanted a boyfriend so you settled for him. But all along you were like, 'I want the whole package. I know he's out there.' And then Tobey comes along, and everything clicks. And now you realize he's what you wanted all along." Maggie taps her pool stick on the table. "That's real love."

"The thing with Tobey and me is . . . we're just so connected."

"Sounds like something real." Laila clears her throat.

"You love that," I say.

Laila smiles. "I'll admit it's sweet. But the whole idea of true love is ludicrous."

"I disagree!" Maggie says. "Anyway, I'm psyched for you! Everything you want is finally happening." She hugs me. "Too bad . . . *my* life is over."

And just like that, she's crying.

Laila shoots me a look.

I hug Maggie back. "What's wrong?"

She sniffs. "I found out something last night. . . ." She starts crying even harder.

I'm paralyzed with fear, imagining what it could be. Laila digs in her bag for a tissue.

Maggie takes a shaky breath. "It's my dad."

"What happened?" Laila asks.

"Is he okay?" I say.

"Sure. He's just great." Maggie blows her nose. "Him and his *whole other family* in New York."

"*What?*" I say.

"My dad has this whole other family in New York. We found out last night. He came back from one of his business trips, and Mom started yelling at him. She knew something was going on the whole time. But she never said anything to me."

"Shit," Laila says.

"They went into their room, and I could hear them fighting. Well, more like Mom was hysterical and Dad was trying to calm her down. Then he left with his suit-case. He didn't even say bye to me or anything."

"That is so messed up," I say.

"And get this. It turns out every time he went to

New York overnight, which was, like, every time, he would stay at his other house with his girlfriend and her two kids." Her voice cracks. "They don't even know about me."

"I'm so sorry, Mags." I hug her again while she cries. Laila shakes her head at the pool table. Eventually, Maggie says, "Let's bail."

So the one relationship I looked up to was a mirage all along. Like what I've had with Dave. And what I hope I never have with Tobey.

CHAPTER 28
different direction
november 10, 10:10 a.m.

While Mr. Perry waxes rhapsodic about derivatives, I'm checking out my new day planner. Ms. Everman gave it to me last week when I was freaking out about getting all my apps done and doing makeup work and writing my audition piece. She said that organization is the key to success. So I'm getting organized. Or at least I'm trying.

"Mr. Beller!" Mr. Perry shouts. "Is there a particular reason your book isn't open?"

Since I have to get straight A's now, a bit of ass-kissing is necessary.

"Sorry. It won't happen again."

Mr. Perry's expression changes from expecting me to retaliate to utter disbelief. "Uh . . . good." He looks at me as if he's never seen me before. "That's good to hear."

I open my book and turn to the page everyone else is on. The book makes this crackling sound like this is the first time it's ever been opened.

One thing I've perfected over the years is appearing to

be enraptured by a teacher's lecture while thinking about other things. Which is probably true for most of us. I take a look around the room. You can tell that half the guys are thinking about sex right this second. Same with me.

Sara's breaking up with Dave at the mall after school. Then she's calling Maggie to pick her up. I can't because I have practice. Battle of the Bands is next week, and we're still arguing about the damn drum solo Josh wants to add. But this afternoon, Dave will finally be out of the picture.

And then Sara will be all mine.

I couldn't sleep at all last night. I feel like I'm wired on thirty cups of coffee and ten Red Bulls.

School is eternal. Too bad Einstein's dead. I'm sure he would have appreciated my latest discovery within the space-time continuum. The closer you are to experiencing a monumental event, the longer time stretches out. It makes you feel alone.

I still feel alone later in practice. Josh is trying to convince Mike and me that there should be a semi-improvised drum solo at the end of the song we're doing. It's "Feel Like Making Love," this old Bad Company song. It was easy to agree on. It has this hard jam session near the end that you could take in a lot of different directions. Only Josh wants to take it in this way different direction.

"It's gonna get out of control." Mike's trying to talk Josh down from the ledge of public humiliation.

"That's the whole point! That's what we want!" Josh springs up from his stool behind the drums. "Out-of-control chaos!" Josh waves his drumsticks in the air. "And the crowd goes wild!" He makes excited crowd noises.

"Dude." Mike wipes his hand across his face. "If the sound gets disorderly, no one will be into it. We have to reel them in slowly, and then build up gradually. We can't just bust out all loud like that."

"I agree," I say.

The song has this strong drumbeat during the choruses, and there's this crashing climax at the end. Josh wants to take the climax over the top and run with it. Like something you'd hear at a Metallica concert. But it's too risky for a high-school showcase that we're trying to win. For a second, I regret shooting down the ideas to do "Heaven" or "D'yer Mak'er." But "Heaven" is this old Bryan Adams song that is way too safe and standard. And Mike's vocals on "D'yer Mak'er" are scary. Let's just say we're not all that with the Led Zeppelin.

"The sound is strong enough just covering it the way it is," I say. "If we OD, it'll blow up."

"He's right," Mike says. "Let's run through it once as is, and then we'll see what's up."

Josh makes a tooth-sucking sound. "Fine." He retreats to the drums, outnumbered.

The song sounds great. It should by now. It's only, like, the zillionth time we've practiced it. I do backup vocals with Mike. The harmonies sound awesome. And Josh totally kills on drums. We're good to go. As we're playing, I imagine blowing everyone away with our performance. Most of the kids at school have never seen us play. More important than winning is impressing everyone. I don't know why I care. I don't usually care what other people think. But for some reason, now I do.

When I pull into my driveway that night, I notice a car parked across the street. Which is kind of weird since no one lives across the street. It's just these woods. I briefly consider investigating, but I want to get some lyrics down that I thought of on the way home.

The anxiety over what happened with Sara and Dave is killing me. Should I call her right now? Or should I wait for her to call me? But that's ridiculous. I'll call her.

But I never get the chance to call her. Because as I'm walking across the yard, someone jumps out from behind a tree. And runs toward me.

finally found

november 10, 5:53 p.m.

The mall is all tacky atmosphere and bad lighting and uncomfortable places to sit. It's awkward. Just like the conversation we're about to have.

I was planning to take Dave to the food court and do it there. But I can't wait anymore.

"Dave?"

"Hmmm?" The window of Victoria's Secret is distracting him. As usual, anything that's even remotely about sex is more interesting to him than I am. The frigid virgin.

"We need to talk."

Dave shifts his backpack. "About what?" he says.

I stop walking near the escalator. "Us."

I guess he can tell from my face that this conversation is about to get ugly, because he goes, "What's with you lately, anyway?"

"That's what I want to talk about." It's occurring to

me that planning out exactly what to say, although it seemed like a good idea at the time, was actually useless. "Look . . ." I don't want to hurt his feelings. But how can he not get hurt? "I don't think it's a good idea for us to go out anymore."

"*You're* breaking up with *me*?" Dave laughs. "That's rich."

"What's that supposed to mean?"

"Caitlin was right about you."

For the first time, I don't care what his friends think. Or what he thinks. So I decide to ignore him.

I'm expecting this huge confrontation with a lot of yelling. And I'm sure Dave wants to know why I'm breaking up with him. But he doesn't even say anything else. He just turns and walks away. And the whole thing is suddenly over. Like we never happened in the first place.

So that's how it's possible to break up with someone without hurting their feelings. It's easy to do if they don't care.

When Maggie picks me up out front, the first thing I say is, "Go."

She swerves around other cars. "Where?"

"Take me to Tobey's."

"Which way is that?"

"Turn left up here. I'll show you."

"So what happened?"

"It's over."

Maggie looks at me. "Was it nasty?"

"It was mainly just weird. And disappointing. It was like he didn't even care. I'm sure he's already scoping out some junior just dying to lose her virginity."

"He's such an ass."

"Oh! And he was all shocked that I was the one breaking up with him. Like any day now he was going to dump me for not sleeping with him."

"He's so conceited."

"I know!"

I feel free. All of these possibilities are becoming reality. It's just like I've been visualizing all along.

"Well," Maggie says, "you're officially the coolest person I know."

"But who's cooler than you? You were the one who rejected the popular clones first."

"Yeah, but you rule."

"Woo-hoo!" I roll the window down. What I just did finally hits me. "Yeah!" I yell out the window. "I did it!"

"Yes, sweetie, you did. Now could you maybe roll the window up? It couldn't possibly be any colder in here."

I roll up the window. I have that giddy feeling like when your life is going exactly the way you want it, and so you feel like asking someone questions about their own life.

"Hey," I go. "What's happening with you and Rick?"

Rick is the guy Maggie's been seeing. They met in Tower when they both reached at the same time for the only 10,000 Maniacs unplugged CD left. Rick let her take it. Then she let him take her to Johnny Rocket's. Rick is in college at Rutgers, but he still lives around here with his parents.

"Not as much as I want," Maggie says. "He only calls me like a couple times a week. I hate when guys play that game."

"You could always call him." I point for her to turn up ahead.

"No. I want to know how much he's into me. If I call him, it gets too hard to tell."

"Maybe he wants to call but he doesn't want to come on too strong."

"I thought of that." Maggie clicks on her blinker to make a left turn. "But it doesn't make sense. When we're alone, it totally feels like he's into me. But then . . . he doesn't call. If he was really that into me, wouldn't he call more?"

"If you feel it, he's into you."

"I feel it. But then I don't know if it's for real or if he's playing me. You know?"

"Yeah." Maggie and Laila and I have wasted so much time talking about the mixed messages of Maggie's many boyfriends. Guys she doesn't even know anymore. But I guess it's not a waste. If we didn't spend so much time talking about what we want, how will we recognize it when it finally happens?

Maggie slows down on Tobey's street. There's woods all along one side and houses on the other. She pulls over across from his house and turns the car off.

"You sure you don't mind waiting?"

"Are you kidding?" Maggie says. "I'll take any distraction from the home life I can get."

Standing in Tobey's dark yard behind a huge tree, I don't even care that I'm freezing. When his car pulls into the driveway, I crouch down. I hear the car door slam. I hear him crunching across the dead grass. I hear his car keys jingle.

When he walks by me, I run out from behind the tree and throw my arms around his back.

Tobey yells. He whirls around.

"Sorry," I say. "Can I walk you to your door?"

I can see Tobey smile in the dark. Light from the streetlamp reflects off his eyes. "Sure."

I hold his hand. We walk to the porch and climb the stairs. Somehow I know I won't be left alone on his porch, waiting for the kind of kiss I want.

I look up at Tobey expectantly.

"So," he says.

"So," I say.

"How'd it go?"

"Okay. Everything's okay."

"Yeah?"

"Yeah."

Tobey smiles at me.

I smile at him.

He brushes my cheek softly with his fingers. He leans down. And then it's happening. *Oh my god. He's actually kissing me he's kissing me and this is for real.*

Then I relax. And it feels like this missing part of me has finally been found.

CHAPTER 30
the only one
november 21, 7:00 p.m.

I try to block out everything about the other bands playing tonight. MindFlame rules. And we'll rule Battle of the Bands. It's simple. So what if Zack has a better guitar than mine. Or if Fred's jeans are cooler than Mike's. We sound better. That's the bottom line.

The gym has been transformed into a semi-cool space. It's all dark with lights changing patterns on the walls. This portable thing our school uses as a stage for stuff that's not in the auditorium is set up against the back wall. The bleachers are pulled out, and snack tables are set up near the entrance. When the bands start playing, everyone will cram in front of the stage.

Eddie comes rushing over to me with a flyer. "Check it out," he says. Eddie's the emcee tonight. He does all this underground rap that actually isn't too bad.

"E, I already have a flyer," I tell him.

"No, man. This one's revised. Check out who's playing last."

I take a look at the list. I see Marco's name last.

"How did he even get past the audition?"

"You got me," Eddie says. "Laters."

Marco is this Nas-wannabe rapper who always says his vocab is scorching. I guess no one's told him that overusing the dictionary can be a bad thing. The other bands are your standard assortment of genres: Fred and Zack are in Jade Elephant and play indie house punk, then there's Julian's band called Zeitgeist who all worship Coldplay, another alternative-type band, a techno group, one band that does all unplugged stuff, a heavy metal band, us, and Marco. And Overlord, with this kid George who's a genius on about five different instruments. There's usually ten bands selected to play, but the tenth had to drop out because the lead singer has mono. MindFlame is listed to go on fourth.

Mike's already tuned up. Now he's outside trying to convince his latest conquest that her life will be incomplete unless she agrees to dance with him tonight. Before the bands play, there's dancing for an hour. This night will rock. Dancing with Sara, then making the crowd go crazy, then winning when the applause for us is way louder than for any of the other bands.

Josh arrives during sound check. "What's good?"

"Same old. Fred and Zack think they're wiping the floor with us."

We look over at them, sitting on the side of the stage. They both have these glazed looks of boredom. Like they're doing everyone a favor by being here. Just because they've gotten gigs at the under-21 club in Stirling doesn't mean they're better than us. The club owner is, like, Zack's uncle or something.

"Whatever," Josh says. "That'll just make it more fun to watch how crushed they are after we finish stomping all over them."

We grab a spot to the side of the stage. Music plays. A few kids start dancing, but most of them sit in groups on the bleachers. People filter in. They reek of self-consciousness. Nervous excitement is in the air. And there's that charge of hope I always feel at these things when I have a girl watching who's into me. But now I have a girl I actually want to be with.

"Whassup?"

I snap out of my trance and there's Marco.

"What's good?" I say.

"What's real good, fam?" Marco mumbles. Then he gives Josh and me pounds. He's such a wigga it's hard to take him seriously sometimes.

"How's Eddie gonna be dissin' me like that, yo?" Marco's medallion slaps against his chest. His jeans are so low and baggy I don't know how he keeps them on.

"Like how?"

"He's tellin' everybody how I'm some kinda lame-ass rapper. That's some cold shit!" Marco looks around like he wants to snuff Eddie.

"Yo," Josh warns. "Be easy."

"Nah, yo, he's gettin' me tight."

"Dude," I say. "He's just jealous of your skills."

Marco considers this. "Ya think?"

"Absolutely."

Marco smirks. "Peace out, homes." He shuffles off.

When Sara comes in, I forget how to act like a normal human being.

Josh notices where I'm looking. "She's gorgeous, isn't she?"

"Yeah. Most definitely."

"I might ask her to dance," he says.

Not like I own Sara or anything, but what the fuck? "I don't think that's a good idea."

"You don't think she'd dance with me?"

"She's taken, okay?"

"Since when?" Josh looks confused.

"Uh . . . since me?"

Josh looks back at the girls. "Dude! I'm talking about Maggie, not Sara! Give me some credit here. I'd never horn in on your girl."

My brain starts to work again.

"Oh. I knew that."

"Do you think she'd dance with me?"

I'm so happy he's not talking about Sara that I say, "Absolutely. What girl would be crazy enough not to dance with you?"

"Yeah, right? Listen, I'm getting a drink. You want anything?"

"No, I'm good."

Then Mike comes back in. I watch him work the crowd. He eventually finds me.

"Hey, man," he says. "Why are you over here and she's over there?"

"I'm watching."

"God, you are so weird. Let's try me watching while you go over and ask her to dance."

Josh comes back.

I say, "Let's go."

"Go where?"

"Didn't you want to ask Maggie to dance?"

"Yeah, but I can do it myself, Dad."

"I'm asking Sara to dance, so I'm going over anyway. Come on."

Walking over, Josh says, "How's my hair?"

"Horrific. It'll give me nightmares for weeks."

"No, seriously."

"Chill, you're fine."

Sara sees me walking toward her. She says something to Maggie. Maggie looks over. She doesn't look too happy to see me. I wonder what that's about.

"Hey," I say.

"Hey," Sara says.

"Hey, Maggie," I say.

Maggie steps away from us a little. "Hey."

Sara hugs me.

"Hey, guys! Great music, huh?" Josh thumps me on the back and looks back and forth between Sara and me. "What's up?"

"Nothing now. You guys know Josh, right?"

Maggie looks like she just swallowed sour milk. "Unfortunately." She is so obviously way out of Josh's league. Then again, look what happened to me.

I look around. A lot more kids are dancing now.

"Do you feel like dancing?" I ask Sara.

"Yeah."

We walk into the crowd a little. She puts her arms around me. I rest my chin on the top of her head. I breathe in her familiar smell, those flowers.

We dance like that for a couple more songs even though they're both fast ones. Then Eddie blows into the microphone.

"Testing . . . testing . . . Let's do this! First four bands, you're wanted backstage."

Sara gives me a big hug. "Good luck," she whispers in my ear.

"Thanks."

"Not that you need it."

Fred and Zack are first up. They have everyone slamming by the third chord. I start to feel intimidated on top of nervous. Mike watches the crowd's reaction with me.

"Don't sweat it," he says. "We're better than those fools."

The next two bands aren't all that. It seems like we have a real chance of winning this thing.

Then I hear Eddie announcing us. "Give it up for MindFlame!" he yells. There's loud applause.

I'm psyched.

When Josh clicks his drumsticks together for the beat, I look for Sara in the crowd. Her eyes lock into mine. *Sweet.*

The song starts out okay. Mike and I are totally on key with vocals. Josh is slamming on the drums like a professional. I scan the crowd for reactions. Most people seem to be in a trance. But not in a good way. Kind of like they're watching commercials. A bad feeling creeps over me that no one gets what we're doing. But I'm sure I'm just being paranoid. We clearly rock. Everything's perfect so far.

I look back at Sara. She's watching me and moving to the beat. This encourages me near the end with the heavy drum-and-guitar jam session. I pour everything I'm feeling into it. Josh is crazy on the drums. I've never heard him sound so hard. I answer back with even more force. The power of it is almost better than sex.

Everything builds to this enormous crescendo. You can see the sweat flying off of Josh's face. Mike's bass shakes the stage. When it's time for the last chord, I nail it.

The last chord reverberates through the gym. I can almost hear it splat against the floor. It dies out.

No one moves. No one claps. No one does anything.

It's completely quiet.

What are we supposed to do now? Stand here looking like morons? Play it off like it was supposed to go down like that? Or get the hell off the stage as quickly as possible?

I vote for the last one.

Then I hear some clapping. And other people join in. And soon there's official applause happening. But it feels kind of forced.

We get our stuff together without talking. Backstage, Josh grabs a towel and mops his face off. He throws the towel on the floor.

"We are so underappreciated." Josh kicks the towel. "I was working my ass off out there!"

"I told you we should have done 'Heaven' instead," Mike says.

"But that is so standard," I say. "Anyone could pull it off."

"That's the point. At least we'd have a chance with something people recognize."

"Bad Company rules," Josh says. "Just because *kids nowadays* have no appreciation for where it all came from . . ."

"We rocked," I say. "Everything was perfect. That jam?"

But Josh just shakes his head. He looks at his towel on the floor.

"Nah." Mike wipes sweat off his forehead. "It was our one chance to show them who we are. And we royally fucked it up."

Josh glares at him. "No we didn't."

"Whatever."

"Remember when *Wild Mood Swings* came out?" I say. "And all the bad reviews it got? But The Cure was still The Cure. We can't let a bunch of ignorant meatheads decide who we are."

Mike looks unconvinced. "Like we're anywhere near The Cure."

We hang out backstage, listening to the other bands. Zeitgeist is good, but someone needs to let Julian know that ripping off Coldplay can only get you so far in life. Marco is hideous. His lyrics don't make sense, and his flow gives me motion sickness. At the very least, we should come in third.

"Okay, peoples!" Eddie announces. "It's voting time!"

Now the audience votes by applause. The two bands that get the most applause will do encores for the title.

"Jade Elephant!" Eddie yells.

The crowd goes wild. I see Fred and Zack high-five each other in the corner.

Eddie announces the other band names in order. Maybe I'm paranoid, but it sounds like we hardly get any applause.

Then Eddie consults with some kids in the front row. He announces the results.

We come in last. Even after Marco.

"Well," I say to Sara. "We officially suck."

"You do not," she says.

We're sitting on the wall outside the front entrance.

"You guys were great." She holds my hand in her lap.

"Yeah?"

"Yeah."

"Then what was up with the applause?"

"Everyone was just . . . shocked by your talent. They had no idea what hit them. It was like . . . like a delayed reaction."

I look over at Sara to see if she's serious. I expect her to start laughing at me any second now. But she's not making fun of me at all.

"Thanks."

"Anytime."

"Sara!" Maggie yells from the parking lot. "Let's go!"

"Oh. I better go."

"You're still sleeping over at Maggie's?"

"Yeah."

"Okay . . . well . . ." I put my hands on the sides of Sara's face and kiss her.

Sara sighs. She slides down off the wall. Then she does this crooked walk like she's dizzy from the kiss. I laugh. She's the only one who could make me feel good right now.

Mike drove Josh and the equipment home already. I stick around for a while. I wonder where I'll be at exactly this time next year. What if the band bites? What if we break up? It's kind of inevitable, anyway. I mean, Mike and I might be in New York, but Josh is probably going around here somewhere. Then what?

I walk to the parking lot. And think about Sara. The way she looked at me, even after we bombed . . . she makes me feel like I can do anything.

So I got the girl. If that's not proof that anything can happen, I don't know what is.

the little things
november 21, 7:00 p.m.

So of course Laila's not allowed to go to Battle of the Bands. Her father is seriously deranged. But at least she's allowed to sleep over at Maggie's later.

Maggie has been getting ready for over an hour. I barge into the bathroom again.

I go, "Are you ready yet?"

Her makeup is spread all over the counter, and she's putting on a fifteenth coat of mascara.

"In, like, two seconds."

I go back to my room and put away my sketchbook stuff. Hopefully she's being accurate this time.

When Maggie's finally ready, I get my coat and key and look into Mom's room. She's watching TV.

"Bye," I say.

"Bye! Have fun," Mom says. She's been in an unusually good mood for the past few days. I overheard her talking to my gram on the phone about how she can't believe I'm going away to college already. Maybe if she'd paid more attention to me this whole time, she wouldn't feel like it's "already."

But I don't want to think about her now. Soon I'll be with Tobey. And he gives me all the affection I need.

❂

Walking to the gym doors, I notice the windows are covered with black construction paper, so we can't see in yet. We giggle about nothing.

The gym has swirling, bubbly lights in all different colors spinning around on the walls. There are black lights right when you come in, so my white sweater glows with that weird purple hue. A lot of kids are here already. "Going Under" is playing. Evanescence rocks.

"What is Caitlin wearing?" Maggie asks. "Don't look."

I look.

"I said don't look!"

I pretend to look for someone else and see that Caitlin is wearing a dress. No one wears dresses to these things. The dress has one shoulder, then cuts diagonally across her chest and goes under her other armpit.

"Maybe she didn't get the memo about this not being a nightclub," I say.

"Like, where does she think she is?" Maggie goes. "Nineteen seventy-eight?"

I wonder how everyone's going to react to Tobey's band. I've gone to a couple of their practices, so I've heard the song they're doing. Josh had to explain the history of it and the band that wrote it, and I don't think anyone here is going to know it. But so what? They're really good, and that's what matters.

Most of the guys are on one side of the gym, and the girls are on the other. We walk over to the girls' side. I look around for Tobey. I see him standing near the stage with Josh. I get the same butterflies I get every time I see him.

"Fabulous," Maggie says.

"What?"

"Your Something Real and Mr. Maturity are coming over."

"Just be nice to Josh, okay?"

"I'll try, but if he stares at my boobs, I'm out."

"Hey," Tobey says.

"Hey," I say.

"Hey, Maggie."

"Hey."

"You guys know Josh, right?"

"Unfortunately," Maggie mutters behind me. I jab her in the ribs.

"Hi, Maggie." It's obvious that Josh is totally infatuated with her.

"Hi."

Then nobody says anything.

"Harder to Breathe" comes on, but it's not the standard Maroon 5 version. It sounds acoustic. I'm loving that the music doesn't suck.

"Do you feel like dancing?" Tobey holds his hand out for mine. I'm someone who gets highly affected by the little things. And this little thing is huge.

I put my hand in Tobey's. We walk to where some other couples are dancing. He puts his arms around me and makes me feel safe. I rest my head on his shoulder and blend into him.

As we slowly turn, I watch all of the unlucky kids standing on the sides with no one to dance with. Maybe they're watching me, wishing they could have someone to dance with, too. The way I used to at so many dances. I'm so relieved to be on the other side.

Everything is perfect. Until I see Dave dancing with some sophomore. I don't even know her name, but I've heard she's easy. Which is the primary quality Dave looks for in a girl now.

A fast song comes on, but I don't let go of Tobey. I wish I could dance like this with him all night.

Feedback from the microphone snaps me back to reality.

"Testing! Testing!" Eddie yells. "Let's do this! First four bands, you're wanted backstage!"

I'm so excited and nervous for Tobey. MindFlame has to win.

I practically strangle him with a hug. I put my lips against his ear. "Good luck," I whisper.

"Thanks." He looks like his usual confident self as he walks to the stage. I feel like such a rock star's girl-friend.

Maggie comes running over to me. "Oh my god!"

She grabs my arm. "Chad is snorting Kool-Aid through a straw. You gotta come see!"

"I think I'll pass on that one."

Everyone starts cramming in front of the stage. I pull Maggie to the front. I want Tobey to be able to see me.

When Fred and Zack start playing, the bass is so strong I feel every beat of it shake my bones. The crowd moves like we're all one big entity. It's a total blast. I've never wanted to come to Battle of the Bands before. Now I'm stoked that I'm here.

But while MindFlame is tuning up, Dave starts a commotion with his people in back of us. I glare at him. He doesn't see me.

"What?" Maggie says.

I point at Dave. He's got the rest of the beautiful people all around him. They're obviously planning something.

"He's such an ass," Maggie says.

And he's going to feel like even more of an ass when MindFlame wins. He just better not throw anything at them.

"Give it up for MindFlame!" Eddie yells. I'm relieved when there's a decent amount of applause.

Josh clicks his drumsticks together. Tobey sees me and smiles. I smile back. They sound great. They sound even better than they did in practice this week. I love how Tobey's arm muscles look when he plays. And how he gets this really serious expression, like he's concentrating so hard.

Near the end of the song, Tobey and Josh do this

jam thing that sounds supercool. I feel all special, knowing the behind-the-scenes truth to what they're playing. How they practiced certain parts over and over. How hard it is for Mike and Tobey to harmonize on one line of the vocals. The part where Tobey always thinks he's going to mess up but never does. I'm so proud of him.

Then I hear this loud cough. Or someone gagging. But it's not just one person. To hear that over the music, it had to have been a lot of people together. Like something synchronized.

Like something stupid Dave would do. And get his people to do with him.

I hear it again. Other kids laugh. It's the kind of suggestive cough you hear in class when someone is making fun of someone else. Usually there's a word under the cough, like "loser" or "homo" or "asshole." It's disguised as a cough so the teacher won't get it.

They keep coughing. And there's more laughing. A lot of people are supporting the interruption. There's none of those harsh *shhhh!* sounds you hear when people want someone to shut up so they can hear. Just laughing. And some conversations are starting.

It's a total disaster area.

I look up at Tobey, expecting him to be noticing everything. But he either can't hear what's happening or he doesn't care. He's playing with his eyes closed. I can tell he's completely focused on the music. All three of them are.

When the song is over, no one claps. Everyone just stands there like they're waiting for something else to happen. Maggie and I clap really loud. Other people join in. It doesn't sound like they mean it, though.

"Dave's a child," Maggie says. "You got out just in time."

"Seriously."

She points at the stage. Tobey is pulling his guitar strap over his head. "Could he *be* any hotter?"

"Not so much, no."

The guys go backstage. I don't know if Tobey's coming out or not.

"Wanna try to get backstage?" Maggie asks.

"Yeah."

As we're pushing past people, I overhear conversations about Tobey's band.

"How queer was that?"

"They suck so bad."

"Do any of you know what the hell that was? Did they write that?"

"Probably."

"They are *so* coming in last."

"Even Marco is better than that shit."

I push past people harder.

"Josh is such a spaz."

"Seriously. Was he playing the drums or having an epileptic fit?"

"Both."

I turn around to see who's talking. I almost die

when I see that it's Joe Zedepski and Robert Garten.

Things are worse than I thought. I just have to convince Tobey that they're not.

❧

"I always miss the good stuff," Laila says. We're in Maggie's living room. I've seen airport terminals smaller than this.

"Don't worry." Maggie sits down next to her on the couch. "I'm about to fill you in on all the details."

"But they came in last? How is that possible?"

"I'm getting snacks," I announce.

"Can you bring the Sun Chips?" Maggie says.

"And is there Crunch 'n Munch?" Laila asks Maggie.

"Yeah," Maggie says.

"That, too," Laila tells me. "Oh and P.S.? I am in dire need of more coffee. Industrial strength."

"But we're going to sleep soon," I say.

"I know." Laila shudders. "Addiction is a bitch."

I go into Maggie's humongous kitchen. The coffee Laila made before smells really good. I take out the snacks and get bowls to empty them into. I kind of wish I was with Tobey right now, making him feel better. I lean against the counter and think about him.

When I finally go back to the living room, I put in the movie we rented. We got *crazy/beautiful* since it has Jay Hernandez, and it was Laila's turn to pick. He's her main man. Which means next time we get to watch *The Good Girl* with Jake.

I turn on the huge flat-screen TV. An old *All in the Family* is on.

"Oooh!" I yell. "Can we watch this?"

"What are you on?" Laila says.

"I'm on life!" I dissolve in a fit of giggles.

"Now you need to chill." Maggie throws a pillow at me. "Okay. Truth. Do you guys think Josh is cute?"

I immediately stop laughing. "What?"

"Josh? Cute? Yes or no?"

"In which solar system?" Laila says.

"Where's this coming from?" I ask.

"I was just thinking. . . . You know when I was dancing with him? He's looking better these days. Not as nerdy as before."

I arrange the floor pillows into two big piles in front of the TV. "Josh was never a nerd."

"You said he was a geek."

"Right. But definitely not a nerd."

"What's the difference?"

"I've explained this to you before. A geek is like a dork. Someone who's on the fringe, who you wouldn't want to hang out with. A nerd is someone too weird and smart to fit in with the masses. Like me."

"You're not a nerd!"

"It's okay. I know who I am. I consider it a compliment. I like when people tell me I'm weird." I cram four Cheez Doodles into my mouth. "I mean, why be normal?"

"Okay, fine." Maggie licks fake orange cheese product from her fingers. "So he's looking less geeky."

"Do you think he's cute?" Laila looks at Maggie.

"Sort of." Maggie looks at the floor.

I'm totally shocked. "Ew! He's, like, the epitome of immature!"

"Get out!" Maggie yells. "I don't mean for me! No, I was thinking about fixing him up with Brenda."

I'm like, "Since when do you know Brenda?"

"Since we got put together for that history project. She's cool."

"Yeah, right," Laila says. "You are so hot for Josh!"

"Uh, well, no," Maggie says. "It's for Brenda?"

I can't decide which piece of information is more astounding: Maggie thinking a geek like Josh is cute or Maggie thinking a punk like Brenda is cool. It must be the full moon.

"I can't believe you thought I liked him," Maggie huffs. *"Jeez."*

"That's why I was like . . . " I make a repulsed face.

"These high-school boys are too immature for me," Maggie announces. "I'm only dating college guys from now on. Guys my age don't know how to handle me!"

"You're too hot to handle." I press my finger against Maggie's arm and then pull it away quickly. "Ouch! Too hot to touch!" I make a sizzling noise. "Stand back!"

"Well, stand back unless your name is Rick."

"Oh, yeah!" I say. "What's the progress in Lovaville?"

"Much improved. He's incredible. He's such a good kisser. Among other things."

"Like what?"

"Huh?"

"Like what other things?"

"Whatever." She shrugs. "Anything I want."

"Are you going to sleep with him?" Laila eyes Maggie.

"Probably."

I say, "But you've only been going out for, like—"

"So what? We're not twelve anymore. I'm eighteen. I'm supposed to be an adult now. What's the big deal?"

"Since when is having sex not a big deal?" I say.

"I'm not exactly a virgin. Anyway. Don't you feel like you want to sleep with Tobey?"

"Maybe."

"Then you're not ready. You'll know it when you are."

Laila goes, "Okay, Miss After-School Special."

I put the movie on and get back into my pillow piles.

Halfway through the movie, we pause it for a bathroom-slash-beverage-refill break. Maggie's upstairs talking to her mom. She told me how her mom's been spending a lot of time in bed lately. I could never just go talk to my mom like that. Or even ask her if something's wrong. It would feel way too uncomfortable.

I look at Laila. "Maggie told you how Dave sabotaged Tobey's band?"

"Yeah. It's classic acting-out. He's still hurt."

"About me dumping him?"

"Yeah."

"Like he even cared."

"Of course he cared! He got dumped. You think he can't feel it?"

"Please. Like I ever knew what he really felt. He was probably fantasizing about every girl on the cheerleader squad while he was telling me how much he wanted to sleep with me."

"Some people just don't know how to act."

"I can't believe I ever wanted them to like me! Uuuuhh!" I smother my face with a pillow.

"So you were going through a phase. It's over."

I come up for air. "How shallow is that?"

"No regrets," Laila tells me. "You found something real."

"Will you quit saying that?"

"You know you love it."

She's right. Laila's always right.

CHAPTER 32

one of those talks
november 29, 4:51 p.m.

"Try not to highlight so much, though," she says.

We're in my room. I spent three hours cleaning it yesterday so Sara wouldn't find out what a slob I am.

So far today, she helped me make a schedule of everything I have to do. She says I'm all cute with my day planner. I also asked her for help with my essays. She seems into it. Which rocks, because now we finally have something substantial in common. Besides the million other little things that make me feel so comfortable around her.

Now she's demonstrating study skills.

"But this whole section looks important," I say. "And using the highlighter is fun."

"Yeah, but you should only be selecting the key ideas."

"This whole section looks key."

We're doing study sessions at my house twice a week. Sara's trying to be patient. I'm sure this is much harder than she thought it would be. My study habits have sucked since freshman year. It's so hard to change, even when you want to. But I promised her I would try. And so far I've been getting all A's.

My parents aren't home. It's hard to focus on this stuff when the knowledge that my parents aren't home is draining my power of concentration.

"It looks like it," Sara says, "but it's not."

"What parts would you highlight?"

Sara picks up the neon orange highlighter. Her chair scrapes against the floor as she slides it closer to mine. We huddle together over the history book on my desk.

"Maybe just . . ." She slowly swipes the highlighter over a sentence. "And . . ." She highlights another one. It's all the same to me. It's like she has this knack for knowing exactly what every teacher wants. Was I zoning out when they explained how to do this in third grade?

"I hate history," I say.

"Same here," she says.

"You do?"

"Totally."

"Then why do you care so much?"

"This stuff doesn't matter. What matters is what you do with it." Sara snaps the highlighter cap on. "I try not to think about how boring it is. I just keep reminding myself about how I want my life to be and what I have to do to get there. Then it's simple."

She is way determined to succeed. My goals haven't inspired the same amount of motivation for me. But now I have some reasons to quit slacking. A few kids came up to me after the Battle and said they liked MindFlame, but it's obvious that most people think we suck. So the band's not exactly going anywhere at the moment. And now I really want Manhattan Music Academy to take me. But mostly, there's Sara.

After an hour of reading and trying to restrict my high-lighting addiction to key concepts, I couldn't be more exhausted. A nap would be good right about now. But Sara's over on my bed, tearing through a pile of physics handouts like I'm going to give her a pop quiz any second. She looks so sexy leaning back against my pillows like that. Mike always laughs that I have so many pillows. He's always joking about, *Where are the stuffed animals?* But he doesn't get it. Girls love my pillows. They make the bed more inviting.

And my parents still aren't home.

I go over and sit on my bed. Sara sorts the pile of paper into smaller piles.

"When do we get a break?" I ask.

"According to our contractual agreement," Sara says, "break time doesn't happen until you're done with your homework for at least one subject."

"I'm done."

"With what?"

"History."

"You were still on history?"

"Yeah, but I'm done now."

Sara looks at me skeptically.

"I'm serious. I'm ready for my break."

"Okay." Sara stretches her arms out. "I guess we could take a break. A short one."

"What should we do?" I attempt to telepathically convince Sara to announce that we should hook up.

"Talk," she says.

"Oh. Yeah. Well . . . okay."

"Is there something you'd rather do?"

"Who, me? Nah. Talking's good."

"Good." Sara pulls her legs against her chest. She wraps her arms around her legs.

"What do you want to talk about?" I try to get comfortable.

"Relationships," she says.

Suddenly things take on a serious tone. I hope this isn't one of those talks where you have to go over the details of every single girl you've ever jerked off to. Sara doesn't seem like the jealous type. But you never know.

"Okay," I say.

"I was just wondering . . ." Sara traces her finger in circles on her knee.

"Yeah?" Maybe we'll be done talking soon and she'll want to hook up. If we still have some break time left. I try to arrange my expression so it appears interested.

"Have you ever . . . I mean I know I'm not your first girl-friend or anything, but . . . were you ever . . . like . . . serious about anyone else?"

I take a few seconds before answering. Girls ask you things that sound one way but really mean something else. What does Sara want to know? If I ever liked anyone else as much as her?

Does she think I'm a virgin?

"Um." I decide clarification is the best approach. "Do you mean did I have a girlfriend for a long time?"

"Yeah."

"Not really."

"Did you ever go out with Cynthia?"

"Sort of." This part can get tricky. Having sex with someone and going out with them are two different things. I never considered Cynthia to be my girlfriend. I don't want to lie to Sara. But I also don't want to tell her a bunch of stuff that's just going to make her obsess and worry. Does she really need to know about every girl I've hooked up with? Not that it's that many. And is this the right time to admit that I slept with Cynthia? I just think it's unnecessary to tell her all of that. At least, it is at this point. "I haven't had a long-term girlfriend, though."

"How long did you go out with her?"

"Not too long."

"So how long was your longest relationship?"

"Uh . . . three months?"

"What happened with *that* girl?"

"You mean why did we break up?"

"Yeah."

"She was kind of neurotic . . . and, like, really goth and depressing all the time."

"Who was it?"

"You know Brenda?"

Sara nods.

"Brenda."

Sara presses her lips together. She nods some more.

"How long did you and Scott go out for?"

"Most of last year."

"What happened with you guys?" I'm sure she didn't sleep with *that* dork.

Sara picks a piece of bubble wrap off the floor. My dad got a new computer last week. I kept the bubble wrap from the box. I like to pop it when I'm stressed.

Sara pops the bubble wrap. "Scott's a great guy. It's just . . . he didn't make my record skip."

I knew it.

I laugh. "Been there."

"Yeah."

"Do *I*?"

"Do you what?"

"Make your record skip."

"Pretty much," she says.

"Yeah?"

"Yeah." Sara smiles. She just looks so cute.

I lean over.

"Don't go there." She holds up her hand.

"Why not?"

"We have to study."

"But—"

"I want to, but we can't. You have to focus, or you'll never get through everything."

"Man, you're harsh."

"Break is over." Sara picks up one of the physics piles. "Back to work."

"Okay . . . well . . . am I allowed to go to the store? We're out of snacks."

Sara gives me a look like I'm trying to get out of studying.

"No, I'm serious! If I'm working insane hours, my body requires very specific types of fuel."

"Like what?"

"Like Mallomars and Oreos and—"

"Oooh! The ones with the mint filling?"

"Those would be them."

Sara bites her lip. "Okay, you can go."

"Thanks. You want anything else?"

"Just those. Thanks."

"Cool." I don't get up. "Can I have a good-bye kiss?"

"Yeah. But just one!"

"Understood." I crawl over to Sara. She giggles.

"Just one," I whisper. Then I kiss her.

The hardest thing I do all week is get off my bed. And leave the house. While my parents still aren't home.

CHAPTER 33
real experiences
december 22, 4:15 p.m.

I have no idea why I'm this nervous.

But I am.

I'm like, "So this is my room."

But what it really feels like is, *Here's my bed and some other stuff.*

"I like it," Tobey says.

Is he looking at my bed? Why does my bed feel like it's the only thing in the room?

"Seriously?" I say.

"Completely. It's so you."

"It's way too small. And this desk is just like . . ." I make a face like, *Who else has a desk like this?*

"It's cool. Is that burlap?"

"Yeah."

"Kickin' it old-school."

"Unfortunately."

Tobey looks at the things on my shelves. "You have a xylophone?"

"Oh. Yeah."

"Random!"

"Totally. Yeah, my old babysitter gave it to me when I was, like, five."

"Can you play?"

"Sort of."

"That's cool," Tobey says. "I haven't mastered the art of xylophone yet. Maybe you can teach me."

"Sure." I quickly check the back of my door to make sure I didn't leave any bras hanging there. "It's an experience you don't want to miss."

Tobey smiles at me. "I have a feeling you'll be showing me a lot of those."

I feel my cheeks get hot. "And . . ." I go over to my bed. I'm desperately trying to divert Tobey's attention away from my burning face. But diverting the attention to my bed was an example of bad decision-making skills in action. Now I'm blushing even more because I'm sitting on my bed. "This is Chez." I pick up my stuffed koala bear I've had since before I can remember. "It's short for Mr. Chester M. Wick."

"I dig his shirt," Tobey says. Chez wears a vintage *Late Night with David Letterman* T-shirt. "I'm a total Dave fanatic."

"Me, too! Whenever there's someone good on, I tape him and watch it after school."

Tobey goes, "Same. Except now I have so much to do . . . it's quite possible I'll never see Dave again."

"That is just not true. You already have straight A's so far. And after your apps are in and your makeup work is done, all you have to do is keep up. It's easy."

"Maybe for you. . . ."

"It will be for you, too. You'll see."

Tobey goes over to my CD rack. I watch him inspect my CDs. I always thought that if a guy really liked me, he'd at least make an effort to see what kind of music I was into. Dave would only pick out the ones he had and then play those. But Tobey's really looking at all of them. I hope he likes what I like. Not that we have to like *all* the same things. I just love how we have so much in common.

"I can't believe you have this!" He holds up The Shins. "The Shins are sick!"

"Why can't you believe it?"

"I don't know. You just seem . . . I didn't know you were into alternative stuff." He picks up another CD. "Who's Nick Drake?"

"Put it on. He's awesome."

Tobey puts the CD on. Then he comes over and hugs me. I lean my head on his chest.

"I want to know everything about you," he whispers.

"Same here," I whisper back.

There's so much I want to say to him. I'm dying to tell him everything I'm thinking. But I don't want to freak him out.

Tobey starts swaying to the music. I sway with him. I love the way it feels like Tobey's really with me, like he's not holding any part of himself back.

The song ends.

"What are you thinking?" I whisper.

"Right now?" Tobey whispers.

"Yeah."

"I'm thinking I can't believe we're finally together." He moves his hand down my hair.

That's when I realize it would be impossible to freak him out with how I feel about him. Because I'm pretty sure he feels the same way.

"What are you thinking?" he asks.

"I think . . ." My heart almost stops for a second. "I think . . . I'm falling in love with you."

Tobey doesn't freak out. He kisses me over and over, barely pressing his lips against mine.

After he leaves, I turn the lights off. I put *Disintegration* in my CD player and lie down on my bed. I listen to the whole thing, replaying what just happened five hundred times in my head, over and over until I don't know how I'll ever be able to think of anything else again.

The next day is the day I agreed to do something totally out of character for me. Tobey said since I turned him on to a new way of life, he wants me to experience part of his old way of life. It will be the first time for me and the last time for him. Since it's the last day before Christmas break and most teachers are doing games and stuff anyway, I don't feel too guilty about our plan.

Plus everyone's all hyper, like wearing tinsel and giving out candy canes and cards, which is annoying and makes me want to leave.

In homeroom, I'm ignoring Caitlin & Co. They've been ignoring me since Dave and I split anyway, so it's not that hard. But it's pathetic that whether Caitlin talks to me depends on who I'm going out with. So I'm focusing on drawing a blue door in my sketchbook. The thing about this door is that it also comes with two blue porch lights. They symbolize a source of pure blue energy. I swear I was a moth in another life. I'm drawn to lights, any lights, especially at night. But blue lights in particular always make me get this intense feeling.

On my way to gym, I throw my stuff in my locker. There's a neon orange Post-it note stuck up. It says:

S-

Meet me here before class.

-T

I peel off the note and stick it inside my sketchbook. It's already obvious that I'm going to do a page about this day. Whenever something major is happening in my life, I mentally design the sketchbook page to document it later. But I'm still in the moment, feeling everything, so I put my sketchbook away.

This is too exciting. And also scary. What if we get caught? I don't know how I'm supposed to function like a normal person until ninth period.

I can't eat my lunch.

"Aren't you hungry?" Laila asks.

"Nerves."

"Relax," Maggie says. "It'll be fab."

"Are you actually going through with this?" Laila squints at me.

"Yes. I promised Tobey."

"I don't know why it's so important to him," Laila says. "Isn't he reformed?"

"The point is to share something about his past life so I can understand where he's coming from better. And he says I'll have a ridiculous amount of fun."

"Hmmm." Laila bites into her soggy cafeteria pizza.

"And it's the last time I'll get to do something like this," I say. "I don't want to graduate and be sitting around on some random porch ten years from now, regretting. You have to live in the moment. You can't let experiences pass you by without doing anything about it."

"Preach it, sister girl." Maggie waves her hand in the air.

"Can I sit with you guys?"

We look up at Josh. He looks like a lost puppy.

"Um." I look over at Laila and Maggie. Sometimes Tobey sits with us, but we haven't advanced to the stage of combining lunch tables yet.

"Uh . . ."

Laila mouths *No!* to me.

Maggie jumps in. "It's just that we're talking about . . . girl stuff. It would be boring for you."

"Oh, I don't think that would be boring at all. In fact, it's one of my favorite topics." He has this big cheesy smile.

"Where's Tobey?" I ask him.

"I don't know. Somewhere with Mike. They like spending quality time alone together." Josh gives me a look. "I'd be worried if I were you, Sara."

I laugh. Josh is such a case.

"Grimy," Maggie says.

There's that big cheesy smile again.

Maggie smiles a little.

He goes, "Anyway . . . later." He lopes off toward the drama geeks' table.

Laila scrutinizes Maggie's face. "What's up with you?"

"What?" Maggie sips her lemonade. "Nothing."

"Nooo," Laila presses. "Something is definitely up. I mean, other than Josh's Mr. Happy."

"Oh my god!" Maggie yells. "I so do not like him!"

"Are you sure? Because it looked to me like—"

"Of course I'm sure. Come on. Josh? *Ew.*"

"Whatever," Laila says.

"Like we don't have more important matters to discuss." Maggie fans her face with a napkin, which is completely ineffective. "What's the story with later on?"

"We're going after eighth period."

A roar of general chaos emanates from the jock table. We look over. Dave is doing something juvenile involving his straw and his nose. How could I have missed the part where he's so fifth-grade?

"Hideous," Laila decides.

"Abhorrent," Maggie adds.

"Ooh!" I say. "More reading of the dictionary?"

"But of course."

My nerves twang for the rest of the day. But in a good way. It's like I'm actually starting to have real experiences. Ones that actually mean something.

By the time I meet Tobey at our lockers, I couldn't be more nervous.

"Ready?" Tobey says.

I used to have this problem with listening to myself. My soul would be screaming directions, and I'd always do the opposite thing. Normally I would back out of a plan like this. And I do feel the old me trying to ignore my heart. But the new me goes with the flow.

So I nod.

I can't believe I'm going to cut class.

I've never cut class in my life.

I love how we walk down the hall, like we own it. Like we can leave anytime we want. It doesn't matter that we have to go out the side door and sneak to the parking lot so no one sees us.

It feels incredible to be outside when I'm supposed to be inside. The sensation of freedom is intoxicating.

We drive until we get to the way-back roads. The

dirt road we turn onto is a dead end. There's nothing but trees everywhere you look.

Tobey turns the car off. He reaches over and takes something out of the glove compartment. It's crookedly wrapped in the Sunday comics.

"Merry Christmas." He holds the gift out to me.

"Wow. Did you wrap this yourself?"

"Of course not. I had it professionally done."

"Impressive."

"You deserve the best."

I take his gift out of my bag. We agreed to exchange gifts today since we'll be stuck doing family things for the next few days. I made him a mix CD and gave him a blacklight bulb.

I unwrap my gift. Of course he made me a mix CD, too. But then he also gave me the new White Stripes.

Tobey pushes around all these tapes and CDs covering the backseat.

I look at them. "Is there any kind of music you don't listen to?"

"No. Well, opera maybe."

"Who's Jane's Addiction?"

"They're phenomenal. You can borrow it."

"Okay. Thanks."

He goes, "Here's that R.E.M. I was playing before."

I love how he said "before." I love how we have this history.

Tobey hands it to me. "Borrow it for as long as you want."

I examine the cover. "Why's the cover orange if it's called *Green*?"

"Stare at it."

"I'm almost positive it's orange."

Tobey takes the CD and holds it in front of my face. "Just stare at it."

I stare at it. I try not to laugh.

"Now look away really fast."

I refocus on the glove compartment. A splotch of green hovers over it for a few seconds.

"Oh! Cool!"

"Complementary colors."

"Yeah."

We both sneak a look at each other at the same time. Then we quickly look out at the trees.

"So, um . . . I hope you like the mix CD," he says. "I put 'You Are the Everything' from *Green* on there— that was the one you liked—and there's some Journey and live James Taylor. . . . Oh, and some of that Led Zeppelin you liked—"

"Yeah!" I love how he always remembers what I like. "Thanks."

Suddenly I feel that pull toward him. A tingly feeling spreads along the back of my neck when he kisses me. My brain fizzles.

"Want to get in the back?" Tobey says.

"Okay." I don't even care that it's freezing.

We climb over the seat into the back. The backseat is huge. His whole car is huge. I remember how Matt made fun of it one day in the parking lot. He was like, "What's this *Titanic* joint supposed to be? His car?"

Tobey says, "I'd turn the heat on, but if my battery dies we're screwed."

"It's okay."

"Wait." Tobey runs out to the trunk. He runs back in with a blanket. "This blanket kind of smells," he says. "Sorry."

The blanket smells kind of like gasoline, but I've always liked that smell.

"It's fine."

Tobey spreads the blanket out on the seat. He kisses me.

"Are you comfortable?"

I forget the word for yes. I nod.

He starts kissing me again. His lips feel amazing.

It seems like five minutes later, but I know it's more like an hour at least. It's getting dark out. Plus the windows are all fogged up and my lips feel puffy.

I love how his hands feel on my body.

"Sara," he whispers. "You feel so good."

I kiss him over and over.

He moans. I want to take his clothes off . . . to know what it feels like. But it's still too scary.

He says, "I can't take it anymore."

I love how I'm making him this crazy. And the best part is that he never pressures me to do anything.

Tobey stops kissing me. I put my arms around him. We lie next to each other for a while.

Eventually he says, "I don't want to do this, but . . . I guess you have to go home."

But I don't want to go, either. I want to stay here with him, like this, forever.

He holds my hand the whole ride to my house.

And now we're supposed to go back to our normal lives. That's what people do. They have these amazing experiences with another person, and then they just go home and clean the bathroom or whatever.

shocking facts
january 5, 10:04 a.m.

Shocking Fact #1: I still do my math homework.

And my grades are still decent. I'm determined to show Sara that I've changed. That I'll be as successful in college as she wants me to be.

I feel so good that I'm also determined to do something crazy in pre-calc. Mr. Perry is picking people to put homework problems on the board.

"Twenty-three?" Mr. Perry growls. "Who wants to put up number twenty-three?"

Five kids are having conniptions, their hands straining to punch right through the ceiling.

Shocking Fact #2: I am currently raising my hand right along with them.

I've never raised my hand in math. Ever. Not even to answer a simple question. I've been doing all my work, but that's as far as it goes. Nothing extra included.

Everyone stares. One girl barks out a laugh.

Mr. Perry thinks I'm joking. "Yes, Tobey? What can I do for you?" he says in this weary tone.

"I'm volunteering to put up twenty-three."

Everyone freezes like they're in a game of Red Light Green Light and I just screamed "Red!"

Mr. Perry is not amused.

"Very funny." Mr. Perry starts to call on someone else.

"No, I'm serious. I did my homework. See?" I wave the paper around over my head. "And I want to do twenty-three."

"Very well." But he still looks uncertain, like I might run up to the front of the room and rip some math posters off the wall. "Twenty-nine? Anyone?"

As I walk up to the board I'm grinning like crazy. I can't help it. It's Sara's influence. Even when she's not around, she's still with me.

I know twenty-three was the hardest problem. And I know I got every step right.

Shocking Fact #3: If I didn't know better, I would think that look in Mr. Perry's eyes is something like hope.

There's been tension between us ever since Battle of the Bands. Our momentum has changed. And we're so stressed out with everything else going on.

"What key is this in?" Mike squints at the sheet music I wrote around two in the morning.

"F-sharp," I say.

Mike squints some more. "Oh yeah duh. I see it now."

Josh is sprawled out on the garage floor. "This floor is cold."

"So maybe you should get up," Mike says.

"I'm trying. My body just hasn't responded yet."

Mike pinches the bridge of his nose. He puts the sheet music on top of the amp. "You sound more exhausted than I feel."

"There's no contest in the exhaustion department," I say. "I already won."

"Now you know how we've felt all year," Josh says. "I can't believe how much effort it takes to maintain a C average."

"That's because you've been smoking the chronic again," I joke.

Josh tries to throw a crunched-up Coke can at me. He slowly lifts his arm a few inches off the floor like it's too heavy to be attached to his body. The can lands next to him with a tinny clank.

"Take that," Josh says. He looks like he's about to fall asleep.

"What's happening to us?" I say. Lately it's like we barely have enough energy to get through half of our set list. And we're not playing up to our usual standards.

I don't want to be here as much as I used to. And I don't think I'm alone.

"We're in a rut," Mike says.

Josh yawns, still on the floor.

"Maybe we should . . ." I want to say maybe we should take a break for a while. I'm still making up work from last marking period, and I only have like a week left to get it all done. Plus now that I'm maintaining an A average, I have to do all of these stupid projects and reports and stuff. And after the Battle of the Bands fiasco, it occurred to me that maybe we're not going to be famous after all.

Maybe we'll even break up.

"Should what?" Mike looks at me.

"I don't know. I was just thinking . . . we're all so busy and tired, and . . . it's not the same. Practice, I mean. Maybe we should . . . take a break?"

This perks Josh up. "You can't take a break if you're trying to make it." He pushes himself up into a semi-sitting position. "You have to work at it all the time."

"I know that," I say. "Don't you think I know that?"

"So what are you saying?" Mike demands.

"Just that maybe—" But then I stop. I haven't even thought about what to say yet. "Forget it. Let's just take a break and . . . How about I play my audition piece? I could really use some feedback."

Mike calms down a little. "What are you playing?"

"You had to write your own piece. I haven't titled it yet."

I swing my guitar strap over my head and strum a few chords. Then I start playing from memory. That's one sweet skill I've always had—being able to play without sheet music. I can also sight-read pretty decently. So at least I have those things going for me. Because diverting the judges' attention away from my lacking academic history is the only thing that will save me.

This song I wrote is definitely my best work. I want to

show them how good I am. It's really technical in some places, but I don't think it's too busy. Just enough to distract them from my transcript.

When it's over, I try to read their faces. "Well? What do you think?"

Mike and Josh exchange a look.

"Ummm . . ." Josh squints and massages his temples like he has a colossal headache.

"What was that supposed to be?" Mike says.

"My song, scumwad."

"So, what? You're playing that in public?" Josh shakes his head. "Bad idea."

"Yeah, maybe you should . . . What do you call it when it's like lip synching, but with a guitar? Strum synching?"

"I think the term you're looking for," Josh says, "is pluck synching."

"Okay, you ass-munchers. Seriously. How was it?"

Josh pushes himself up off the floor. "Incredible."

"Seriously?"

Mike nods. "They won't know what hit 'em."

Maybe this can really happen. And maybe there's a real chance that Sara and I can stay together next year.

"Let's bounce." Josh starts to pack up.

"Are we still on for tomorrow?" Mike says.

"Why wouldn't we be?"

During the ride to my place with the dark trees moving past us, I think about Sara. I wanted to tell her the whole truth about Cynthia before, but I couldn't. I don't want to scare her off. But it has to come up sometime. Especially if things keep going the way they are. The couple of times we've hooked up since my car have been just as intense, even more. But here's the thing. I don't want to hurt Sara. If she knows there was someone before her, would that scare her away? Would she think I'm like Dave, just using her for sex? And if she knows it was Cynthia, will she still like me?

CHAPTER 35
shocking discoveries
january 11, 9:18 a.m.

When Mr. Perry turns back to the board, I throw the note on Laila's desk.

Yesterday when I was over at Tobey's, we were studying and he went out for his usual snack-break provisions. I always let him go as long as he gets Oreos with mint filling. So while he was out, I kind of snooped around his room. I found condoms in his nightstand drawer. And then under some laundry on the floor there was this notebook with all these lyrics about girls. The last thing he wrote was this really intense song about having this really intense sex with some mystery girl. It couldn't have really happened, though. Tobey said he's never had a serious girlfriend before me, so there's no way he's had sex. He's not the kind of shallow guy who would sleep around. Just the thought of him with another girl is infuriating enough.

But that song. It was so real. Like it already happened.

The note lands on my desk again. I cover it with my hand. Mr. Perry babbles about the Chain Rule. I slide the note to the edge of my desk. I transfer it to my lap. I unfold it slowly to minimize crackling sounds. So far it says:

Lai-

What if the lyrics weren't about me?
-S

S-

Who else would they be about?
-L

You-

Yo no sé. Am I being paranoid?
-Me

Me

It's all you. He's fantasizing like crazy. He wants you so bad.
-You

Bert-

Why do you think he was weird that time I asked him about his old girlfriends?
-Ernie

John Mayer

He's probably embarrassed because he doesn't have a lot of experience. He wants to come off like he's all that with the ladies. Guys tend to think that makes them more attractive. Gag me.
-Jon Stewart

Wallace-
It's getting so hard not to sleep with him. I'm turning into a total slut.
—Gromit

Pokey-
That's true. But you're still the good girl we know and love. For now.
—Gumby

I'm just about to write back something particularly X-rated when I notice how quiet the room is. And that Mr. Perry is standing right by my desk. Looking down at me.

He snatches up the note in one spastic move.

"Perhaps I should share this with the class?" he threatens.

I'm paralyzed with fear. He absolutely cannot read this note. There's just no way.

"Please don't," I whisper.

"I'm sorry? I can't quite hear you, Sara."

I look up at him. He's still glaring at me with a look of disgust. I never want to develop that look. I want to be full of life and light and inner peace. Mr. Perry is a test.

The bell rings.

Mr. Perry strides up to his desk. He shoves the note under the homework pile. The next minute is everyone packing books and notebooks into their bags and shuffling out and Joe Zedepski picking his calculator up off the floor and Scott glancing back at me as he leaves the room when he thinks I'm not looking and the grinding whirr of the electric pencil sharpener and three kids surrounding Mr. Perry at the board with a question and the next class coming in. So it's not that hard for Laila to walk by Mr. Perry's desk and rescue our note without him noticing.

☯

The next day is a teacher conference day, so we don't have school. Which means I get to spend the whole day at Tobey's. While his parents are at work.

"Do you want something to drink?" Tobey says.

"You're just trying to divert attention from the fact that I'm winning."

"You're winning? I don't think so."

"Excuse me. Look at my guys, and then look at yours. What does that tell you?"

"That I currently hold the Guinness Book World Record for backgammon wins?"

"Uh, no."

I get up from the beanbag and stretch. I make it look casual, but it's a totally strategic move. With this shirt I'm wearing and the way I'm stretching, my shirt pulls up over my stomach. Tobey's eyes are immediately riveted.

In the kitchen, I point to his blender and protein-shake mix sitting on the counter. "Isn't that stuff gross?"

"If I don't breathe through my nose, it's not so bad."

Tobey's wearing my favorite shirt. It's red with white glittery letters. It says I'M BIG IN EUROPE. There's just something about him when he wears it. He rocks my world in that shirt.

I lift myself up to sit on the counter. My head cracks against the cabinet.

"Ow!" I yell.

"Are you okay?" Tobey comes over and puts his hands on my knees. "Where does it hurt?"

"Here." I point.

He puts his hand on my head.

"And here." I touch my lips.

He kisses me. And kisses me. I wish we could be alone like this forever.

Eventually Tobey says, "I was just getting that drink."

"You're supposed to ask me what I want first."

"Right. What would you like? We have orange juice, milk, seltzer, iced tea—" And then he takes out the iced tea. He already knows what I want.

I go, "Does anyone drink milk straight?"

"Straight? You mean like a shot?"

"Like, plain. As in not in cereal. I mean, who sits around drinking a glass of milk? Unless you have chocolate cake with it or something."

"Hey, yeah. What's up with that?"

"It's outrageous."

"It's out of control," Tobey says. "Want to go to my room?"

I've been waiting for him to ask me that all day. The anticipation was driving me insane.

It's almost dark now. I usually hate that about winter. How the only time I ever get to see daylight is through a classroom window. But Tobey puts music on and turns off the light, and now the darkness is a good thing. He flicks on the lamp next to his bed. It has a blue light-bulb in it.

"That's so cool!" I say. "Blue lights are my favorite." It's a sign. They're everywhere.

"There's something I want you to hear." Tobey goes over to his stereo.

Just being in his room is exciting. And it smells like him. I remember the first time I opened his closet. That soothing feeling of *Here are all his clothes.*

Tobey puts a CD on. Then he lies down next to me. I look over at him and think, *How did I get here?*

He brushes my hair away from my face.

"Hey," he says.

"Hey," I say.

I have no idea how much time passes. When I'm with Tobey, an hour seems like a second. I just want to kiss him and kiss him forever. I never want to leave his room. I try to remember how everything feels while it's happening. When we're apart, I miss the feel of his hands on my body. Then I need to remember how it feels when he touches me.

At one point I hear something downstairs.

"What was that?" I say.

"Probably the porch door. It's always banging open."

Now I'm on top of Tobey. I only have my bra and panties on. His shirt is off, but his jeans are still on. I wonder how long he's going to wait to take them off. I've already decided I'm getting completely naked tonight.

"Tobey, didn't you hear me?" His dad swings the door open without bothering to knock. He takes in the scene.

He stares at my bra.

"Oh," he says. "You must be Sara."

"Dad!" Tobey yells. "Can't you knock?"

"I was honking my horn, but I guess you didn't hear me." He's apparently attempting to have a normal conversation like this girl he's never seen before is not lying on top of his son in her underwear. "I need you to move your car. We can't get in." Then he leaves.

I'm like, "Oh my god."

I am mortified. This is the worst.

That did not just happen.

"Oh my god." I get up. My arms are shaky as I pull on my clothes. "That did not just happen."

Tobey sits up. "Don't worry, it'll be okay. I don't know why they're home so early." He comes over to hug me. "I'm so sorry about this. I'll run down and see if we can sneak out."

"What should I do?" I look out the window and try to estimate how far up we are. There's no way I'm going downstairs.

"Don't worry," he says again. Which is easy to say if you weren't the one who got caught like a skank. "I'll be right back. Then we'll go."

I stand in the middle of his room, trying to think clearly. What can I tell them? What do you say in this kind of situation? "Hey, people, what's good? Thanks for not coming in ten minutes later, Mr. Beller. My bra would have been off, too!"

I don't think so.

A few minutes later, Tobey's mom comes in.

"Sara?" She holds out her hand. "I'm Mrs. Beller. It's great to finally meet you. I'm sorry Mr. Beller forgot how to knock."

"I'm so sorry about this." I'm trying really hard not to cry. "This is really embarrassing."

"I know, but I think Mr. Beller has recovered. We've never met any of Tobey's girlfriends." She smiles. "Until now, of course." She puts her arm around me. "Mr. Beller really has been wanting to meet you, so why don't you say hi and then Tobey can drive you home. Okay?"

I nod gratefully. Imagine if I had to stay for tea or something. But now I'm pissed. Tobey's *girlfriends*? As in more than one? As in he's had girlfriends, even though he told me he hasn't been in a serious relationship before me? I won't ask him about it, though. I don't want to be the nagging, jealous-girlfriend type. I just want to trust him. And his mom just said they've been wanting to meet me, so Tobey obviously told them about me.

When I get downstairs, Mr. Beller is in the kitchen making coffee.

"Hi, again." I try for the humorous approach.

"Oh!" Mr. Beller says. "You look much different with your clothes on!" He laughs at this.

He did not just say that.

"We should really get going, Dad." Tobey takes my hand. I guess hand-holding is nothing compared to catching us practically doing it.

"All right, now," he tells the coffee beans. "Take care, Sara. Hope we see you again soon."

We walk outside.

"Right," I say to Tobey. "With clothes on."

Tobey laughs.

I swat his arm. "It's not funny! I am so mortified I could die right now."

"Oh, don't worry." He opens the car door for me. "In a few weeks you'll be laughing about this."

"Your parents must think I'm a total sleaze."

"Are you kidding? My parents love you. They always say how you're the reason my grades rock now. They're probably in there celebrating that I finally have a serious girlfriend. I'm sure they were wondering when I was going to come out."

We dissect the encounter for the entire ride home. I can't imagine ever being able to laugh about this one day. Then again, the old me wouldn't have been able to imagine living my life on my own terms, regardless of what everyone else thinks. And now here I am.

points

february 9, 3:02 a.m.

My audition for Manhattan Music Academy is this Tuesday. I'm afflicted with anticipation of the unknown combined with that horrible Sunday-night feeling of having school the next day. Where you can never sleep because of noisy brain. No matter how tired you are. It's impossible to accomplish anything but lying here in bed. Frustrated and victimized at three in the morning.

So a few hours later when Sara gets to her locker to put her bag away, I'm already there. I've been waiting here since the doors opened. I think this is the earliest I've ever been in school.

"Oh my god," Sara says when she sees me. "You're actually here this early?"

"I think so. Although it's too early for me to be sure

about anything. So maybe it's not really me." I'm so drained that I don't even know what I'm saying.

Sara scrutinizes my face. "Are you okay?"

"I couldn't sleep."

"Because of the audition?"

I nod.

"Listen to me." Sara presses her hand against my cheek. "You have absolutely no reason to be nervous. You rock. You got straight A's last semester! And didn't Mr. Hornby say your piece is perfect?"

"Yeah . . ."

It doesn't sound like she's just trying to be nice or make me feel better. It sounds like she really believes I'm that good.

"Can you go out after school?" I put my hands around her waist. "I need to unwind."

Sara puts her hands in my back pockets. "I think I have an idea."

I press my forehead against hers. "You have really good ideas sometimes."

"Sometimes."

"So what is it?"

"It's a surprise."

"Can I have a hint?"

"Um . . . it's something we both like to do."

Wild scenarios of extreme sex flash through my mind. Is she bringing me back to her place?

She whispers, "Think . . . lots of hand motion."

"Now I'm definitely looking forward to later."

When the surprise turns out to be going to the arcade to play Skee Ball, I'm a bit disappointed. But anything to take my mind off the audition is a good thing.

Sara rules at this game. I don't know how she does it, but she gets every ball into either the center hole (fifty points) or the ring around it (forty points). I'm lucky if my ball lands in the third ring (a whopping thirty points). It usually barely makes it into the outside ring (a humiliating ten points).

"What's your technique?" I say.

"With this?"

"Yeah."

"It's all in the wrist."

"Oh, man. Don't torment me."

If she only knew what she does to me.

This weekend is Valentine's Day. I'm asking Sara to go on a road trip with me. We've been on two so far. They're these day trips where we drive down Route 78 and get off at random exits. The last time we went, we ended up at this truck stop near Newark. Sara loved it. So this time I planned something even better.

"What I mean," Sara says, choosing to ignore me, "is that you kind of skim the ball along the fabric until you feel it . . . like, catch, or something. It's like the felt picks up the ball at one point, and if you don't let it go right then, it rolls too slowly."

I try. But to no avail. Sara has a steady stream of tickets

whirring out of the box every time she rolls a ball. Whereas I might have ten tickets by the time we're finished.

During an exceptionally impressive round, I reach down to rip Sara's tickets off.

"Don't!" she yells.

"I was just ripping off your tickets. The strip is getting really long."

"I like it long. It looks like I have more that way."

"Like you need more?" At this rate, she'll be able to trade in her tickets for a big-money item. She'll probably pick one of the giant stuffed animals that float above all the loser prizes in the display case. Me, I'll be lucky to walk away with a Superball and rock candy.

Sure enough, Sara picks out a giant stuffed penguin when we're done. I get a Superball and hide the rest of my tickets. When Sara goes to the bathroom, I trade them in for a glittery plastic ring. To go with my Valentine's Day plan.

I sleep better that night. But the second I wake up way before the alarm goes off, there's that anxiety, punching me in the gut again. And for the whole train ride to New York, all I can think about is how much better all the other applicants probably are. I'm no longer Mr. Applied Guy. Now I'm Mr. Rampant Insecurities Guy.

What I was expecting the audition to be like was all bright

lights on a big, empty stage. A row of anonymous judges would be in the audience, but I wouldn't be able to read their expressions. Even the air would feel empty. I would play in a blur and then leave, with no idea how they're deciding my fate.

What I wasn't expecting was a sunny rehearsal space with friendly-looking people sitting behind a table. Which is exactly what I see when the door is opened.

"Tobey Beller?" the official-looking woman standing in front of me says.

"Yes."

"I'm Jenna Segal, the—"

"Director of Admissions," I say. I remember her name from the letter telling me when my audition was.

She smiles. "That's right." We shake hands.

The three people at the table smile. Ms. Segal introduces them to me.

I set up my stuff. There's a stool and a music stand and some other equipment already there.

I balance on the stool. The judges already have my sheet music I sent in last week, but I don't even need a copy. It's just me and my guitar.

"Whenever you're ready," Ms. Segal says.

While I play, I practice a visualization technique Sara taught me. I see myself here in September, playing in this room, writing the best music of my life. Walking down to NYU every day to see Sara. Music. And Sara. The only things I need in life to be happy.

"Thank you," Ms. Segal says. "We'll be in touch."

I look over at everybody. They're all smiling at me again.

Either they're happy people in general or they like what I did. I think I did okay, but it's hard to say since I kind of zoned out.

"Thanks for your time," I tell them. "This really means a lot to me." I pack up my guitar and smile at them on the way out. Happy people like other happy people.

In the hall, I see the next two applicants waiting on the bench. One's this hardcore punk rock chick with pink spiky hair and leather pants and severe-looking studs in her lip. Then there's this guy with glasses and a T-shirt that says VOTE FOR PEDRO with a clarinet case on his lap. I guess Manhattan Music Academy is into diversity.

Back on the train, I lean against the window and listen to my iPod. I watch the lights come on in people's houses, beyond the tracks, through the trees.

This is the hardest part. Waiting to know what my future is.

CHAPTER 37
probability
february 12, 8:10 a.m.

Maggie's eyes are majorly bloodshot. Her dad told her that he's moving out. He did it while they were having breakfast.

"I can't deal with gym," she whispers. "Let's go to the bathroom."

We sneak in and stand at the sinks.

"This is so freaking horrendous," Maggie says in a raspy voice. "I'm sure they're getting divorced."

She lets the cold water run and splashes her face a few times. I'm mad at myself for being petty enough to actually feel jealous. I could never just splash some cold water on my face in a time of stress. Then all my concealer would wash off and I'd have to put it back on and I don't have my moisturizer here so my skin would get dry and it's this whole complicated thing with me.

"I think he's staying in a hotel. How pathetic is that?"

"He deserves it," I say. "He should suffer for a while and think about what he did."

"Yeah, whatever. He's not gonna change. My mom told me that she tried doing all these different things to make him happy and nothing worked. That's why they were always fighting." She turns the water off. "Guys don't change. They just get worse with age." Maggie stares at herself in the smeary mirror. "This is not happening."

I'm trying to think of something profound to say that will make her feel better. Something that will take away all of her pain. But of course there's nothing.

Maggie takes a shuddery breath. "Anyway."

"I'm really sorry, Mags."

"I know."

I'm in a sad mood the whole morning, feeling bad for Maggie. So when Laila and I are walking to lunch and Cynthia comes up to me, I'm not ready to deal with her. Even though I know she went out with Tobey last year, I still can't believe he would like someone like her.

Cynthia walks right up to me. She stands there, blocking me.

"Sara?" she asks. As if she's not sure that's my name.

"Yeah?"

"Can you say hi to Tobey for me?"

Laila's looking at her like she just escaped from the psych ward.

"Uh . . . yeah," I say.

"Thanks. See ya!" Then Cynthia struts off down the hall.

"What was *that*?" Laila says.

I don't say anything. Because what it looked like was someone a little too interested in my boyfriend. And I don't want to say that out loud.

At lunch, it's me, Tobey, Laila, Maggie, Mike, and Josh all at one table now. Laila and I put our stuff down. No one else is here yet.

"Are you going to tell Tobey?" Laila says.

"No," I say. "She's just trying to create drama. I'm sure she'll be watching to see if I get mad at him."

"Fascinating. I hope the quality of social interactions improves between now and college."

Tobey comes in and puts his notebook down.

"Hey, beautiful," he says.

"Hey." I look into his eyes, searching for changes. But it's the same intense gaze I always see.

In line, Tobey's like, "Whoa. Déjà vu."

"Why?"

"Don't tell me you forgot about the dime!"

At first I don't know what he's talking about. But then I remember when Tobey and I bumped heads picking up that dime I dropped. Back before I got a clue.

"Never," I promise.

Back at our table, everyone's complaining about Mr. Carver.

"He's obviously been smoking the weed," Josh says.

"Seriously," Mike slurps his drink. "The man is mentally disturbed."

"He needs to reevaluate his career choice." Josh looks at Maggie.

"Drill sergeant would be a good one," Maggie offers.

I sip my iced tea and look around at my new lunch surroundings. Everything seems completely different on this side of the world. I can finally relax instead of being concerned about what Dave's friends think of me. Sitting with Tobey and our friends all together feels like the most natural thing in the world.

Tobey takes my napkin and writes something on it. He slides it back to me.

It says:

I think you're cute.

I immediately turn pink.

He writes something else. He slides it back to me.

It says:

You're even cuter when you blush.

Mike's ranting about how long it took to do his college essays.

"I swear, this one was like, 'Write page two hundred

eighty-seven of your autobiography.' Who comes up with this stuff?"

"Oh my god," Maggie says.

"What?"

"Where was that one from?"

"The New School."

"I had the same one from Florida State!"

"Dude," Mike says. "That's scary."

"You guys don't know from essays," Laila starts.

They actually have onion rings today. Tobey and I reach for our mustard packets at the same time. We give each other a weird look as we open them.

I stare at Tobey as he squeezes mustard onto his plate. "What's the mustard for?" I say.

"This." Tobey dips an onion ring in the mustard.

I'm like, "No way."

"So way."

"You do *not* like them that way."

"I do, but there's no way you can."

"Why not?"

"Because the probability of two people sitting at the same table who both like their onion rings with mustard is too small. The stratosphere would ignite, and life as we know it would cease to exist."

"That's hot."

"That's boiling."

"Let me get this straight," Laila says. Everyone's oblivious to the monumental event that just occurred between us. "You want to be an actor?"

"Definitely." Josh smiles all big.

"That's your career goal."

"Uh-huh."

"Do you have a plan B in mind?"

"Laila, you like John Mayer, right?"

She hesitates. "Right."

"Well, I forget what song it's from, but you know when he says how everyone always told him to stay inside the lines? And how there's so much more on the other side?"

Laila smiles. "Point taken."

Josh is gassed. "Does anyone want more cake?" he says.

"No, thanks," Maggie says.

"Oh, well . . . Can I get you something else?"

Maggie looks toward the door, as if planning her escape. "Uh . . . no thanks."

"Are you sure?" Josh is all wide, hopeful eyes.

"I'm all set," Maggie says. I get the feeling that Maggie is starting to like Josh. She finally dumped Rick because he's a manwhore. He went back to his game-playing and didn't call her for like a whole week. Meanwhile, Josh is always paying attention to Maggie, and they've even talked about her parents. Josh isn't her type, though, so she's in denial. But now I know that eventually those feelings take over, and it won't matter if he's her type or not.

I catch Maggie's eye to see if she's feeling better from this morning. She winks at me.

Now my napkin wants to know:

So, what about that road trip this weekend?

Here's our version of a road trip. Tobey drives us down the highway, and we get off at a random exit and eat rest-stop junk food and experience city life. It's awesome.

At first I remember this inhumane problem set I have to do for calc and the scads of other homework I'll have over the weekend. But then I remember how frustrated I feel when I miss out on the living part of life. I don't want my life to go places without me. Plus, this weekend is Valentine's Day.

So I write on his napkin and slide it back to him.

How soon can we leave?

CHAPTER 38

room 523: the right words
february 14, 6:41 p.m.

I rented a room for us at the Short Hills Hilton. I didn't tell Sara where we're going. Just that she won't be sleeping at home and she had to think up an excuse for being gone tonight. Sara told her mom she's sleeping over at Maggie's, and my parents think I'll be at Mike's. So they're all oblivious to the fact that we're about to spend the night together for the first time.

There's a slight chance that Sara will hate me for this. I might have to stay at Mike's for real. But I don't think so.

"No peeking," I say.

"Are we almost there?" Sara's fidgeting in the passenger seat. Blindfolded with the only tie I own.

"We'll be there in, like, ten minutes."

She giggles. "Where are we going?" she says in a please-tell-me voice.

"Ten minutes," I say, "is all the information you get."

I park the car and grab our bags from the backseat. I go

around to Sara's side to open her door. I consider leaving her blindfold on until we get to the room, but I don't want to draw attention to the fact that we're still in high school. I felt ridiculous enough making the reservation. But I decide to leave the blindfold on until we get to the front door.

I hold her hand while we walk.

"Tell me if I'm about to step off a cliff or something," Sara says.

"That's what I'm here for."

In front of the glittery entrance, I take off the tie.

"Oh my god," she says.

I examine her face for signs of disgust. But all I can see is excitement.

"We're staying in a hotel?" she says.

"Only if it's okay with you."

Sara smiles. "It's okay."

I push open the door to our room and say, "After you, *ma chérie*," as if I own the entire hotel. "As you can see, I'm still renovating the kitchen. Excuse the mess." I pull Sara into the room. The door swings shut behind her. "But the living room is done. I've expanded it to twice the original size."

"Impressive." Sara goes over to the windows. "I love what you've done with the place." She moves the curtains apart.

I go over and stand next to her. You can see city lights for miles. Just being away seems to make Sara come alive.

She told me that she feels better in a city atmosphere. More like herself. I know she'll love being at NYU. I just hope I get to be there with her. I won't know how my audition went for at least another month. Sara keeps saying I have to visualize the outcome, imagine getting the acceptance letter, see the exact words that tell me I'm in. Only sometimes when I try to do this, I visualize the letter saying how much I suck and how they wouldn't take a reformed slacker like me if I were the last applicant on earth.

We order room service and watch movies until midnight. We're both in a good mood, laughing a lot and making up alternate story lines for the characters in the movies. Sara already opened her gifts. I made her another mix CD of all the songs she likes now from us listening to them so many times. I also gave her the plastic ring I won at Skee Ball. I put it in a ring box, all serious. She loved it.

Sara gave me a scrapbook. She said it's to document us. There's one page covered with song lyrics. Another page has stuff from Music Theory, like Dots. Then there's a black-and-white photo of us that someone on yearbook took. Sara wants me to do the next few pages and then give it back to her. Then we'll keep handing it back and forth until the whole thing is done. Mike and Josh would tease me about it for the rest of my life if they ever found out. But it's a cool idea.

After the movie we're watching ends, there's a shift between us. Night. Possibility.

I try to act casual. Since Dave was such an asshole about sex, I want to make sure I'm not.

We're both lying back against the pillows. I have to tell her. It's now or never.

I open my mouth to say it, and all of a sudden Sara pulls me on top of her. And after a while, she's only wearing her underwear. I just wish that wasn't the only thing in my way.

CHAPTER 39

room 523:
this horrendous jealousy
february 15, 12:41 a.m.

I'm totally freaking out.

I thought we were sleeping over at Tobey's house, like maybe his parents were going away for the weekend or something. So this hotel room is way more than I expected. And I'm freaking right now because everything was so relaxed and I felt so comfortable all snuggled up against him watching movies and then I just *had* to kiss him. And now he's trying to take my panties off and I've never been that naked with a boy. But if there was ever a good time to do it, now works for me. And I was going to do it that night his dad walked in on us anyway. And of course I'm nervous, but when won't I be?

But then Tobey pulls away from me. He moves over to his side of the bed and puts his hands over his face.

"What's wrong?" I say.

"I just . . . I'm getting too worked up." Tobey turns on his side to look at me. "You get me all worked up."

"Isn't that the point?"

"Yeah, but . . ." He holds my hand so his fingers are in between mine. "I have to tell you something. Something hard."

"Okay." But it's not okay. I'm scared and nervous about what he's going to say.

"I'm not . . . I've . . ."

"Tobey. Whatever it is, it's okay. Just tell me."

"I've had sex before."

Did he just say that? He didn't just say that. I can list at least ten different reasons why he didn't just say that. One, he told me he's never felt this way about anyone before. Two, we haven't even had sex yet. Three, so it doesn't make sense that . . .

"I don't understand," I say.

"Huh?"

"How is that possible?"

Tobey squints at me and shakes his head. "Is it that hard to believe someone would want to have sex with me?"

"What? No! It's not—no! It's because you said . . . I thought you said you've never felt this way about anyone before."

"I haven't."

"Well . . . then . . . how could you sleep with someone if you felt less than this?" I feel like I'm going to cry.

"Oh," Tobey says. "No, it's . . . it wasn't like that. It didn't mean anything."

I never get when guys in books or movies say it didn't mean anything when they talk about sleeping with someone. It means *everything*. What could be more personal and intimate and enormous than that?

"What do you mean it didn't mean anything?"

"It was just sex," Tobey says. "No emotional attachment."

"Then why did you do it?"

Tobey looks at me. "Come on. I'm a guy."

"Oh, so you're a guy so . . . you'd have sex with just anyone?"

"No. It's different now." He squeezes my hand. I pull my hand away. "I'm with you now. You mean everything to me."

"How many girls did you sleep with?"

"Just one."

"Was it just one time?"

"No."

"Like, how many times?"

"I don't know. I already told you I was seeing someone for a while."

"Yeah. You just forgot to mention that you were also sleeping with her."

This horrendous jealousy builds up inside my chest, right next to my heart. It makes it hard to breathe. I want to know who. I need to know who.

"Was it Cynthia?"

Tobey looks at the wall. "No."

"Who was it?"

"No one you know."

"From school?"

"Sara."

"Was she from school?" My voice is loud, panicked at the possibilities.

"Look . . . that part of my life is over. I just wanted to be honest with you."

Um, yeah. So now he feels better after dumping that all over me. And I get to feel hurt and jealous.

I *hate* that there was someone before me.

I move over to my side of the bed and get under the covers. I know I shouldn't be mad and I know he did the right thing telling me this. But I still can't believe it. I've always imagined what our first time together would be like for both of us. Now I have to imagine what it's going to feel like to be with a boy who's already had his first time. Without me.

If it wasn't Cynthia, who was it?

That's the thing with jealousy. It chews at your soul. And it doesn't stop until you let it go.

"Hey," Tobey says.

I don't answer him. I spend the rest of the night on my side of the bed. Far away from what I eventually have to deal with.

CHAPTER 40
so much more
march 13, 5:25 p.m.

The fact that I'm in Sara's room studying for my history midterm is astounding enough. But the fact that being with Sara still makes me want to study is incredible. Since it's the middle of March, I'm assuming the Manhattan Music Academy people have pretty much made up their minds about me. What I do from here on out isn't going to have much of an impact on their decision. But Sara's making me keep my grades up anyway. And I'm fine with that, as long as I take frequent breaks.

Sara got over the whole sex scandal thing after a while. It wasn't like there was this whole big makeup scene. She just gradually warmed up to me, opening back up a little more every day. Now we're back to where we were before the hotel fiasco . . . but we still haven't gone all the way.

I still feel bad about lying to her, but she doesn't need to know it was Cynthia. Especially because Cynthia has a reputation for being easy. Sara wouldn't understand. Plus,

Cynthia asked me out last week. The girl is relentless. Sara doesn't know this, either, and I intend to keep it that way. I've had to spend the past month convincing her that I don't care if we don't have sex. And I really am okay with it. Even though sex takes up the largest allocation of my pie-chart brain.

I take a surreptitious peek at her clock. We've been studying for over an hour. Time for a break.

"Hey," I say.

"Hey," Sara says. She doesn't turn around from her desk.

"We didn't even have a snack."

"How old are you? Five?"

"You know I always have a snack after school."

"Well, I'm not hungry," Sara says. "But you can get something if you want."

"How can you not be hungry?"

"I'm just not."

"Jeez. Well then . . . let's take a break."

"We can't."

"Why not?"

"Tobey." Sara puts her pencil down. She turns to look at me. "Do you have any idea how long it's going to take to be ready for midterms?"

"So . . . what, we can't take breaks anymore?"

"Not after only an hour!"

"Oh. I wasn't aware that we were following an itinerary."

"There's no—" Sara turns back to her pile of papers and books and notebooks and tons of other boring things.

If we don't do something fun in the next five minutes, I may snap.

"Look, let's just go to the playground real quick. We could play with that ball-catcher thing."

"Huh?" She shuffles some papers.

"You know. That thing on the pole where you throw the ball in it and it has those four tubes the ball comes out of? And the tubes are all different colors?"

"I think—"

"It's the best. It's the most exciting thing ever. There's no way to know which tube the ball's coming out of, and the suspense is the best part. I'm going. You have to come with me. You must come with me." I go over to her chair and scrunch down next to her. "Please come with me?"

Sara sighs. "I just don't think it's a good idea."

"Why?"

"It's not very responsible."

"Responsible?" Why can't she ever be more spontaneous? It's like we can never do anything unless it's been penciled in her day planner for a week. She's always studying. Like she'll even remember this stuff by next year. But the things I want to do are experiences she can remember for the rest of her life. "Fuck that! What do you really want to do?"

"I want to ace my midterms! NYU's going to look at these grades."

"You're still worried about that?" Sara is so getting into NYU. They'd be absurd not to take her. But ever since she sent in her application, she's been stressing. She tried to

apply early decision, but they didn't get her SAT scores in time or something. Sara was devastated because she did everything she was supposed to, but someone else messed up. So now she's paranoid other things might go wrong. As if worrying about something you have no control over helps anything.

"Okay, *that*? Is my future. It's my first-choice college, Tobey. I think you know what that feels like."

I get up and stand there, uncertain. Should I leave and let her work? Or should I stick around and try to smooth things out?

"You're stressing too much. I think you'd feel better if you took a break with me. That's all."

"No, *you'd* feel better because you'd get out of studying." Sara shakes her head. "I should have known you weren't serious about doing this for the rest of the year."

"Yes I am!"

"So then why are you slacking again?"

"I'm not!"

"I know about the English paper." Sara crosses her arms.

We had this huge report due for English. I was too exhausted to care. I figure with all the other work I've put into the class, I should still come out with a B. B-minus, worst.

"We had extra practices that week." The band took a break for a while. Then Josh lined up more gigs for us. Now we're back to practicing almost every day.

"What are you guys going to do next year?"

"I'm not thinking about later," I say. "I'm living in the moment."

"You're forgetting about your priorities."

"But the band's taking off again. And if we don't stay together I can put together a new group in New York and—"

"Everybody's in a band!" Sara yells. "Don't you get it? Anybody who wants to be a musician or an actor or a writer goes to New York. And sorry to be the one to tell you, but there aren't that many job opportunities for starving artists. Unless you like being a waiter."

"Don't you think I'm good?"

"You know I do. But it doesn't matter what I think. It only matters what the right people think. And they're already swamped with everyone else who wants to do the exact same thing as you."

"You know how dedicated you are to school?"

"Yeah."

"That's how I am about my music. I have dreams, too, Sara. Just because they're not the same as yours doesn't make them less important."

"I'm not saying they are. But college needs to be your priority. Anything can happen."

"Exactly. And I know it's going to happen for me."

"God!" She jumps up and walks to the other side of the room. Her optical-fiber lamp moves its stringy fingers up and down, red bleeding into purple bleeding into blue bleeding into— "Why are you doing this to yourself?"

"What?"

"You're so much more than you're letting yourself be."

"And life is so much more than you're letting it be."

"Don't do this. You're like—if you screw this up now, you know what you're going to be saying when you're thirty?"

"What?"

"'You want fries with that?'"

"So? What's wrong with working at McDonald's?" I know it's the wrong thing to say right after I say it. Unfortunately, they haven't invented a verbal delete button yet.

"If you don't know how wrong it is, there is no way I can even begin to explain how wrong it is." Sara flings her door open and stomps down the hall. The bathroom door slams.

I wonder what this means. Do I stay? I know I won't be able to study anymore tonight and she'll get mad. Do I leave? Then she'll think I'm pissed, and she'll get mad. And I guess I am, sort of. But she's also sort of right. Either way, I lose. So I sit back down on her bed. And wait for her to make the next move.

just not good enough
march 17, 3:47 p.m.

I've been trying to be okay with the fact that there was another girl in Tobey's bed before me. And I've been trying to be okay with the fact that Tobey's first time wasn't with me. But I'm not okay with the fact that he won't tell me who she was. Or anything about her. Even though he denied it, I can't get rid of this pressing feeling that it was Cynthia.

Tobey's waiting for me at my locker while I pack my bag. I want to ask him about it again, but at the same time I don't want to act so jealous and like I can't trust him.

I slam my locker and turn around. And that's when I see her.

Cynthia. Walking right toward us.

I look at Tobey to see how he's reacting, but he looks normal.

"Hi, Tobey," Cynthia says. Like I'm not even there.

"Uh. Hi."

"How's it going?" She doesn't even glance in my direction.

Tobey looks annoyed. He's like, "Yeah, we were actually—"

"Tobey," Cynthia says. "Do you remember the time we went kayaking? Wasn't that almost a year ago?"

"Why?"

"No, I was just thinking of it. . . ."

Then they exchange a look. It only lasts a second, but I can feel the history in that look.

"That's nice, but . . . we have to go."

"Whatever," Cynthia says. "You don't have to be so cold. You weren't this cold last year." She saunters off.

Now I know what it feels like when people say they were so mad their blood was boiling.

"What was that about?"

"Insanity. It runs in her family." He's obviously trying to be laid-back.

"What happened last year?"

"Nothing."

"Seriously," I say. "Did you sleep with her? In a kayak?"

Tobey glances behind me. "Do you really want to do this in the hall?" Which I know is bullshit, because he's the last person who cares what other people think.

"Did you sleep with her or not?"

Tobey sighs. He reaches out to hold me, but I step back.

"Well?" I say.

I can tell from Tobey's look already. "It was only a couple of times . . . but, yeah. We slept together."

So it *was* Cynthia. I immediately feel inferior. She's, like, the worst possible girl for it to be. Everyone knows she's been doing guys since she's fourteen. But she's gorgeous and sexy, and any guy would die to be with her. I can't compete.

"But you said—"

"I know what I said. And I'm sorry I lied to you." Tobey reaches for my hand. I pull my hand away. "I didn't want to hurt you. I know what you think about Cynthia."

"Why'd you say it wasn't her?"

"I didn't think you'd understand. I—"

"So those lyrics were about her? She's such a slut!"

"You read my notebook?" Tobey says.

Okay. So he lied and I snooped. But we're nowhere near even.

"You said those things were only things you felt about me."

"I thought I felt those things at the time. But it's different now. I was in a different place then." Tobey tries to hold my hand again. I still don't let him. "Everything I said to you is true, Sara. Cynthia didn't mean anything."

"I just don't get how you can sleep with someone and not have it mean anything."

"It's different for guys."

"Oh! So, that's how it would be with me? Just sex?"

"Of course not. You—"

"You know what?" I'm so furious it's not even funny. "I changed my mind. I don't want to hear anymore."

I run down the hall. I can't believe that Tobey is like every other guy, skanking around with whoever. I thought he was different. But I was wrong. He's just another man-whore, like all the rest of them.

When I get home, I put on my Sade CD and play "By Your Side" on repeat mode. I cry for a really long time. When the phone rings, I hope it's him.

"It's me," Tobey says. "Can we talk about this?"

"Fine. Talk."

"I'm sorry."

I wait for more. Because that's just not good enough.

"Hello?"

"Yeah?"

"I'm sorry."

"Congratulations."

"Can you tell me why you're so upset?"

The thing is, Tobey should get this. I mean, he's gotten everything else about me. And I don't want to explain it all. So much of it has to do with jealousy, and I know it's stupid to be mad at him because he had a life before me. But I am anyway.

"I can't talk to you right now," I say.

"Can I call you later?"

"I don't think so." If I talk to him anytime soon, I'm going to say a bunch of things I'll regret. And I'm just so mad. "I need some space."

"What?"

"I need some time alone. To think."

Tobey's quiet. I can hear him breathing. Then he goes, "What do you mean by space?"

"I have to take a break for a while."

"What? From me? Why?"

"I just do."

"Are you . . . You didn't just break up with me, did you?"

"No."

"Are you sure?"

"Yes."

I need to make sure this is the last time he lies to me. Maybe if he thinks I might leave him, he'll realize what he has. And he won't keep anything else from me ever again.

The next day in drafting while we're doing photographic etchings, I put my stick down. I'm making a list on the DL.

Reasons Why I Should Be with Tobey
1. I love him.
2. I still think he's my soul mate.
3. He gets me.

4. He makes me feel alive.
5. Everything we do together is new and feels like I've never done it before. Even everyday things like watching TV.

And then I have this other list I've been trying to do.

Reasons Not to Be with Tobey
1. He lied to me.
2.

I can't think of anything else to add. Occasional slacking relapses aren't a big enough reason. I decide to ask Mr. Slater about it. I wonder when he's going to start charging me for being my personal counselor.

I raise my hand.

Mr. Slater comes over. "Etching issues?"

"Actually? I'm doing something else I'm not supposed to be doing."

"Ah." He sits down next to me.

I slide my paper over.

"Hmm," he says. "Interesting."

"Really?"

"Yeah."

"What's interesting about it?"

"That you wasted your time making lists that didn't need to be made."

"Lists help me figure out what to do."

"Yeah, but you didn't have to make these. You already knew what you wanted before you started."

"How do you know?"

Mr. Slater picks up a purple marker. He circles item number two on the second list, which never got filled in. "It's right here."

He's right. Nothing else is on that list, because I didn't want anything to be there in the first place.

After school I put on my fuzzy pajamas and park myself in front of the TV and contemplate calling Tobey. I was the one who said they needed space. So that would imply that I'm the one who should let him know when I'm over it. And now I'm starting to miss him. But it'd be so much more romantic if he begged me to take him back. And I'm still mad.

Okay. If I click up three channels and there's a commercial on, that's a sign to call Tobey.

Click-click-click.

The Frugal Gourmet is doing something alarming with breadcrumbs.

Okay. If I click over to HBO and there's something good on, that's a sign to call Tobey.

Legally Blonde Two is on. I loved the first one, but this one bites.

Okay. If I hear the refrigerator kick on in the next five minutes, that's a sign to call Tobey.

After waiting for the humming noise for fifteen minutes—which of course is totally annoying and all up in my business whenever I need extreme quiet, but won't come on now—I get in the shower. I decide that if the phone rings while I'm in here, that's the universe telling me we're meant to be together.

The phone never rings.

CHAPTER 42
space
march 22, 12:33 p.m.

It's lunch, but we're not in the cafeteria. Mike and I are in the gym, shooting hoops. Ever since Sara said she needed some space, I haven't exactly had a killer appetite. Everyone knows needing some space is, like, the kiss of death.

"Are you guys still in a fight?" Mike says.

"Yeah."

Mike passes me the ball. "Dude. Sucks to be you."

"Tell me about it."

"She's probably just waiting for you to apologize."

"I already tried that." I bounce the ball. "It didn't work. I blew it." How could I have been so stupid? Why didn't I tell her about Cynthia right from the start?

I didn't realize how angry I was. But suddenly I'm so furious I don't know what to do with myself. I slam the ball against the backboard.

"I hate when chicks pull that space shit. It's like, you already said you're sorry. What more does she want?"

"I wish I knew."

"It would suck if she broke up with you."

I've only been worried about that this ∖
Hearing it out loud from my alleged best friend
story.

"Yo. Can I have the ball?"

I whip the ball at him so hard he stumbles back∖

"Hey!" Mike yells. "What's your problem?"

"My problem? My problem is that you are suppose
be on my side. But for some twisted reason, you've dec
ed to be a fucking asshole instead."

"Jesus. I'm only—"

"Don't you think I already thought of that?" I run my
hands through my hair. "She just said she needs some
space."

"Fine. Sorry, man."

I bounce the ball.

"We're never gonna understand women," Mike says.
"They're way too complex. You've got too many variables to
consider. PMS, bad hair days, miscellaneous mood swings...
there's no way to tell what's causing their attitude."

I sigh. "So what should I do?"

"Sorry to tell you," Mike says. "But this time? The guru
is fresh out of plans."

If you looked up "desperation" in the dictionary, there
would be a picture of me. Lying on my bed. Staring at the
ceiling. Thinking about what to do.

I can't eat. I can't sleep. I'm entirely unable to concen-

trate on anything. Even writing music. The band is the only thing that's been keeping me from calling Sara every second.

I reach over and pick up the phone. I dial.

I slam the phone back down.

If I call her, I won't be respecting her need for space. She tells me she needs space and then I call her? That would be wrong.

But if I don't call her, she'll think I don't care.

I have to call her.

When her answering machine comes on, I almost hang up. But then I start talking.

"Hey. It's me. I know how you said you needed some space and I respect that but I also want you to know that I miss you. A lot. And I'm sorry I lied to you but I didn't want to hurt you and I was so wrong. I swear it won't happen again. And when you said you needed space I should have said this and I just wanted to say that . . . I love you."

I slam the phone down. I realize I'm sweating.

And then suddenly I have an idea. I grab two CDs and my boom box.

I almost dislocate my knee racing downstairs. I fling the door open and run out into the night.

time
march 22, 8:18 p.m.

I just got Tobey's message. He told me he loves me. It's only like the third time he's said it. Which is kind of weird because Tobey's the most sensitive guy I know. But I've always thought it was because when he says it, he really means it and it's a big deal to him. My stomach is all butterflies. I want to call him back, but I must have said I need space for a reason.

I get up and open my window a little. The cool air calms me down.

I get into bed and stare at the ceiling. I think about living in New York City. Maybe even with Tobey.

And then I hear it.

At first, I don't know what it is. It sounds like the neighbors are playing music. But when I recognize the song, I know where it's coming from.

I get up and look out into the backyard. Where Tobey's standing. Holding his boom box over his head.

Playing a song about the light and heat in my eyes.

I open my window all the way and watch him. He must be the only boy who actually remembers the details of his girlfriend's life. Not only does he remember my favorite movie scene, but he gets it enough to do this. And he's doing it today because he also knows how I've been waiting for spring all winter and today is the vernal equinox.

As usual, Mom is out late with Howard. So it doesn't matter when Tobey climbs through my window.

I hug him as tightly as I can. He hugs me back. Then he pulls a box out of his coat pocket.

"Make-up gift number one," he says.

It's a blue lightbulb. Just like the one in his room. It's just like that John Mayer lyric about blue lights on a black night, how there's something about them that makes you feel more.

"I've had this for a while." Tobey unscrews the regular bulb from my lamp and twists the blue light in. My entire room glows blue. Now my room is just like his.

Tobey takes off his coat and sweater. "I brought that live Dave Matthews I was telling you about." He puts the CD in my stereo. "There's this one song you have to hear."

"Which one?"

"'Say Goodbye.'"

"Oh my god! I love that song!"

Tobey puts one hand on my waist and holds out his other hand for mine. "Wait till you hear it live."

We dance in the blue light. And we kiss in the blue light. And most of my clothes come off in the blue light. Time disappears. . . .

And then I remember how I visualized all of this, exactly how it's happening right now, way back in October. So the universe obviously decided that we belong together.

All of the reasons why we belong together come racing back. And right then, I forgive him. And I believe that he won't lie to me again.

When Tobey takes off his T-shirt, he has a gray tank top on underneath. He's wearing that and jeans. I'm only in my bra and panties. The universe told me to avoid my ratty old ones when I got out of the shower. Now I know why.

In this new world where anything is possible and dreams really do come true, we dance. And when it gets to that point of no return, the place I've been so scared of, it doesn't feel scary anymore.

And I let him take me there.

CHAPTER 44

heavy info—part one
march 23, 4:09 p.m.

"Have you noticed," Josh says to Mike, "that Tobey looks suspiciously happy today?"

"I have. Wanna fill us in, man?"

We're working on some new song lyrics at Jim's, but so far we're blocked. Jim is not a guy. It's this coffeehouse that rocks. They have the strongest coffee anywhere, and you can stay for as long as you want, even after you're done with your drink and it's obvious you're not getting another one anytime soon.

"Not really." I try to hide a smile.

"Is he smiling?" Josh says.

"It would appear so."

They look at me.

"What?"

Josh smirks at Mike.

"What happened last night?" Mike says.

"Nothing. I mean, I was at Sara's. . . ."

"Did you guys make up?" Josh says.

"Oh yeah." I can't hide the smile this time.

Mike looks at Josh. "Our boy is concealing some heavy info. I wonder what it could be?"

"Haven't got a clue," Josh says.

"You can give it a rest, because I'm not talking."

Josh is about to press me, but then two girls who he's been eyeing ever since we got here get up to leave. As they pass us, Josh says, "What's up, ladies?"

The girls don't even look at him.

Josh leans back and stretches his arms over his head. "Oh yeah, they want me."

"So," Mike says. "Did you finally—"

"What's the story with you and Maggie?" I ask Josh.

"I'm asking her out tomorrow. No—I'm doing it now!" He takes his cell phone out and presses buttons.

"Whoa!" Mike says. "When did you decide this?"

"Just now. This whole thing . . . it would make an awesome song."

"Brainstorm!" Mike yells. Which is what he always yells when someone has an idea for a song.

I click my pen. "Okay . . ."

Josh listens and snaps his phone shut. "Voice mail."

"Okay," Mike says. "You see this girl across a room or a club or whatever, and you don't even know her, but she gives you a look, and you know you have to know her . . . and you can't explain why or anything. . . ."

"Yeah," Josh says. "It's, like, magnetic . . . and then she's, like . . ."

They tell the story and I take notes. I wonder if they realize they're telling my story. But it doesn't even matter. Because finally, we have one of our own that's good enough to tell.

CHAPTER 45

heavy info—part two
march 23, 4:09 p.m.

"You mean you're not dating for the rest of the year?" I whisper.

"No," Maggie whispers back. "I mean I'm not dating again *ever*. As in ever again in my life. What's the point? It never works out."

We're in the library doing homework. But I haven't had a chance to talk to Laila or Maggie all day, so they still don't know about last night. I was going to tell them when we got here, but Maggie started talking right away. The deal with her fatalistic attitude is that her parents are going though their divorce proceedings and they're being nasty about it. She's given up all hope of finding something real.

"You're just dating the wrong guys." I scooch my chair closer. "You'll find the right one."

Laila leans over. "Or maybe it can be arranged."

"What? Like a blind date?"

"No. Like an arranged marriage."

"Where are we?" Maggie says. "Beirut?"

"I recently discovered news that is both hilarious and disturbing." Laila motions for us to lean in across the table. Then she whispers, "My parents still have sex!"

"No way!" I go. I'd be less shocked if Jake Gyllenhaal emerged from the stacks and asked me out. Laila's been referring to her parents' celibate lifestyle for years.

"Unfortunately. Remember how I was supposed to sleep over at your place last Saturday? Well, they thought I was there but I was really studying in my room. And then I went to the kitchen for a caffeine fix, and I heard them."

"Oh my god!" Maggie yells. Some girls at the next table snap their heads up and grill us with these irritated looks. "They were doing it in the kitchen?"

"Ew! No! I heard them in their room."

"Bad times," I say.

"Wow," Maggie says.

"I know. I'm damaged for life. It's too offensive for words. We need to talk about something else now."

"Hey," I say to Maggie. "I was trying to call you last night. But then—"

"Oh, sorry. I was IMing with Josh."

"What?" I go. "Since when?"

"Um . . . since he started IMing me?"

"I knew it." Laila turns the page of her calc book. "You so like him."

"Have you been listening to me at all? I just told you I'm not dating anymore. Hello!"

"So you say . . ." Laila sets up a new problem in her notebook.

I go, "Do you . . . like, feel it with Josh?"

Maggie opens her notebook. "I feel . . . something. I don't know what I feel. And anyway, we're just friends."

"For now," Laila says.

"It's just that he understands about the divorce. His parents got divorced a long time ago."

"Hmmm."

Maggie gives up. It's almost impossible to win an argument with Laila. Especially when you know she's right. Even if you don't want to admit it.

Maggie's cell phone rings. The girls grill us again.

"Sorry!" Maggie yell-whispers to them. She takes her phone out and turns it off, looking at who called.

"Who was that?" I say.

"Jake called. He wants to know if this weekend's good for you."

"Duh, he already knows I have a date with Marshall."

"Who's Marshall?" Laila says.

"Hello!" I yell-whisper. "As in Mathers!"

She still has this blank look.

"As in Eminem!"

"Oh right," Laila says. "Naturally."

"No, really." I glance at Maggie. "Who was that?"

Maggie picks up her pen. "Um . . . Josh?"

"Aha!" Laila says. "Admit it already. The two of you have been secretly dating since sophomore year, and now you're planning to elope to Mexico."

"No way," I say. "We have to be in the wedding."

Maggie writes in her notebook like we're not even there.

We all go back to doing homework. But I can't concentrate. I have to tell them.

"You guys," I whisper.

Laila keeps working. Maggie looks up.

"Something happened last night," I say.

Laila looks up. "What?"

"Well . . . Tobey came over . . . and we . . ."

"Oh my god," Maggie says. "I knew it!"

"What?" Laila says.

"Start from the beginning," Maggie instructs. "And don't leave anything out."

Which is exactly what I intend to do.

into the night
april 23, 12:32 p.m.

Josh runs over to our table. He slams his backpack down. He yells, "I got into Rutgers!"

"Genius!" I hold my hand up for him to slap.

"Was that your first choice?" Sara asks.

"No, my safety. But I didn't even think I'd get in there!"

"So you'll all be near New York!" Maggie says.

"We don't know for sure yet." Sara stresses. "Don't jinx it."

I keep trying to convince Sara that nothing else will go wrong with NYU. She's usually so good about staying positive and her whole visualization stuff, but she's been majorly stressing this. She just wants this one thing so badly.

"We'll be neighbors," Mike tells her. "The New School's right next to NYU."

"And Manhattan Academy's, like, three subway stops away." I got my acceptance letter last week. My parents still haven't stopped smiling.

Now that it's real, I'm kind of stoked about college. And not just to impress Sara or my dad. I'm excited for myself.

Mike looks at Laila. "Are you psyched about Penn?" Laila got her acceptance letter a while ago because she applied early decision.

"Of course. But only because I find Yale way too pretentious."

I laugh. Laila's a trip.

"What about you?" Mike says to Maggie.

"Oh," Maggie says. "I'm still waiting to hear from Florida State. It's either that or California."

Josh comes racing back from the lunch line with this huge piece of chocolate cake. "They have cake!" he announces.

"So we see," Laila says.

"Yeah, but is it any good?" Maggie scrunches up her face.

"Let's see." Josh peels the plastic wrap off the cake. Icing gets stuck to the wrapper. He swipes his finger through the icing and tastes it. "The icing's good." He holds the plate out to Maggie. She shakes her head.

"You better watch your cake fetish," Mike tells him. "You're at serious risk of the Freshman Fifteen. And I hear Rutgers has an outstanding cafeteria."

"Do you want a piece?" I ask Sara.

"Okay, but only if you're getting one."

"Yeah," I say. "I was getting more iced tea, anyway."

In line, I inspect the cake section. I want to make sure I pick the biggest piece with the most icing. It's the little things that make Sara happy.

After school, Mike and Josh and I are up in our old tree house. We used to have really important meetings here about which CDs were missing from our collections and which girls might possibly be wearing training bras.

Somehow I remember it being a lot bigger than this.

"How did you talk me into this again?" I say.

"Dude!" Mike yells from inside the secret compartment. "I found my old Etch-A-Sketch. Righteous!"

I shift my weight on a rotted-out board. "I think I'm too tall for this."

"Come on," Josh says. "Live a little."

I sit down on a stool that's older than me. "So what's the latest with Maggie?"

"I don't know. We've only gone out twice. It's like she's avoiding me or something."

"Imagine that." Mike shakes his Etch-A-Sketch.

"What if . . ." Josh walks over to the tiny window.

"What if what?" I say.

"No, it's just . . . what if I tell Maggie how I feel about her, and she doesn't feel the same way?"

"You have to take the risk. If I didn't, there's no way I'd be with Sara now." I want them to know exactly how Sara's changed me in ways I never thought possible. But instead I say, "Just go for it, man. Whatever happens happens."

"You know what? Yeah. I'm calling her." Josh takes out his cell phone. "And I'm telling her exactly how I feel. I'm nice, yo!"

"Don't call yet," Mike says. "Let's plan what you're saying first."

Josh looks at me. We crack up.

"*What?*" Mike says.

The garage door is open. Light spills out into the night.

"When's your mom coming home?" Josh says.

"Late," Mike says. "We have time."

During our tree-house meeting, we decided that the band is on an unofficial hiatus. Lately we've been getting together only to jam and stay sharp. I finally realized that it would be impractical to continue this as if it were going somewhere. So this is our last jam.

"From the top," Mike says.

We're playing this old Bob Seger song called "Night Moves." It's a good song for us because the guitar and bass and drum parts are equally fierce. The song's all about being young and free and making out in your car with the girl you love. The things that matter in life.

CHAPTER 47
into the unknown
april 24, 4:25 p.m.

Technically, it's not spying if you're looking into your neighbor's window—and you can see stuff inside—if they don't even have their curtains closed. It's like, come on. How are you not going to look? But I have a valid purpose here. I'm sitting in my yard, working in my sketchbook. My neighbors have the best windows for miles around. Each window has this little crank inside and you turn the crank to open or close the window. I wish I thought of that first.

I love these warm spring days. The anticipation of everything.

I switch to a thinner pastel stick. Drawing the angle between the windowsill and the side of the open window is harder than it looks.

Mom drops my mail on top of what I'm doing. Don't mind me. I'm only trying to prepare for my future career.

She goes, "Here's your mail."

"Hm."

After she leaves, I sift through a catalog and a letter from my pen pal from camp and something from NYU and—

Oh my god.

It's here.

I hold the NYU letter in front of me and stare at it, hoping for a telepathic message. It's thick. That's supposed to be a good sign. I hold the envelope up in front of the sun. I can't see through it. Of course I can't. *It's too thick!* I have to open it. I'm dying to open it. But I can't do this alone.

Mom's in the living room.

I sneak into her bedroom and close the door. Then I dial.

"Hello?"

"It's here," I tell her.

"Did you open it?"

"I can't."

"You have to open it," Laila says.

"I know."

"Is it thick?"

"It's thick."

"Yes! You totally got in! Open it!"

"Okay," I breathe.

I slide my finger under the seam of the envelope and rip it open slowly. I peek inside.

"Well?" Laila goes.

"I'm still opening it."

"You're in. You're so in."

"Okay," I tell her. "I'm taking the letter out." I'd be less flushed if I'd just run twenty miles.

"Well?" Laila screams.

I scan the first sentence of the letter.

"I got in!" My eyes tear up. "I got in!"

"Congrats! But, like, obviously."

"Yes!" I'm jumping all around like a maniac.

"It would appear that we're destined for greatness. But this we knew."

I sit down on the bed to catch my breath.

"If they didn't take you, they'd be seriously wrong."

"I can't believe it."

"Why? You earned it."

"No, it's like . . . it's all working out."

"Not while we still have all this calc," Laila complains. "Could this homework be any longer?"

"No," I tell her. "It definitely couldn't be."

But I don't have to care anymore. I've already gotten into college. High school is now officially irrelevant.

Tobey's coming over in half an hour. He says he wants to take me out to celebrate. Of course I don't have anything to wear. It's going to take me at least that long to get something together. I briefly consider stealing that fierce halter top I like since I'm already in Mom's room, but she'll see me leave with it on.

I open the door. Mom's standing right there.

"Were you listening?" I say.

"No."

"Well . . . I just found out I got into NYU."

Mom says, "Really?"

"Yeah."

And then something really weird happens.

She hugs me.

Okay, so it's not one of those warm and fuzzy hugs where you bond and cry and go make s'mores around the campfire. But at least it's something. At least she's trying.

"I have to figure out what to wear. Tobey's coming to pick me up."

"Well, here," Mom says. She goes over to her closet and takes out the halter top. "You liked this when I showed it to you before, right?"

"Yeah?"

"You can borrow it." She holds it out tentatively.

"Thanks."

Getting ready in my room, I put on this old Chicago song, "If You Leave Me Now." It's so overwhelmingly romantic, which is exactly how I feel right now. And I feel good. I'm thinking that it might actually be possible for things to work out sometimes. Definitely not everything and maybe not the way you imagined. But sometimes, when you least expect it, life surprises you.

end of familiar
june 15, 5:10 p.m.

"Like, what kind of sadist invented these hats?"

Josh is struggling to keep his mortarboard on. He tried to do this thing with hair product today, and it's not exactly working for him.

"Someone who obviously didn't graduate from high school," Mike says.

I'm sitting in the row of wobbly chairs behind Mike and Josh since I'm taller. It's crazy hot out here on the football field. The person who invented these ridiculous hats also forgot to come up with a material for these gowns that lets air circulate.

I search the girls' side for Sara. She's focused on Laila's speech, which is a lot more interesting than the fifteen hours of other speeches. Laila was valedictorian by some absurdly microscopic quantity of GPA points. The rumor is that Michelle tried to OD on Tylenol when she found out she was only salutatorian.

When they start calling our names, I'm relieved that it's almost over.

"Sara Tyler!"

There's applause from the bleachers. I clap, too. I watch her walk across the stage, with her NHS rope. When she put it on, she joked about how it looked like a tie for curtains. Watching her get her diploma, all of these images flash in front of me like a blur. The prom, the senior luncheon, the awards ceremony . . . it's like we've just been through so much so fast. I'm suddenly overwhelmed by everything. Maybe it's exhaustion from cramming for finals. Or maybe it's the heat.

I stand up straight. I'm next.

"Tobey Beller!"

There's less applause for me, but that's cool. The important thing is that it's over.

I walk across the stage and shake hands and grab my diploma in a haze. And when I'm walking down the stairs on the other side, I see Mr. Hornby and Ms. Everman sitting together. They're both smiling at me. And I feel something I've never felt before. I'm proud that they're proud of me. And I'm proud that my hard work really did pay off.

After it's over, parents start filtering across the field to take pictures and stuff. Our group is hanging out, waiting.

"All I want to do is go home and take a cold shower ten minutes ago," Maggie whines.

"The best part of graduating is the knowledge that I will never have to take gym again," Sara says.

"We also don't have to subject ourselves to any more of Mr. Carver's ties," Laila adds.

"Damn, yo," Josh says. "What was it with those ties?"

"I know," Maggie says. "How can people have such different tastes? What, is taste genetic?"

"Clearly," Laila says. "Name one possible environmental influence that could make someone like those ties."

"Early head trauma?" I guess.

"Seriously," Maggie agrees. "It's like, nineteen forty-seven called and they want their wardrobe back."

I'm going to miss this. I finally have a decent group of friends beyond Mike and Josh and it's already over.

Sara's mom comes over. She fans her face with the program.

"Sara," she says. "Well . . . congratulations . . ." Then her mom gives Sara a quick hug.

"Oh," Sara says. "Thanks." She looks embarrassed. I guess I would be, too, if my mom was so out of it she didn't even know what to say to me right now.

We all stand there, shifting awkwardly in the hot sun.

But then all our parents come over, and it's a whirlwind of hugs and kisses and pictures.

Dad hands me a small box wrapped in gold foil.

"Congratulations, Tobey," he says. "We're . . . very proud of you."

Mom dabs under her eyes with a tissue.

I open the box. It's a really expensive-looking pocket watch.

"It belonged to your great-grandfather."

I get that overwhelming feeling again, like it's all too much when really it's no big deal. I don't know what's wrong with me.

"Thanks," I tell him.

Mom keeps dabbing.

I look around at everyone else. It seems like half the people here are related to Laila. Everyone swarms around her, fighting for the chance to stand next to her and have their picture taken. Mike and Josh and their families all look happy. Josh is jumping around like a lunatic, hamming it up for the camera. Maggie's talking to her mom, but I don't see her dad anywhere. And Sara's mom is trying to make small talk with some of the parents, looking off into the distance sometimes. Sara looks miserable.

"Hey, Dad?" I say.

"Yeah?"

"I'm going over to talk to Sara, okay?"

"Sure," he says. My parents can't stop gushing about Sara. They think she's the best thing that ever happened to me. I was kind of scared they wouldn't like her after the time Dad walked in on us, but it's like they forgot all about it once I got into MMA.

Sara watches me walk over. She smiles a little.

My parents are taking me out to dinner. Everyone else is going out to dinner with their parents, too. Except for Sara.

"Hey," I say.

"Hey," she says.

I look at her mom. We've only spoken a couple times. She knows that I'm Sara's boyfriend, but she hasn't made much of an effort to get to know me. It's so weird.

"Hi, Tobey," her mom says. "Congratulations and all."

"Thanks. Um, I was wondering? If Sara could come to dinner with me and my parents tonight."

"I think that sounds fine," she says.

"Okay. Good. Well um . . . bye." I grab Sara's hand and take her away. It occurs to me that I didn't ask my parents if it's okay with them. But I know it will be.

"If you hadn't rescued me just now, I don't even know," Sara says.

"What else would I do?"

"You're my hero."

"That's what I'm here for," I say.

Seeing everyone I grew up with for the last time, leaving this school and never coming back . . . it all feels really strange. But I'm ready to make things finally happen.

CHAPTER 49
edge of possibility
july 11, 7:23 p.m.

"The Boys of Summer" plays through the Putt-Putt Mini Golf speaker system.

"Exclusive!" Josh yells. "Check out this huge Slurpee! Did you guys know they're only seventy-nine cents right now?"

"It's changed my life." Maggie is so obviously love-struck. Even though she's still pretending to be aloof.

We're all here to celebrate Laila's last day with us, since she's moving to Philly tomorrow for her summer internship. And Maggie's leaving for Florida State in two weeks.

"Could it be any bigger?" I ask.

"The correct answer," Laila says, "is no."

"Dumb big!" Josh yells.

Laila also got a drink at 7-Eleven on our way over. I can't remember the last time I saw Laila drink something other than coffee.

I go, "Why are you drinking that?"

"Didn't you hear?" Laila says. "It was only seventy-nine cents."

"No, like, there's this huge Starbucks right across from 7-Eleven."

"I'm off coffee."

"What!" Maggie and I yell together.

"If I don't start training myself to stay awake without artificial stimulants, they're going to have to keep me hooked up to a caffeine IV drip at Penn."

"Sounds delicious," Mike says.

"It's normal to get tired," Tobey tells her.

"If I got tired like a normal person, my dad would probably bribe my roommate to sneak crushed up NoDoz into my dinner every night," Laila says. "That is, before I become wildly famous for inventing a cure for sleep."

It's my turn. I smack my ball way out. It lands in some bushes by the fence overlooking Route 78.

"Bummer," I say.

"Yeah," Tobey says. "Weren't you winning?"

"I still am."

"What? No way," Josh says. "Your ball's like in Greenland. You'll never find it."

"I Just Want To Be Your Everything" comes on.

"Who is this?" Laila says. "The Bee Gees?"

"God!" Maggie says. "It's Andy Gibb!" She rolls her eyes.

"Wish me luck," I say. At least my ball is neon orange.

"Wait," Laila says. "You don't have to look for it. Tobey's going."

"I don't think so," Tobey says.

Laila goes, "I'm cashing in on a deal we have."

"Oh?"

"Yeah, see, we have this deal in which you said if I did something you'd be my personal slave for the rest of the year—well, life, if I remember correctly—and I did it. And I haven't even mentioned it until now so I figure you have no choice."

Tobey told me about Laila's personal-slave deal for trading partners in Music Theory, so I go, "Hey, yeah! How could you let the whole year go by without offering to do anything?"

"She should have asked!"

"Well," Laila says. "I'm not asking. I'm telling. I'm in charge here."

Tobey groans. He salutes Laila.

"Go fetch," she orders.

"Demanding!" Mike yells. "I like that in a woman."

"Oh, please," Laila says. "You like breasts in a woman. Preferably somewhere around a C-cup."

"Bye!" Josh yells after Tobey. "Send me a postcard!"

"Me, too!" I yell. "I hear Greenland is beautiful this time of year!"

"Ow!" Josh yells. "Brain freeze!"

"So why'd you have to guzzle the whole thing in like two seconds?" Maggie says. They're like an old married couple already. I wonder what Maggie will do if she finally realizes how she feels about Josh in Florida.

The next course is the windmill one. The one that gave me a sign last summer.

Josh jumps onto the fake grass and does this vintage disco John Travolta move, waving his golf club all around. We just stand there looking at him.

He notices we're not laughing. "Play it off. . . ." he mumbles. He puts his ball down and whales it. It bangs into the windmill and comes rolling back.

"Nice try, slickness," Maggie teases. "Let me show you how it's done for future reference." She puts her ball down.

"Does that mean we have a future together?" Josh says.

"Maybe." Maggie smiles coyly. "If you're lucky."

Josh just stands there, mesmerized.

"Watch," Maggie says, "and learn." She gets ready to hit the ball. "Are you watching?"

Josh, who is staring at Maggie's butt, goes, "Huh—oh, yeah!"

Maggie's ball rolls through the windmill slats. She smirks at Josh.

Tobey comes running back with my ball. He looks over the course. He says, "This is too easy!" He puts his ball down, takes an inventory of the windmill, and swings. The ball bangs one of the windmill's arms and zings off toward the batting cages.

"Okay, then," Tobey says. "I guess it would be your turn."

I position my ball the same way as before. I don't need a sign this time. I own the windmill.

I want to tell Tobey about when I was standing in this exact same place last summer, wishing for him to be real. But it's hard to remember life before Tobey. He makes everything seem possible. Like whatever you feel is true, really true in your heart, you can make happen. And you just know, when it happens, it's for real. And there are a million possibilities.

Like the possibility of going separate ways.

Together.

35674045727030